Botulinum Toxin in Clinical Dermatology

Botulinum Toxin in Clinical Dermatology

edited by

Anthony V Benedetto DO FACP
Clinical Assistant Professor of Dermatology
University of Pennsylvania School of Medicine
Philadelphia
PA, USA

and

Dermatologic SurgiCenter
1200 Locust Street
Philadelphia
PA, USA

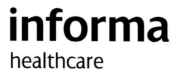

Informa Healthcare USA, Inc.
Telephone House
69-77 Paul Street
London EC2A 4LQ, UK

International Standard Book Number-10: 1-8421-4244-5 (Hardcover)
International Standard Book Number-13: 978-1-8421-4244-8 (Hardcover)

Visit the Informa Web site at
www.informa.com

and the Informa Healthcare Web site at
www.informahealthcare.com

Dedication

This book is dedicated to all those who have mentored and supported me throughout my past endeavors. Also to those who have given me the confidence and their invaluable assistance which has helped bring this challenging project to fruition, including friends, colleagues, family, and most of all Dianne.

CONTENTS

Foreword   *Jean Carruthers*   xi

Preface   *Anthony Benedetto*   xiii

Prologue   The psychology of cosmetic treatment   1
            Matthew Silvan

Chapter 1   Pharmacology, immunology and current developments   15
            Roger Aoki

Chapter 2   Facial anatomy and the use of botulinum toxin   33
            James Spencer

Chapter 3   Cosmetic uses of botulinum toxin A in the upper face   45
            Anthony V Benedetto

Chapter 4   Cosmetic uses of botulinum toxin A in the mid face   121
            Anthony V Benedetto

Chapter 5   Cosmetic uses of botulinum toxin A in the lower face, neck
            and upper chest   163
            Anthony V Benedetto

Chapter 6   Muscle contouring with botulinum toxin   207
            Michael S Lehrer

Chapter 7   Other dermatologic uses of botulinum toxin   219
            Kevin Smith and Francisco Pérez-Atamoros

Chapter 8   Dysport®: a European botulinum type A neurotoxin   237
            Gary Monheit

Chapter 9   Botulinum toxin B   247
            Neil Sadick

Chapter 10   Botulinum toxin in the management of focal hyperhidrosis   261
            Oliver Kreyden

Appendix 1   The preparation, handling, storage and mode of injection of Botox®   295

Appendix 2   Consent to have botulinum treatments for facial and body wrinkles   299

Appendix 3   Patient treatment record   301

Appendix 4   Muscles of facial expression   303

Appendix 5   Side-effects and contraindications to BOTOX® injections   307

Index   309

CONTRIBUTORS

K Roger Aoki PhD
Vice President, Neurotoxins Research Program
Biological Sciences
Allergan, Inc
2525 Dupont Drive
Irvine
CA 92612
USA

Anthony V Benedetto DO FACP
Clinical Assistant Professor of Dermatology
University of Pennsylvania School of Medicine
Philadelphia
PA
USA

Oliver P Kreyden MD
Praxis Methiniserhof
Baselstrasse 9
Muttenz 4132
Switzerland

Michael S Lehrer MD
Clinical Assistant Professor
Department of Dermatology
Hospital of the University of Pennsylvania
3400 Spruce Street
Philadelphia
PA 19104
USA

Gary D Monheit MD
Monheit Dermatology Associates
Ash Place, Suite 202
2100 16th Avenue South
Birmingham
AL 35202
USA

Francisco Pérez-Atamoros, MD
Centro Dermatologico Tennyson
Tennyson 241
Polanco
Mexico City 11550
Mexico

Neil Sadick MD
Sadick Dermatology & Aesthetic Surgery
772 Park Avenue
New York
NY 10021
USA

Matthew E Silvan PhD
Department of Dermatology
St. Luke's-Roosevelt Hospital Medical Center
1090 Amsterdam Avenue
New York
NY 10021
USA

Kevin C Smith MD FACP FRCPC
Suite 201 – 6453 Morrison St.
Niagara Falls
Ontario L2E 7H1
Canada

James M Spencer MD MS
Professor of Clinical Dermatology
Mt. Sinai School of Medicine
1 Gustave L. Levy Place, Box 1047
New York
NY 10029
USA

FOREWORD

Botulinum toxin A is the most exciting new drug from the past century. Dr Alan Scott deserves the credit for the originality of his idea to use a drug rather than a surgical procedure to repair misaligned eyes. Alastair and I have seen our idea of using it for a cosmetic treatment flower from a rather strange 'fringe' idea to seeing BTX-A injections becoming the world's most frequently administered aesthetic procedure. Groups of physicians who were once skeptical of its rationale and effects now are ardent users and supporters.

In the wake of the wildly unsafe use of a non-human-approved botulinum neurotoxin in Florida in late 2004, this book is a very timely addition to the scientific literature. Safety and predictable efficacy are of paramount concern to aesthetic physicians. None of these goals can be reached without the knowledge of anatomy, aesthetics, physiology, injection technique, numbers and placement of units of BTX-A which are all stressed in this excellent book. The aesthetic physician authors who have contributed to this work are well respected and authoritative and deserve to be read and studied. One of the great results of the cosmetic revolution started by BTX-A is that many physician groups who did not traditionally learn from each other now greatly value the modern hybrid aesthetic approach – as exemplified by this book.

Jean Carruthers
Clinical Professor
Department of Opthalmology
University of British Columbia
Vancouver
Canada

February 2005

It is quickly becoming very difficult to remain up to date with what is being published about botulinum toxin. This small instructional manual was written to organize what dermatologists and other physicians need to know about treating patients for cosmetic purposes with injections of botulinum toxin A. Recently, several therapeutic indications for the use of botulinum toxin in dermatology have also been proposed. Many of these indications have been included in this text.

Currently, the only FDA approved botulinum toxin A for ***cosmetic*** use in the USA is BOTOX® Cosmetic. It is approved only for the treatment of glabellar frown lines. However, the majority of the cosmetic corrections that are done with BOTOX® Cosmetic are performed on an off-label basis. Consequently, prior to the printing of this book, there has been no established text detailing the many different injection techniques presently available.

Who are the patients who seek cosmetic enhancement, and why should we treat them? Dr Matthew Silvan presents us with a glimpse into the psychological aspects of someone seeking to cosmetically improve their outward appearance. Why does one seek the help of others to modify, and hopefully, improve upon their natural appearance? Is it a means to create a façade of deception for others, or is it a way to transform themselves inwardly and improve their self image? With some insight into the mind of the 'cosmetic patient', this textbook begins with a historical perspective on the development of the medical use of botulinum toxin presented by Dr Roger Aoki, Vice President of Neurotoxins Research Program in Biological Sciences at Allergan, Inc. Over the years, Roger has helped me and a score of others understand the essential concepts concerning the pharmacology and immunology of botulinum toxin.

There is much emphasis on anatomy in this text. No one should attempt to administer botulinum toxin unless they possess a solid working knowledge of the mimetic muscles of the face. Ideally one should be able to visualize the functional anatomy of a particular facial muscle or set of muscles while gazing upon a patient and deciding where to place the needle and inject the next unit of botulinum toxin. Not only is there a full chapter dedicated solely to the muscular anatomy of the face by Dr James Spencer, but anatomy is again discussed in the 'Functional Anatomy' section of the individual chapters dealing with how to inject BOTOX® Cosmetic.

Many physicians have their favorite manner in which they inject botulinum toxin, some of which are reliable and reproducible, others of which are not so reliable and reproducible. This text attempts to cull the many different techniques of well-known physician injectors who use botulinum toxin regularly, and who get excellent and reproducible results. By emphasizing the proper way to inject BOTOX Cosmetic®, we can alert the neophyte injector on how to carefully select the appropriate patients, produce acceptable results, and avoid complications.

The chapter written by Dr Michael Lehrer describes a technique of reducing muscle bulk and girth with botulinum toxin. These techniques are practiced by physicians in areas of the world where oversized muscles create an unacceptable cosmetic dilemma for which invasive interventions occasionally are performed. Botulinum toxin now provides a non-invasive way to accomplish similar results. Drs Kevin Smith and Francisco Pérez-Atamoros then give us a glimpse of what may be in store for us in the future. They discuss controversial uses of botulinum toxin A that are in the purview of a practicing dermatologist, some therapeutic, and some cosmetic, but they all seem to work and produce remarkable outcomes.

Next Dr Gary Monheit gives us an overview of Dysport®, the other botulinum toxin A that is currently being used in other parts of the world outside the United States. Soon Dysport® will be available for use by physicians in the United States under the tradename of Reloxin®. A chapter on the comparative uses of botulinum toxin serotypes B and A is presented by Dr Neil Sadick, who puts into perspective our understanding of the currently available botulinum toxins. Dr Oliver Kreyden, one of the first and foremost users of botulinum toxin for hyperhidrosis in Europe, concludes our compilation of dermatologic uses of botulinum toxin by contributing a detailed chapter on the pathophysiologic rationale and the therapeutic use of botulinum toxin in suppressing localized hyperhidrosis.

Finally if it were not for Drs Jean and Alastair Carruthers, many of us in dermatology would not be injecting botulinum toxin for cosmetic and therapeutic purposes. It is because of them and their many disciples that most of us continue to learn and develop different ways to treat various problems in different areas of the body with botulinum toxin. Thank you Drs Carruthers for your insight, genius, and encouragement.

Anthony V Benedetto DO, FACP
March 2005

Notes on the text

Chapters 2, 3, 4, 5 and 9

Please note that each line drawing of facial muscles in the above chapters depict superficial muscles on the left hand side of the diagram, and deep muscles on the right hand side of the diagram.

Prologue

THE PSYCHOLOGY OF COSMETIC TREATMENT

Matthew Silvan

Introduction

A consideration of the psychological issues related to cosmetic treatments, from surgical face lifts to non-invasive procedures such as BOTOX®, forces us to look at ourselves in a deeper way. It makes us confront our vanity and look at who we are and who we want to be. In addition, since cosmetic treatments are often used to stave off the effects of aging, their usage is intimately connected to our sense of our bodies, our sexuality, and even to our mortality. But how can we understand the differences between vanity and wanting to look our best? What does it mean to grow old gracefully? To pathologize the search for beauty and any effort to make one look younger, healthier, or just be more physically attractive seems contrary to a physician's clinical and personal experience. However, to see the use of BOTOX® and other cosmetic treatments as divorced from psychological meaning is also problematic and avoids the complex and subtle nuances of how we think about ourselves and how we look at our patients. Ultimately, the individual decision to change one's looks is complex and multidetermined. It is influenced by our culture, our sense of our selves, and the ubiquitous wishes, fears, and conflicts that are in all of us.

As the reader of this book is primarily concerned with the science and therapeutic uses of botulinum toxin, the following comments are applicable to that specific population. However there are currently no experimental data yet published in peer review journals that can tell us specifically who are seeking BOTOX® treatments. We do not know what their psychological motivations are, with what conflicts they struggle, or what psychiatric diagnosis they carry. We may presume that, since BOTOX® is a less invasive medical intervention than cosmetic surgery, this group of patients may differ somewhat from the cosmetic surgery population. However, more than likely psychological factors are present in all patients who seek even the least invasive cosmetic treatments. Placing cosmetic treatments in a psychological and social context, illustrates that regardless of what one actually does there are core motivations and pressures that drive our patients to us to alter their appearance. Individual differences may exist, but the central psychodynamics that drive us and our patients are still quite generalizable. In addition, this chapter will describe how psychopathology may be assessed and, more importantly, how the presence of conflict and motivation is distinguishable from the pathology that may preclude cosmetic treatment.

Let us begin with some anthropologic and historic observations about beauty, age, and the use of cosmetics. Culture, in terms of how it values and defines beauty either directly or indirectly, influences behavior. By exploring the use of cosmetic treatments in more depth, dermatologists can more effectively understand patients and the often complex and subtle expressions of the needs and wishes that bring them to the office. By articulating a more comprehensive and complex understanding of a patient's psychology, dermatologists are in a better position to assess whether the treatment they are offering will be what their patient actually wants and needs. By listening more acutely to their patient's words, dermatologists are also better able to recognize those patients for whom cosmetic treatment is contraindicated and even dangerous. In covering this wide range of issues it behooves the cosmetic practitioner to recognize the psychological complexity of the work s/he is doing, the multi-determined motivations with which patients arrive, and the way in which this perspective can enhance the practice of their profession.

History

The search for beauty is not new or specific to this time in history. These concerns have been with us for millennia, although how they are expressed may shift from one extreme to the other. A review of sociologic, anthropologic, and literary sources can be extremely useful in helping us reflect on who our patients are today. Fossil records show that Neanderthals used ochre as a deodorant and later primitive man used vegetable dies and mineral pigments for adornment and make up[1]. So even before Narcissus looked at himself in a pool of water we have been concerned, consumed, and even obsessed with beauty. Simon[2] reports on a seventh century physician from Alexandria who practiced a form of cosmetic surgery. De Gama sought the fountain of youth and Oscar Wilde's *Dorian Gray* was willing to sacrifice much to look young and beautiful. As Kligman[3] notes, Cinderella was probably the first 'extreme makeover'. In the mid 1900s Pope Pious XII said that cosmetic procedures used to increase the powers of seduction or vanity were sinful and morally unlawful[4]. Today you cannot turn on the television or open a magazine without reading about beauty, cosmetics and which star had what plastic surgery. While it may be tempting to think that the media is driving this issue, history tells us otherwise.

However, it is true that far more people are having cosmetic treatment. Yet this seems more a function of an improvement in technology, an increased availability of affordable options for invasive and non-invasive procedures, and a change in the social acceptability of cosmetic treatment than a change in who we actually are. While our conceptualizations of what is beautiful may have changed over time, the psychological motivations that drive us to alter our appearance have not. While some might long for the imagined simplicity of the past, others race full speed into the future. Yet, as Sullivan[5] said, 'we are all more human than otherwise' and it would appear that an aspect of being human is to be concerned about one's appearance.

Cultural influences

Surveys have shown that some cultures or groups seem far more focused on their appearance than others[6]. For example, 61 per cent of Brazilians think that physical attractiveness is very important as compared to 32 per cent in the US and 27 per cent in France. Even within the US, regional variations are noted. Southerners are far more concerned with their appearance than Northerners. Moreover, cultural factors profoundly influence what is considered beautiful and what people are willing to go through to make themselves that way. In some cultures, at some times, foot binding, grinding and blackening the teeth[7], as well as scarring and piercing[8], have all been considered acceptable body modifications that increased attractiveness. Are the cosmetic procedures we do today in our culture such as breast augmentation and rhinoplasty any different? On a conceptual level, the smoothing out of a few wrinkles does not seem like such a big thing. In fact can this even be considered body modification since it does not fundamentally change the way we look but only returns our skin and our appearance to a previous state? In this sense one could place cosmetic procedures along a continuum. At one end is the use of make up, at the other, complex cosmetic surgery that changes and modifies the body. In between are things like dieting, going to the gym, whitening teeth, and treatments such as BOTOX®.

However, the search for beauty is more than skin deep. Data show that there are distinct advantages to being beautiful aside from being asked to the prom. Researchers have found that people with good looks are more likely to be hired[9,10], promoted faster[11], and paid more[12]. In a dramatic study about the benefits of being beautiful, Hamermesh and Biddle[13] found that men with above-average looks are paid 5 per cent more than those with average appearance, while those with below-average looks are paid 9 per cent less. Finally, Graham[14] reports on studies that show that good looks improve one's chances in court, make you less likely to get referred to a therapist and generally mean you will get treated as different or special by the world around you.

Age

Maybe our cultural obsession with beauty and cosmetics is due to the unconscious drive of the species to propagate. Those who look beautiful are thought to be more youthful and thus more fertile. Maybe this is a reflection of a change in society such that age and wisdom are no longer revered in the way that they were. Nevertheless, agism is quite evident in the US. For example, single women of a certain age still despair of being able to find a partner and older workers frequently are fired or treated less favorably than younger ones. In an interesting and relevant study, Johnson[15] looked at perceptions of the elderly. Analysis of the data revealed that attractive features are associated with youthfulness and unattractive features are associated with aging. His findings also indicated that, even in the elderly, beauty is associated with more socially desirable personality characteristics, more positive life experiences, and greater occupational status. He concludes that 'maintaining or recapturing youthful vigor is an important determinant of judged attractiveness'.

Growing old is something that few people do without some degree of psychological conflict. In part it may be that focusing on one's wrinkles, receding hairline, or growing paunch is a displacement for no longer being fertile or able to hunt effectively. As we age, doubts about one's ability to work or make love appear even in the absence of any 'real' evidence to the contrary. In addition, there is an almost universal fear of death and dying which all of us deny to a greater or lesser extent. As we struggle with getting older, most people try a variety of surgical and non-surgical measures to stave off the inevitable.

Anne, a 53-year-old executive with a large textile firm, dressed in elegant suits by a famous designer. Trim and fit, with understated gold jewelry, she began jogging after the birth of her daughter, now 20. She thought the highlights in her hair softened her face, although she was having second thoughts on whitening her teeth. 'The Hollywood look just isn't me.' She sought BOTOX® for some wrinkles around her eyes after seeing what the procedure had done for a friend. 'It just made her look better. I can't explain it. It's not fake or too dramatic.' Anne easily admitted she didn't like getting old and while she knew she couldn't turn back the clock she wished to 'slow the process down some'.

For Anne there seemed to be the unspoken hope that what she was doing would help recapture lost time. While this is obviously untrue, it does seem that looking younger helped her feel younger. For those patients who choose non-invasive treatments like BOTOX®, the dermatologists I spoke with report that few are interested in major cosmetic surgery but, like Anne, seem to want to 'take a few years off'.

However, what are these cosmetic treatments, either face lifts or BOTOX®, actually treating? Is it an illness? A medical condition? Is aging pathological? What are the moral and ethical implications of trying to combat a normal process of human development? Ringel[16] raises some of these questions in a very provocative paper that questions the morality of cosmetic treatment. She notes that in defining aging skin as an illness we imply that life itself is an illness. In her view, doctors instead have a responsibility to fight agism and the stigma attached to getting old. She argues that all cosmetic treatments promote an inauthentic enhancement of the self. In doing so they promote a false sense of who one is and serve to perpetuate the denial of the true self. For Ringle, self esteem is clearly better served by embracing maturity rather than denying it.

However, while considering this viewpoint is useful, there can be a temptation to fall too quickly not only into pathologizing but dichotomizing. To say that cosmetic treatments, including BOTOX®, are either moral or immoral, bad or good, indicative of a psychiatric illness or not simplifies the issue and misses the point. Focusing on one side of the debate or the other only obscures the more subtle but infinitely more important question of what is best for the patient. These psychological and philosophic questions are both relevant and useful to orient clinicians in assessing patients who come for BOTOX® treatment. They also help to place these specialized medical efforts in the larger context of how to help the 'whole person'. It is critical to find out what our patients want and whether their goals are realistic and within our power to gratify.

Part of the cosmetic dermatologists' moral, ethical, and professional responsibility is to co-operatively work with patients to determine when treatment is appropriate. To do so, practitioners must enhance their ability to better understand the complex motivations of patients and assess when treatment will actually address the concerns they have. This is crucial to developing and maintaining a good doctor–patient relationship and assuring that patients come away satisfied with the treatment they receive. Patients like Anne abound, but others are unlikely to be pleased with the outcome of their treatment if their expectations and motivations are not well clarified.

Motivation

In simple terms, the majority of those who choose to have cosmetic treatment are motivated to look younger, healthier, and sexier and, by extension, feel better about themselves.

Jim, a 48-year-old lawyer, was determined not to be outdone by the young hotshots coming into the firm now. Since getting divorced three years ago he had been a beast at the gym and had taken two inches off his waist and added them to his chest. 'Fixing all my suits was a pain but it was worth it. You should see the women I meet now'. He showed up like clockwork every three months to get his BOTOX® shot. When he did, he had already circled in black ink any age spots or moles he also wanted lasered off. He told his dermatologist he made a day of it by spending the rest of the afternoon at the spa getting a haircut, massage, and manicure, and generally pampering himself.

People like Jim care about how they look and are invested psychologically in their bodies. As they worry about the effect of age, they are beginning to doubt they can still compete with their younger colleagues at work or in the dating game. They hope that making some change in their appearance will increase their self esteem, lift their low mood, and make it easier for them to interact with others.

This interest is not necessarily pathologic. In fact, its absence is often one of the first signs of psychiatric illness. Those with major psychiatric illness frequently have little or no interest in their appearance. Yet there is also a tendency to say that such concerns about appearance are shallow. That professional success or a loving family is the true measure of one's worth. It may even be that a more intense concern about appearance represents a displacement of other thoughts and feelings. It is probably true that worries about the skin and the face can often represent deeper unconscious thoughts, feelings and fantasies about ourselves. Although concentration on physical flaws may reflect deeper psychopathology, it is also reasonable to be upset with the blotchy skin or acne breakout that one sees in the mirror.

The desire for cosmetic intervention from the mildest to the most dramatic is motivated by the subjective experience of how one feels about oneself. One may feel young but perceive oneself to look old. Such individuals seek treatment to recapture a feeling they once had. They have the sense that they are still vibrant, energetic, and sexy inside but that their outsides no longer seem to reflect this. At a more subtle level they may even have the experience that how they look is beginning to reflect how they feel instead of the other way around. Thus, they seek cosmetic treatment in the hope that, if they make the wrinkles disappear, so too will the feeling of getting older. Some will express these hopes in more magical ways. The middle-aged woman who believes that cosmetic treatment is the only way to keep her husband from leaving her is quite likely to be disappointed in the outcome. Yet for others, cosmetic treatment is part of a coordinated effort to 'do something' in their lives. Data support the idea that some who seek cosmetic treatment are 'doers'[17,18]. These are people who take action in their lives. Thus, cosmetic treatment may be integrated into a characterologic approach towards life which results in not just a new face but also meaningful and long-lasting changes.

The psychological profile of cosmetic patients

The existing data have focused almost exclusively on surgical procedures. Thus, there is reason to wonder whether the results can be applied to non-surgical procedures such as BOTOX®. It seems that psychological and social pressures previously described are present in all patients who seek to improve their looks. Core motivations remain constant even as the way these motivations are expressed may vary. In addition, researchers have not found differences between individuals based on the types of procedures performed. As such, if there is no difference between groups of patients who get face lifts as compared to those who get nose jobs, perhaps there is little difference between these surgical patients and those who get BOTOX®. Finally, there are also overwhelming data to support the high rates of psychiatric symptomatology in dermatology patients as compared to the general population or other medical specialties. Therefore, we can reasonably assume that many cosmetic patients will present with some type of psychological symptomatology. While we must await empirical confirmation for our contention that there is more uniformity than not amongst cosmetic patients when it comes to BOTOX®, there is still much to be learned from examining the psychological studies that do exist.

Many of these studies have been reviewed elsewhere in more detail[18], so highlights of a few of the major findings from some of the more empirically rigorous studies will be discussed.

Edgerton et al, in one of the first such studies conducted in 1960[19], found that almost 70 per cent of his sample were psychiatrically impaired, with many suffering from depression and personality disorders. Thirty years later he conducted a second study[20] and found similar rates of psychiatric disturbance. Meyer et al[21] found 70 per cent of the face lift patients he interviewed suffered from some type of personality disorder, while Napoleon[22] found that according to the Diagnostic and Statistical Manual of Mental Disorders, 4th edition (DSM IV), 70 per cent of his sample met the criteria for personality disorder and 19.5 per cent had a major psychiatric diagnosis.

Some of these studies have been criticized because they relied on interviews and there was a perception that the researchers were biased towards the presence of psychopathology. It has been argued that a slightly different picture emerges if one looks at the results from studies that have relied on 'paper and pencil' or psychometric measures. Several of these studies have not found such severe levels of psychopathology in patients seeking cosmetic surgery. Goin conducted two studies[23,24]. In one, he found no significant levels of psychopathology as measured by the MMPI in 50 face lift patients . In the other, 121 rhinoplasty patients scored in the normal range according to the Brief Symptom Inventory. However, similar psychometric studies have supported the notion that cosmetic patients suffer from underlying psychopathology. Micheli-Pelligrini and Manfrida[25] found 'marked psychopathology in 65 rhinoplasty patients according to scores on the MMPI and the Rorschach while, Kisley et al[26] found patients presenting for cosmetic treatment were nine times more likely to have high scores on measures of body concerns and psychiatric morbidity than a matched control group.

In an especially rigorous study that employed both types of assessment procedures and was conducted in several sites, Meningaud et al[27] evaluated 103 patients scheduled to receive a variety of different cosmetic procedures. These included blepharoplasty, face lifts, liposuction, rhinoplasty, baldness surgery, and otoplasty. Patients were assessed using both structured interviews and psychometric scales. The subjects were assessed on their level of depression, and the degree of social phobia and social anxiety and were given a generic test that measured quality of life. The study employed three control groups. The first was based on normative scores in a larger study of European populations; the second, a group of patients scheduled for non-cosmetic surgical procedures of similar severity or intensity; and the third, individuals randomly chosen from the phone book.

The structured interviews indicated that 50 per cent of the patients had taken psychotropic medication, of which 27 per cent was antidepressants. The study population was significantly more depressed ($p < 0.01$) than the composite control group and had greater social anxiety ($p < 0.001$). Further analysis of their thoughts and feelings about social interactions revealed that this group was preoccupied with appearance and what other people thought about them. On quality of life, the findings were a bit more equivocal. Although there was no significant difference between the two groups, a more detailed analysis of the individual items revealed that the study population was overly represented by subjects with anxiety/depression and only 53 per cent considered themselves neither depressed nor anxious.

Thus, how are we to understand this mixed set of data? It may be that the psychometric measures are not tapping into the type of psychological vulnerabilities and concerns that are most applicable to the group of patients who are seeking cosmetic surgery[28]. Psychometric measures are unlikely to delve as deeply as clinical interviews and so it may be that on the surface there is less evidence of psychopathology and conflict, but that a more intensive examination of these patients reveals more deeply held concerns and conflicts. Despite the higher rates of psychopathology that are apparantly evident in their patients, most plastic surgeons[29] and certainly most dermatologists do not report that their patients present as more noticeably depressed or anxious. Confirming this, Meningaud et al[27] made a point of saying that in most instances the depression documented in their patient sample had not been noted by the treating physician. Thus, it may be that many patients seeking treatment do have some underlying psychopathology but that it is not being picked up by the dermatologist. This may be due to the fact that the patient's psychiatric symptoms are not sufficiently severe enough to be noticed during a brief clinical encounter, or that dermatologists are not directing their attention to this aspect of their patient's presentation and of course are less clinically trained to perceive what may be subtle psychological clues. Moreover, if they are sensing something, they may not think this is an issue to assess further or be concerned about.

In summary, we may be unable to say definitively which psychological symptoms or disorders are present or how severe they are in patients seeking cosmetic surgery. By extension, we are also unsure as to the degree to which we can apply these findings to patients requesting non-surgical procedures such as BOTOX®. However, the empirical data seem unequivocal in that individuals who present for cosmetic treatments can and do present with a broad range of psychological symptoms and conflicts that may not be clearly apparent to the cosmetic practitioner. The findings are relevant to the clinical practice of cosmetic dermatology and the implementation of BOTOX® because they help us understand who our patients are psychologically, what they may be struggling with emotionally, and how treatment can be helpful. More specifically, these findings can help alert the dermatologist to particular psychological conditions or symptoms that may preclude BOTOX® and other cosmetic treatments. These include body dysmorphic disorder (BDD), certain acute phases of psychiatric illnesses, and those patients who obsessively seek multiple cosmetic procedures.

Body dysmorphic disorder and problem patients

The DSM IV[30] lists three criteria that must be met for the diagnosis body dysmorphic disorder (BDD). These are

1. The person is preoccupied with an imagined or barely perceptible defect in their appearance.
2. The preoccupation causes marked distress and impairment in their social and occupational functioning.
3. Their concern is not better accounted for by another mental disorder.

Grossbart and Sawyer[31] argue that many cosmetic patients could be seen as meeting the criteria for item one since 'imagined or barely perceptible defect' is quite subjective and what may be distressing for one person barely registers for another. While some more objective criteria may be available for dermatologists to use in assessing the degree of wrinkles or lines in a person's face, to a great extent the decision to seek treatment is a purely subjective one. Still, it can be helpful to consider whether the flaw is one that is noticeable to the untrained eye or, as Phillips and Dufresne[32] suggest, 'not noticeable at a conversational distance'.

Regardless of the size of the physical defect, BDD patients are far more distressed and disorganized by their perceived flaw. Therefore, many authors[33–35] focus on the degree of preoccupation and impairment in functioning as the hallmark of this disease. The defect with which they present has become an obsession and is described as ruining their lives. In addition,

BDD patients frequently display a rigidity and concreteness in thinking often associated with more severe psychiatric disorders. As Philips and Mckelroy[36] note, while insight can vary amongst these patients, many can be quite delusional.

When I walked into the consulting room, Frank was perched silently on the examining table looking downward and rubbing absent-mindedly on the backs of his hands. A casually dressed, white man of about 40, he seemed unremarkable in all outward appearances. He looked up, smiled wanly and at my general query about why he was here began to talk. He said that three years ago his hair had begun to fall out and he was now going bald. He bowed his head and showed me several areas on his scalp. To both my eyes and those of the dermatologist there was nothing whatsoever noticeable and our physical exam confirmed this. In fact, Frank's hair was rather long and carefully combed, with no evidence of thinning or loss. Frank quickly admitted that he could not go out and was unable to work because of his hair. He spoke about how going bald made him feel ugly and unattractive to woman and unable to go on interviews for jobs. 'Who would ever hire me looking like this' he exclaimed. He went on to say that he felt just like Samson, weak and 'just not a man'. After a bit more history he admitted that he had been saving the hairs in a jar by the side of his bed and was convinced something dreadfully serious must be wrong with him. We reassured him that we did not think this was the case. We offered to do some tests, which despite numerous consultations had not been conducted, and to try to help him solve this dilemma. We also took photos to document his status since he said he lost 'tons of hair each day'. Over the next several weeks we saw him regularly and continued to work with him on understanding his experience of the problem. We reported that the tests and our close monitoring of his scalp indicated there was nothing wrong with him and gently suggested that, as the photos documented, it appeared that he was not actually losing much hair. I explained that people frequently attributed emotional worries such as depression, anxiety, and low self esteem to physical complaints and offered some medication that might improve his mood and decrease his constant worry that he was gravely ill. Although unconvinced that he was not rapidly balding, he was now sufficiently comfortable with us to accept our recommendation, especially when we assured him we would continue to work together.

The prevalence of BDD is thought to be 1–2 per cent in the general population[32]. However, this is considered to underestimate the actual occurrence as many patients report they are too embarrassed to tell their doctor about their concerns[37]. Surprisingly, studies have shown that BDD occurs equally in men and women[38]. The illness often begins in adolescence with the appearance of puberty and the increase in bodily concerns and anxieties about sexuality. BDD frequently occurs co-morbidly with other psychiatric disorders such as depression, obsessive compulsive disorders, social phobias, substance abuse, personality disorders, and other somatic illness such as hypochondria and eating disorders. Several studies have documented that the prevalence in dermatology practices is far higher, with rates varying between 6 per cent and 15 per cent[32]. Thus, this is not a minor problem for the cosmetic practitioner. It is of particular concern because several studies[32,39] indicate that cosmetic treatment is of either no help or actually makes the patients worse.

When Jenny, a 20-year-old secretary, walked into the office Dr S's first thought was that she was a model. He was stunned when she began to cry that she was too ugly to ever get a date. When she indicated the virtually non-existent mole on her upper forearm as the culprit for her despair he was incredulous. Despite his reassurances that 'it was nothing' she kept crying and saying that it made her feel terrible. She was afraid she would die alone and went on to say that her job was in jeopardy because of 'how she looked'. Dr S tried to talk her out of the procedure, adding that the risks from the laser might outweigh the benefits. However, he finally relented, hoping that treatment would make her feel better, only to have her become enraged and depressed at the hyperpigmented mark that was left after the procedure.

This type of reaction makes intuitive sense. For these patients, the cosmetic concern is thought to mask more intense feelings of self loathing or other unconscious conflicts that are not able to be expressed in words but have been displaced on to the skin. It has been my experience that self destructive impulses related to the need for self punishment and problems in self soothing and the ability to manage intense affective states are easily observed. As McDougall has noted[40], these patients are often extremely regressed and have suffered significant trauma that has affected their body integrity at a very early age. This has interfered with their psychological development and their ability to reflect on their own experiences and to form meaningful attachments with others.

Because of the level of distress and impaired thinking, BDD patients often engage in a variety of compulsive behaviors related to their bodily concern. These can include hours of time checking themselves in the mirror, applying camouflage make up, and excessive grooming. These compulsive behaviors can sometimes become destructive, frequently worsening a mild or non-existent condition. In addition to skin picking and excessive scratching, several authors,[35-37] also describe patients who remove their own moles, scour their skin with harsh household chemicals, and perform other 'do it yourself' procedures with catastrophic results. Clearly these behaviors can move beyond the realm of self destructive into the frankly suicidal and there are some data[41] to suggest that these patients have high rates of suicidality.

BDD is thought to be present in many, if not all, patients who seek multiple cosmetic procedures. The patients who have multiple treatments are often recognizable simply by how they look. There do seem to be some natural limitations to what cosmetic treatments can accomplish. Many magazine covers offer excellent examples of people who have sought multiple treatments. Michael Jackson and the Bride of Wildenstien are two of the more famous examples. It seems quite clear that cosmetic treatment with this group is unlikely to turn out well. Thus, for these patients, the seeking of cosmetic treatment really is an example of surgical treatment for a psychological problem that is bound to fail. These are people who end up looking worse despite their efforts to look better. Their need to stay young and their fears of aging and death drive them to make physical changes that are no longer effective. Ironically, in some of the more dramatic cases the intense fear of looking older results in one looking more like a corpse than less so. Treating these patients can be quite difficult as they often have little insight and frequently refuse a psychiatric referral. Their image of themselves is distorted by powerful unconscious forces and they are convinced that changing their outsides will address the sense of disatisfaction or self loathing that they feel inside.

Before concluding this section a brief word should be made about those situations in which a patient in the acute phase of a psychiatric illness comes for cosmetic treatment.

Joan, a 35-year-old grade school teacher, appeared for her appointment dressed in old sweatpants. Dr James, who had known her for several years, noticed that she was also not wearing make up and had not even combed her hair. She told the doctor that she had been feeling tired lately. She was hoping that by smoothing out the laugh lines she hated so much, along with a week's vacation in Florida during the school break where she could work on her tan, things would get better. A few quick questions by Dr James revealed that she had felt too depressed to go to work the last two days and had not been sleeping or eating in a couple of weeks. After ruling out the flu or other organic cause for her behavior, Dr James asked whether she was feeling depressed. She immediately began to cry and admitted that yes, she was. Dr James gently said that fixing her face right now seemed unlikely to help her feel better and instead suggested she might want to call a colleague to make sure that her depression did not get any worse. When she started to balk that she was really fine, Dr James more firmly stated that this was just a precaution but in his professional opinion it was really something she needed to do for herself. Once she was feeling a bit better he promised he would fit her into his schedule and complete the work she requested.

The issue is not that when these patients are no longer depressed they might not want cosmetic treatment. It is that since their desire for treatment is being driven by their depression and a sense of self distorted by this change in mood state, the surface change is almost certainly going to be ineffective and perpetuate a denial of a potentially more serious medical condition. These are patients whose psychological state renders them momentarily unable to make good decisions for themselves. They need their doctor to recognize this and act accordingly by getting the treatment they need and delaying any other decisions until their mood and judgment have improved.

What to do

The good news is that it is possible to recognize these patients and there are several ways to get them the psychiatric help they need. While self report measures are available that have been shown to reliably detect the presence of BDD[41], more useful are good, basic interview skills and the development of a good doctor–patient relationship. Preprocedure interviews should begin with basic questions as to what concerns the patient has about their appearance. Patients should be able to clearly articulate what they do not like about their appearance and what they hope BOTOX® or the cosmetic procedure will accomplish. Their goals should be realistic and within the scope of what the doctor's work can accomplish. Patients who report they are devastated by their problem and have been unable to work or see friends because of the physical defect should immediately alert the physician of the need to explore the appropriateness of cosmetic treatment in more detail. In addition, those who describe spending hours in front of the mirror examining or grooming themselves are describing behavior which may indicate the presence of a more severe psychiatric disorder. It is also wise to always question whether the patient has sought cosmetic treatments before and what their reactions to the procedures have been.

As illustrated in the previous example, when a patient is describing being depressed or anxious about their appearance, further inquiry about the presence of these psychiatric symptoms is warranted. Patients who balk at this type of inquiry are, by their reaction, indicating a greater emotional investment and psychological sensitivity to their appearance and the request for cosmetic treatment. As a rule, overly intense emotional reactions or defensiveness often suggest that an issue is highly charged psychologically. An extreme reaction to a relatively neutral and standard question about a patient's medical history may indicate that other thoughts or feelings are fueling the response. If, after a thorough exploration of the patient's motives, goals, and expectations, the dermatologist is still concerned s/he may wish to seek a consultation. To this end it is useful for cosmetic practitioners to develop a relationship with a psychologist or psychiatrist who is well versed in these issues and with whom they can establish a good, collaborative working relationship. At the point in which a referral becomes indicated it is essential to approach this like any other referral. Explain to the patient that because cosmetic treatment changes the way one looks it almost always impacts on how they feel. In fact, a change in mood or self esteem is usually the motivation for treatment in the first place. The consultation is being sought to assess whether this is the right decision for the patient at this moment in time. Take solace in the thought that sensible patients with whom you can work collaboratively and who want to take the best care of themselves will likely see the wisdom of this. Those who get angry and storm out of the office are likely illustrating that they are not good candidates for cosmetic treatment.

For those who can be referred, or who can be treated within the confines of a dermatologic visit, a number of treatment options do exist. The literature has shown that a variety of psychocutaneous disorders respond well to psychological intervention. Depending on the types of illness and symptoms displayed, individual and group psychotherapy, medication, hypnosis, psychoeducational counseling, and psychoanalysis have all been shown to be extremely useful.

Outcomes

In those patients for whom cosmetic treatment is assessed to be appropriate, outcome studies clearly show that it is effective. Post-procedure interviews and psychometric measures reveal that patients are generally pleased with the results of their cosmetic procedure. Edgerton et al[42] found 86 per cent of his 'aging face' patients reported an improved sense of wellbeing. Marcus[43] found 25 patients who underwent rhinoplasty were pleased with the results, felt more confident in social situations, and were better able to enjoy life. Rankin et al[44] found that depression is lifted and quality of life improves after cosmetic surgery. Meningaud et al[45] also found that social anxiety lessens after surgery and 87 per cent of his sample described positive changes resulting from the procedure. Certainly the anecdotal reports from the dermatologists that I have spoken with about BOTOX® confirm these empirical findings. All report that their patients are almost universally pleased with the results. The only outcome study that assesses patient satisfaction with the use of BOTOX® to treat facial lines also indicates a high level of satisfaction[46]. We can surmise that these satisfied patients did not expect treatment to change their lives but only wanted to look and feel a little bit better about themselves. These do not seem to be people who are pathologically focused on their bodies, or have distorted body image. In fact, studies have shown (see Sawyer et al[28] for review) that while individuals who seek cosmetic treatments may be more dissatisfied with their appearance, they tend to be specifically unhappy with the part of their body they are coming to have changed, not with their appearance as a whole. That is, they do not generally come in saying 'I hate my body', but rather, 'I don't like these wrinkles' or 'my nose is ugly'. They have specific aspects of themselves that they do not like and they wish to have changed. These types of specific complaints may be even more typical of patients requesting BOTOX®. Since this is exactly what cosmetic treatments such as BOTOX® can do, these are the patients who are happy and satisfied with the treatment they receive.

Summary

So far the data seem to suggest that a number of patients seeking cosmetic surgery do have some type of co-morbid psychiatric diagnosis or psychological symptom and that the rates seem to be higher than that of the general population. In addition, there is a smaller group who appear to have the type of severe psychiatric illness that would preclude them from having cosmetic treatment. For this smaller sample the psychological motivation and their goals for cosmetic treatment are likely to be more intense and pervade their whole sense of being. Cosmetic treatment is not experienced as relatively unconflicted but is frequently seen as something that 'will change my life'. For many of these patients, more complex issues of dissatisfaction and conflict have been displaced onto a single physical characteristic and the fantasy is that remedying this physical flaw will alter what is unconsciously a much more profound sense of distress and unhappiness.

However, for large numbers of patients the presence of psychiatric symptoms or conflict does not preclude cosmetic treatments such as BOTOX®. For these people, their wish for cosmetic treatment is not necessarily a consequence of psychiatric disorder and thus pathologic. The uniquely individual choice to have a cosmetic procedure has been integrated into a sense of self that is functionally adaptive. These are people for whom cosmetic treatment represents a decision about their lives and their bodies, not a life-altering or magical experience. For most of these patients, many of the cultural and psychological pressures described earlier are present but not all-consuming. They are influencing but not driving the person to live in a certain way. For these people, cosmetic treatments are not only justified and medically sound but can be very effective.

In closing, I hope that the cosmetic practitioner, especially one who plans to use BOTOX®, has a greater appreciation for the complexity of the work in which s/he is engaged. While it may seem as if the average BOTOX® patient is requesting a simple procedure with little psychological meaning, a more thorough analysis clearly shows that this is not necessarily the case. The choice to change one's body is complex and multidetermined. It is influenced by the culture we live in and the way we feel about ourselves, our bodies, and our sexuality. It clearly involves subtle shifts in how we think about aging as well. The fact that there is more psychological meaning in this choice does not mean that cosmetic procedures are pathologic or morally wrong. Moreover, by listening to our patients and even engaging them in thinking about their decisions more deeply, dermatologists need not fear talking their patients out of something they have already decided to do. However, physicians may learn when the procedure would be dangerous and what steps a patient might take so that they could go forward at a later date. In establishing a thoughtful and collaborative relationship with patients, physicians are in a better position to advise them and have them take their advice.

I am not suggesting that every dermatologist or cosmetic surgeon become a psychologist. That is not who you are, what you are trained in, or what your patients come to you for. At the same time, taking a psychological approach to your work, listening to your patients, and learning a little bit about what makes them tick is an invaluable tool of every good doctor. It is bound to make you better able to assess your patients and determine who needs the treatment you are offering and who does not. It is also certain to aid in the establishment of a good doctor–patient relationship and may even make your work more interesting and rewarding.

References

1. Cordwell JM. Ancient beginnings and modern diversity of the use of cosmetics. In: JA Graham, Kligman AM, eds. *The Psychology of Cosmetic Treatments* 1985:37–44
2. Simon BE. Body image and plastic surgery. In: Graham JA, Kligman AM, eds. *The Psychology of Cosmetic Treatments* 1985:238–46

3. Kligman JA. Overview of psychology of cosmetics. In: Graham JA, Kligman AM, eds. *The Psychology of Cosmetic Treatments* 1985:26–36

4. Grossbart TA, Sarwer DB. Psychosocial issues and their relevance to the cosmetic surgery patient. *Semin Cutan Med Surg* 2003;22:136–47

5. Sullivan HAS. *The Interpersonal Theory of Psychiatry*. New York: WW Norton and Co, 1953

6. American Society for Aesthetic Plastic Surgery. Cosmetic survey national data bank, 2002 statistics

7. Pruzinsky T, Edgerton MT. Body image change in cosmetic plastic surgery. In; Cash, TF, Pruzinsky T, eds. *Body Images: Development, Deviance, and Change* New York: Guilford Press, 1990:217–36

8. Stirn A. Body piercing: medical consequences and psychological motivations. *Lancet* 2003;361:1205–15

9. Cash TF, Gillen B, Burns DS. Sexism and 'Beautyism' in personnel consultant decision making. *J Appl Psychol* 1977;62:301–10

10. Dipboye RL, Fromkin HL, Wiback K. Relative importance of applicant sex, attractiveness, and scholastic standing in evaluation of job applicant resumes. *J Appl Psychol* 1975;60:39–43

11. Frieze I, Olsen J, Russell J. Attractiveness and income for men and women in management. *J Appl Soc Psychol* 1991;21(3):1039–57

12. Dipboye RL, Arvey RD, Terpstra DE. Sex and physical attractiveness of raters and applicants as determinants of resume evaluations. *J Appl Psychol* 1977;62:228–94

13. Hamermesh DS, Biddle JE. Beauty and the labor market. *Am Econ Rev* 1994;84:1174–94

14. Graham JA. Overview of the psychology of cosmetics. In: Graham JA, Kligman AM, eds. *The Psychology of Cosmetic Treatments* 1985:26–36

15. Johnson DF. Appearance and the elderly. In: *The Psychology of Cosmetic Treatments Overview of Psychology of Cosmetics*, New York: Praeger Publishers, 1985:152–60

16. Ringel EW. The morality of cosmetic surgery for aging. *Arch Dermatol* 1998;134:427–31

17. Sawyer DB, Wadden TA, Pertschuk MJ, Whitaker LA. The psychology of cosmetic surgery: a review and reconceptualization. *Clin Psychol Rev* 1998;18:1–22

18. Goin DIM, Goin MK. Psychological understanding and management of the plastic surgery patient. In: Georgiade NG, Georgiade GS, Riefkohl R, Barwick WJ, eds. *Essential of Plastic, Maxillofacial, and Reconstructive Surgery*, Baltimore, MD: Williams & Wilkens, 1987:1127–43

19. Edgerton MT, Jacobson WE, Meyer E. Surgical–psychiatric study of patients seeking plastic (cosmetic) surgery: ninety-eight consecutive patients with minimal deformity. *Br J Plastic Surg* 1960;13:136–45

20. Edgerton MT, Langman MW, Pruzinsky T. Plastic surgery and psychotherapy in the treatment of 100 psychologically disturbed patients. *Plast Reconstr Surg* 1991;88:594–608

21. Meyer E, Jacobson WE, Edgerton MT, Canter A. Motivational patterns in patients seeking elective plastic surgery. *Psychosom Med* 1960;22:193–202

22. Napoleon A. The presentation of personalities in plastic surgery. *Ann Plast Surg* 1993;31:193–208

23. Goin MK, Rees TD. A prospective study of patients' psychological reactions to rhinoplasty. *Ann Plast Surg* 1991;27:210–15

24. Goin MK, Burgoyne RW, Goin JM, Staples FR. A prospective psychological study of 50 female face-lift patients. *Plast Reconstr Surg* 1980;65:436–42

25. Micheli-Pellegrini V, Manfrida GM. Rhinoplasty and its psychological implications: applied psychology observations in aesthetic surgery. *Aesthet Plast Surg* 1979;3:299–319

26. Kisley S, Morkell D, Allbrook B, Briggs P, Jovanovic J. Factors associated with dysmorphic concern and psychiatric morbidity in plastic surgery outpatients. *Aust NZ J Psychiatry* 2002;36:121–6

27. Meningaud JP, Benabida L, Servant JM *et al*. Depression, anxiety and quality of life among scheduled cosmetic surgery patients: multicentre prospective study. *J Cranio-Max Surg* 2001;29:177–80

28. Sawyer DB, Crerand MA. Psychosocial issues in patient outcomes. *Facial Plast Surg* 2002;18:125–33

29. Rohrich RJ. The who, what, when, and why of cosmetic surgery: do our patients need a preoperative psychiatric evaluation? *Plast Reconstr Surg* 2000;106:1605–7

30. American Psychiatric Association. *Diagnostic and Statistical Manual of Mental Disorders*, 4th edn. Washington, DC: APA Press, 1994
31. Grossbart TA, Sawyer DB. Psychosocial issues and their relevance to the cosmetic surgery patient. *Semin Cutan Med Surg* 2003;22:136–47
32. Phillips KA, Dufresne RG. Body dysmorphic disorder: a guide for dermatologists and cosmetic surgeons. *Am J Dermatol* 2000;1:235–43
33. Cotterill JA. Body dysmorphic disorder. *Dermatol Clin* 1996;14:457–63
34. Koblenzer CS. The broken mirror: dysmorphic syndrome in the dermatologist's practice. *Fitz J Clin Dermatol* 1994;March/April:14–9
35. Phillips KA. The Broken Mirror: Understanding and Treating Body Dysmorphic Disorder. New York: Oxford University Press, 1996
36. Philips KA, McElroy SL. Insight, overvalued ideation, and delusional thinking in body dysmorphic disorder: theorectical and treatment implications. *J Nerv Ment Dis* 1993;181(11):699–702
37. Veale D. Outcome of cosmetic surgery and 'DIY' surgery in patients with body dysmorphic disorder. *Psychiatr Bull* 2000;24:218–21
38. Phillips KA, Diaz SF. Gender differences in body dysmorhic disorder. *J Nerv Ment Dis* 1997;185:570–7
39. Castle DJ, Honigman RJ, Phillips KA. Does cosmetic surgery improve psychosocial wellbeing? *MJA* 2002;176:601–4
40. McDougal J. *Theaters of the Body*. New York: W.W. Norton & Co., 1989
41. Dufresne Jr RG, Phillips KA, Vittirio CC, Wilkel CS. A screening questionnaire for body dysmorphic disorder in a cosmetic dermatologic surgery practice. *Dermatol Surg* 2001;27:457–62
42. Edgerton MT, Webb WL, Slaughter R et al. Surgical results and psychosocial changes following rhytidectomy. *Plast Resconstr Surg* 1963;33:503–21
43. Marcus P. Psychological aspects of cosmetic rhinoplasty. *Br J Plast Surg* 1984;37:313–18
44. Rankin M, Borah GL, Perry AW, Wey PD. Quality of life outcomes after cosmetic surgery. *Plast Reconstr Surg* 1998;102:2139–47
45. Meningaud JP, Benadiba L, Servant JM et al. Depression, anxiety and quality of life: outcome 9 months after facial cosmetic surgery. *J Cranio-Max Surg* 2003;31:46–50
46. Cox SE, Finn JC, Stetler L, Mackowiak J, Kowalski JW. Development of the facial lines treatment satisfaction questionnaire and initial results for botulinum toxin type-A treated patients. *Dermatol Surg* 2003;29:444–9

1 PHARMACOLOGY, IMMUNOLOGY, AND CURRENT DEVELOPMENTS

K Roger Aoki

History

Botulinum toxin type A stands alongside digitalis, atropine, and paclitaxel as natural compounds that, although first noted for their toxic properties, are now routinely used as medicines. The recorded history of botulinum neurotoxins dates back to human encounters with improperly stored food, which caused the sickness known as botulism when ingested. In the early 1800s, the German physician Kerner provided one of the earliest descriptions of food poisoning caused by botulism that followed ingestion of smoked sausages[1]. In the late 1800s, Professor van Ermengem, a Belgian microbiologist, identified botulinum neurotoxin as the cause of botulism in a group of Belgian musicians who had eaten inappropriately prepared sausages.

The events of the Second World War stimulated research and study into the activity of botulinum neurotoxins. Much of this research was conducted by Drs Lamanna, Schantz (Figure 1.1), and colleagues at Fort Detrick, Maryland, where botulinum toxin type A was purified, obtained in crystalline form, and synthesized in sufficient quantities for research[1]. A number of other investigators, including Burgen and Brooks, made much progress throughout the late 1940s and 1950s in understanding the mechanism of action of botulinum neurotoxins. By the late 1960s, the inhibitory effects of botulinum toxin type A on acetylcholine release at the neuromuscular junction had been well characterized in experimental animals[1] (Figure 1.2).

Working at the Smith-Kettlewell Eye Research Institute in San Francisco in the 1970s, ophthalmologist Alan Scott was investigating alternatives to surgery for his patients with strabismus, a condition of ocular misalignment. Dr Scott believed that a substance that could chemically weaken the extraocular muscles pulling the eyes out of alignment might prove a useful alternative to surgical excision of the muscles. On the advice of a colleague, Dr Scott

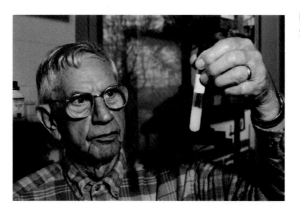

Figure 1.1   Professor Ed Schantz in his laboratory

contacted Professor Schantz to ask whether he had a substance that might be used to produce such chemical denervation. Schantz suggested botulinum toxin type A and Scott soon reported that this protein was able to correct strabismus in an experimental model[1]. The minute quantities of botulinum toxin type A injected directly into its site of action (in this case, extraocular muscles) prevented systemic absorption of clinically significant amounts.

Following this initial success, Schantz, now working at the University of Wisconsin, began developing botulinum toxin type A for testing in humans, focusing on purification, high potency, and preservation. Because no protein drugs of this type had ever been developed, the methods and requirements were novel. Schantz selected the Hall strain of *Clostridium botulinum* for type A toxin for production because it yielded a good quantity of high quality toxin, which was necessary for further purification and regulatory requirements. Scott went on to successfully use the botulinum toxin type A that Schantz had produced for the treatment of strabismus and blepharospasm in humans[2]. The batch of botulinum toxin type A developed by Schantz was eventually approved for human use (Figure 1.2) under the name Oculinum™. Oculinum™ was later acquired by Allergan Inc. and, under the name, BOTOX®, has been the primary treatment for focal dystonias since the late 1980s and, over the past decade, has become an important adjunctive treatment worldwide for adult spasticity and juvenile cerebral palsy.

Although initial studies focused on the effects of botulinum toxin type A in conditions of skeletal muscle hyperactivity, it has become clear that its action extends to other classes of disorders. Botulinum toxin type A is being actively investigated for the treatment of many smooth muscle conditions such as achalasia, anal fissure, and overactive bladder and is an

Bacteria identified as cause of botulism

Studies of BTX-A in animal muscle

| 1822 | 1895 | 1940s | 1960s |

Neurologic effects first noted from sausage ingestion

BTX-A isolated, purified

First FDA approval

Studied for treatment of dystonias, spasticity, selected other conditions

FDA approval for primary axillary hyperhidrosis

| 1970s | 1989 | 1980s and 1990s | 2000 | 2004 |

First tested in strabismus patients

Strabismus, blepharo-spasm

FDA approval for cervical dystonia

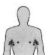

Figure 1.2   History of botulinum neurotoxin development

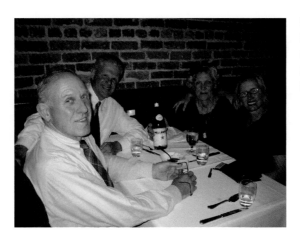

Figure 1.3   From left to right: Drs Alan Scott, Alastair Carruthers, Mrs Ruth Scott and Dr Jean Carruthers at one of their catch-up sessions

accepted treatment for some autonomic disorders such as primary hyperhidrosis. It has also demonstrated utility in migraine and certain other painful conditions, leading to the exploration of possible additional mechanisms of action outside of its inhibition of acetylcholine release. Botulinum toxin A was approved for temporary improvement of moderate to severe glabellar (frown) lines associated with corrugator and/or procerus muscle activity in adult patients aged 65 years or less by the United States FDA in 2002 (BOTOX® Cosmetic) and subsequently in other countries (Vistabel® or Vistabex®). This first approval for an aesthetic indication was due to the early observation by Dr. Jean Carruthers while she worked with Dr Alan Scott during the early clinical evaluation of Oculinum (Figure 1.3).

The majority of clinical studies on botulinum neurotoxin have been conducted with the type A preparation produced from the Hall strain of *C. botulinum* (BOTOX®). This was the original preparation used clinically and continues as the most widely studied and used botulinum neurotoxin therapeutic in the world today. In 2000, a botulinum neurotoxin preparation based on the B serotype was introduced into clinical use in the United States and Europe for the treatment of cervical dystonia. Additional preparations based on the A serotype (based on a different strain than the US product) are also available in Europe and other countries outside of the United States. As biologic products, doses of botulinum neurotoxins are given in units of biological activity as opposed to weight in milligrams as is commonly used for chemically synthesized drugs. However, unlike most other medicinal biological products, units of botulinum neurotoxins are not standardized, and thus doses of one product do not apply to any of the others.

Manufacture of botulinum neurotoxins for clinical use

Botulinum neurotoxins are complex biologic products that must be manufactured according to strict regulatory requirements in order to be approved for clinical use in the United States and other countries. The method of manufacture determines not only the purity of the final product but also the reproducibility of labeled units. The process used to stabilize the neurotoxin protein (e.g. lyophilization, vacuum drying, low pH) can also affect the product's clinical pharmacology, as can excipients added during the manufacturing process. The general process by which botulinum neurotoxins are manufactured is shown in Figure 1.4.

Botulinum neurotoxins are produced by several different clostridial bacterial species and strains. *Clostridium botulinum* is the best known species, although *Clostridium butyricum*,

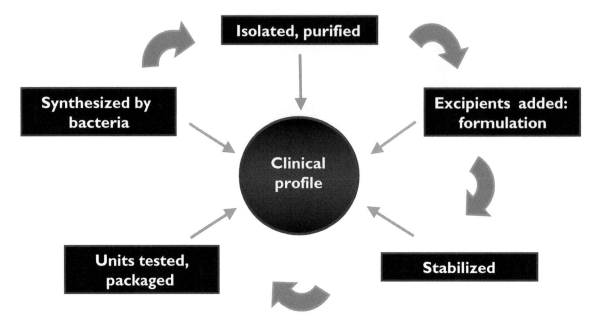

Figure 1.4 General methods of manufacture of botulinum neurotoxins for therapeutic use. Each step in the manufacturing process has the potential to affect clinical profile

Clostridium baratii, and *Clostridium argentinese* also produce botulinum neurotoxins[3]. The different strains of organisms that produce botulinum neurotoxins exhibit variable characteristics, such as temperature needed for growth and proteolytic activity[3]. The particular bacterial strain from which the botulinum neurotoxin is obtained determines many of its properties, including neurotoxin complex size and extent of nicking[3]. Each preparation of botulinum neurotoxin designed for clinical use is synthesized by a different strain of bacteria.

For all botulinum neurotoxin preparations approved for clinical use in the United States, the neurotoxin complex is isolated and purified from the bacterial media using state of the art, pharmaceutical level techniques. Next, excipients are added that comprise the formulation of the botulinum neurotoxin preparation. As shown in Table 1.1, the commercially available

TABLE 1.1 FORMULATIONS OF DIFFERENT BOTULINUM NEUROTOXIN PREPARATIONS[4–7]

BOTOX® (Allergan) (100-U vial)	Dysport® (Ipsen) (500-U vial)	Myobloc® (Elan) (10,000-U vial)
• ~5 ng botulinum toxin type A 900-kDa protein	• ~12.5 ng botulinum toxin type A 900-kDa protein	• ~100 ng botulinum toxin type B 500–700-kDa protein
• 500,000 ng serum albumin	• 125,000 ng serum albumin	• 0.05% serum albumin
• 900,000 ng sodium chloride	• 2,500,000 ng lactose	• 0.1 M sodium chloride
• Vacuum dried	• Lyophilized	• 0.01 M sodium succinate
		• Liquid formulation, pH 5.6

botulinum neurotoxin products have different formulations and vary according to serotype and amount of neurotoxin complex protein, sodium chloride or lactose, and serum albumin. As can be seen from the table, the amount of neurotoxin complex protein that is present in these products is extremely small compared with the amounts of other ingredients.

Each product's distinct formulation results in a unique interaction with biologic systems following injection. The system is exposed to different ingredients and different numbers of molecules that likely influence local osmotic gradients and diffusion. The precise effects of such potentially different interactions have not been adequately studied, but the identity and amount of the diluent used can alter biologic potency[8,9].

The preparation is then stabilized using one of several different available methods, depending on the manufacturer. All botulinum toxins begin the finished product manufacturing process as solutions that must be converted into more stable forms for therapeutic use. Botulinum toxin type A BONT-A. (Allergan) is vacuum dried in a lyophilizer, BONT-A (Ipsen) is stabilized by freeze-drying in a lyophilizer, and BONT-B (Elan) is stabilized as a low pH (5.6) solution.

The units are then tested. For all botulinum neurotoxin preparations, 1 unit (U) is defined as the amount of neurotoxin complex protein administered intraperitoneally in a biological assay I.P. LD_{50}) of a group of 18- to 20-gram female Swiss Webster mice[10]. Even though the same definition of units applies to all botulinum toxin preparations, it is now widely accepted that units of the various preparations are not equal[11,12]. This is most likely due to differences in the way the lethality tests are performed (especially the diluent used) and differences among serotypes.

For the final potency testing step, BONT-A (Ipsen) is dissolved in gelatin phosphate buffer, whereas BONT-A (Allergan) is dissolved in saline. For clinical use, the product labels for both BONT-A preparations recommend dilution with sterile unpreserved saline. The addition of gelatin to the diluent affects the number of LD_{50} units obtained, which may be one reason that more units of BONT-A (Ipsen) than BONT-A (Allergan) are needed for clinical efficacy.

Structure

There are seven serotypes of botulinum neurotoxins (A, B, C_1, D, E, F, and G) produced by different strains of *C. botulinum* with serotype C_2 being cytotoxic and not neurotoxic. All of the botulinum neurotoxins are synthesized as single-chain proteins of approximately 150 kDa that must be nicked or cleaved by proteases into di-chain molecules of approximately 100-kDa and 50-kDa subunits in order to be active[13] (Figure 1.5). Cleavage results in a di-chain molecule consisting of an approximately 100-kDa heavy chain and an approximately 50-kDa light chain, linked by a disulfide bond[14]. Botulinum-producing organisms may be classified as proteolytic or non-proteolytic, denoting the presence or absence of endogenous enzymes that cleave the 150-kDa single-chain neurotoxin into the active di-chain neurotoxin[15]. Type A-producing strains are proteolytic and nearly all of the toxin recovered from these organisms (>95 per cent) exists in the di-chain form[16].

Type B-producing strains may be either proteolytic or non-proteolytic. Proteolytic type B strains have been found to cleave approximately 30 per cent of the single-chain proteins, although the percentage nicked in the commercial product based on the B serotype may be significantly higher[17]. Clostridial strains that synthesize toxin serotypes E and F are non-proteolytic and the toxin they produce must be exposed to exogenous proteases in order to exert its activity[15,18,19].

Inactive single-chain neurotoxin protein

Activated di-chain neurotoxin protein

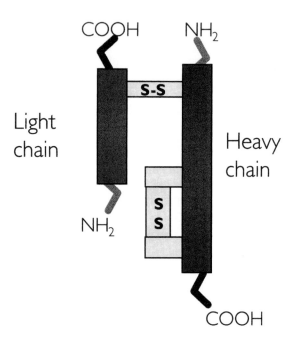

Figure 1.5   Structure of botulinum neurotoxin unnicked, inactive single-chain protein (150 kDa) and nicked, activated di-chain protein (100-kDa and 50-kDa chains)

Botulinum neurotoxins are produced as part of a multimeric protein complex consisting of the neurotoxin and associated hemagglutinin and non-hemagglutinin proteins. The number and identity of the associated proteins vary by serotype and organism[13]. The associated proteins serve to stabilize and protect the neurotoxin molecule from degradation[20].

The crystal structure of botulinum toxin type A was first reported by Professor Raymond Stevens and colleagues[21], which confirmed many of the predictions gleaned from studies of physiology and pharmacology. The protein structure is flat and comprises three modules: the endopeptidase (light chain), the translocation domain (N-terminal half of the heavy chain), and the binding domain (C-terminal half of the heavy chain). The crystal structure of type B is similar to that of type A[22]. The crystal structures of the other serotypes have not yet been reported, although work is proceeding toward this end.

Pharmacology

Mechanism(s) of action

Botulinum neurotoxins exert their activity through a multistep process that involves binding to nerve terminals, internalization, and inhibition of calcium-dependent neurotransmitter release[23].

The heavy chain (~100 kDa) subunit of the botulinum neurotoxin molecule binds to acceptors on nerve terminal membranes[23], located primarily but not exclusively on cholinergic neurons[24,25]. The specificity of these acceptors appears to be different between different botulinum serotypes[24–26]. Although the precise identities of the botulinum neurotoxin acceptors are not known, they are thought to comprise proteins and gangliosides. Progress in identifying the type B acceptor has recently been reported: in PC12 cells and rat diaphragm motor nerve terminals, the entry of botulinum toxin type B (but not type A or E) appears to be mediated by the secretory vesicle proteins synaptotagmins I and II[26]. A recent study has identified two critical carbohydrate interaction sites on the Hc fragment of tetanus toxin that participate in the binding and uptake process of this protein into neurons[27]. Mutation of residues in the binding pocket markedly decreases the binding affinity of tetanus toxin in vitro and significantly attenuates the effects of tetanus toxin on exocytosis[27]. In comparison, botulinum toxin serotypes A and B bind only a single molecule of ganglioside GT1b, with critical residues located within the carboxyl terminal half of the Hc fragment[28].

Following binding, botulinum neurotoxins are translocated into the neuronal cytosol via acceptor-mediated endocytosis[29]. There appear to be two distinct internalization processes: a rapid uptake which may utilize the vesicle recycling system and a slower uptake requiring hours, which may be a less specific endocytotic process. This internalization process is energy dependent and is critical for the activity of botulinum neurotoxins[24]. Upon acidification of the endosome, it is hypothesized that a pH-dependent change in the translocation domain of the heavy chain facilitates the translocation of the light chain to the cytoplasmic compartment. The exact mechanism of this translocation process is not known, but it has been speculated that the heavy chain can form a pore through which the light chain can pass[29]. Inside the endocytotic vesicles, the neurotoxin structure undergoes a conformational change in the presence of a low pH, and the L chain is released into the cytosol accompanied by reduction of the disulfide bond that linked it to the heavy chain.

Once inside the cytosol, the light chain cleaves one or more of the SNARE (soluble *N*-ethylmaleimide-sensitive factor attachment protein receptor) proteins necessary for vesicle docking and fusion, thereby reducing exocytotic neurotransmitter release (Figure 1.6). Each serotype cleaves a specific peptide bond on one or more of the SNARE proteins[29]. The enzymatic activity of the light chain requires the presence of the intramolecular zinc.

Botulinum neurotoxins reduce quantal neurotransmitter release elicited by action potentials, as well as spontaneous quantal acetylcholine release, as determined by an inhibition of miniature endplate potentials[30]. In response to reduced neurotransmitter release, sprouts appear at motor-nerve terminals and nodes of Ranvier, which have been noted within 2 days after injection of type A into mammalian soleus muscles. These sprouts persist and become more complex for at least 50 days following intramuscular injection of type A[30]. Sprouts may establish functional synaptic contacts[30,31]. Eventually, exocytosis is restored, the original terminals recover and the sprouts regress[32]. After re-innervation is complete, the target tissue is fully functional[30] and there is no clinical indication that post-botulinum re-innervation produces functionally substandard synapses.

Botulinum neurotoxins act not only on efferent motor pathways but also on autonomic efferent pathways, which also utilize acetylcholine as a neurotransmitter. The inhibitory effects of botulinum toxin type A on autonomic terminals have led to its successful use in conditions of autonomic hyperactivity such as hyperhidrosis and gustatory sweating[33]. Although the effects

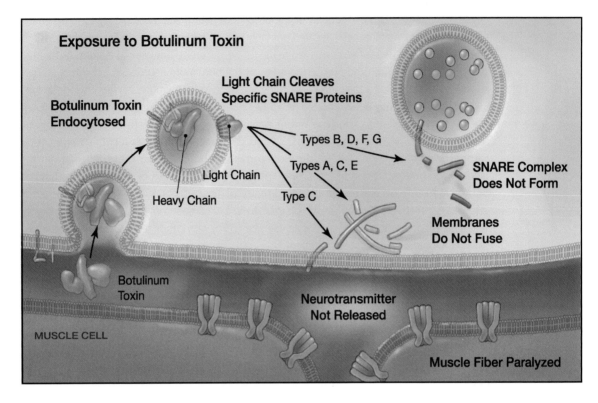

Figure 1.6   Mechanism of action of botulinum neurotoxins
Amon *et al.* JAMA 2001, 285;8:1059–70; copyright© 2001, 285;1059 American Medical Association

on autonomic and motor terminals are thought to occur by a similar mechanism (i.e. binding, internalization, and inhibition of neurotransmitter release), the clinical effects are of longer duration in autonomic conditions than in neuromuscular conditions[33]. The reason for this difference is unknown.

Direct evidence from preclinical studies and indirect evidence from clinical studies indicate that botulinum toxin type A affects afferent pathways via inhibition of neural input to intrafusal fibers[34,35]. Intrafusal fibers are encapsulated fibers that make up muscle spindles (Figure 1.7), or the proprioceptive organs located among skeletal muscle fibers (extrafusal fibers). Extrafusal fibers are innervated by alpha motor neurons, whereas intrafusal fibers are innervated by gamma motor neurons and Ia sensory afferents. The inhibition of gamma motor neurons decreases activation of muscle spindles, which effectively changes the sensory afferent system by reducing the Ia traffic. Filippi *et al.*[34] confirmed this hypothesis by establishing that local injections of botulinum toxin type A directly reduce afferent Ia fiber traffic in rats, thereby modulating sensory feedback. Histologic support for the direct effect of botulinum toxin type A on the rat muscle spindles supported the electrophysiologic results[35]. Thus, the overall effect of botulinum toxin type A therapy is a combination of a direct effect on the primary nerve-end organ communication coupled with an indirect effect on the overall system.

In recent years, there has been an upsurge in research focus on possible actions of botulinum neurotoxins on neurotransmitters other than acetylcholine. The current developments in this area are discussed in the last section of this chapter.

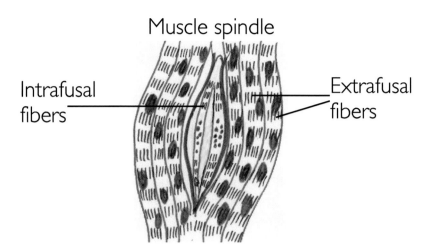

Muscle spindle

Intrafusal fibers

Extrafusal fibers

Figure 1.7 Muscle spindle structure showing intrafusal and extrafusal fibers

Clinical pharmacology

The initial preclinical studies conducted with botulinum toxin type A formed the basis for our understanding of its actions at the neuromuscular junction, including mechanism of action, potency, onset and duration of action, and recovery of function[36,37]. The well-characterized nature of this protein in inhibiting neurotransmitter release at the neuromuscular junction ultimately led Professor Schantz to suggest to Dr Scott that it might be useful for weakening the extraocular muscles of his patients, as previously described.

Neuromuscular injection

In the clinic, botulinum toxin type A is most often injected into overactive muscles that vary depending on the condition to be treated and the patient's individual presentation. Onset of action following intramuscular injection is approximately 3 to 7 days[38]. The beneficial effects of each treatment with botulinum toxin type A last approximately 3 to 5 months in neuromuscular conditions[38–40]. The duration of botulinum toxin type B (Elan) is somewhat shorter than that of type A[41,42], and has been reported as 6 to 8 weeks with 1000 units and 10 to 12 weeks with 2000 units in the management of facial lines[38].

Due to the chronic nature of most of the neuromuscular conditions that botulinum neurotoxins are used to treat, repeated injections are typically required over the course of many years. The results of numerous studies indicate that most patients respond to botulinum toxin type A for many years without decrements in safety, responsiveness, or quality of life, and without increased doses[43–48]. Some studies have reported enhanced benefits with botulinum toxin type A following repeated injections, showing increased duration[49,50], decreased adverse events[50], or greater functional improvements (e.g. gait in children with cerebral palsy[51]) with successive injections. In the case of improved gait, this may be due to adaptation of the patient to reduced tone. However, the increased duration and other benefits may also be due to altered sensory feedback from the periphery to the central nervous system[52]. The effects of botulinum toxin type A on gamma motor neurons that innervate intrafusal fibers lead to changes in muscle spindle activity[34] that may ultimately lead to central nervous system adaptation[53].

Intradermal injection

In the treatment of focal hyperhidrosis, botulinum toxin type A is injected intradermally instead of intramuscularly[54]. The onset of action of botulinum toxin type A in various forms of hyperhidrosis is within 1 week[55], and benefits last approximately 7 months[56]. Benefits are maintained following repeated injections for at least 16 months[56]; longer studies have not yet been conducted for this indication, although there is no a priori reason to expect that patients with hyperhidrosis would not continue to respond over many years given the results in other similarly dosed indications[43,44,50].

Several studies have examined the use of botulinum toxin type B for axillary hyperhidrosis[57,58]. These studies have found that type B significantly reduces sweating, but with distal autonomic side effects that are not observed with type A such as visual accommodation difficulties and dry mouth[57,58].

Immunology

Like most foreign proteins introduced into the body, botulinum neurotoxins can be antigenic and, under the right circumstances (i.e. dose and frequency), elicit immune responses designed to inactivate the protein.

The antigenicity of botulinum neurotoxins has been recognized since the late 1800s when an inactive form of the substance produced by van Ermengem's cultures was subsequently injected into goats and found to elicit antitoxin[1]. During the next decade, differences in the antitoxins produced to botulinum neurotoxins from various clostridial strains led to the discovery and identification of different botulinum neurotoxin serotypes[59,60]. Subsequent studies have identified some similar epitopes within the sequences of different botulinum neurotoxin serotypes[61], suggesting a basis for cross-reactivity.

Only antibodies formed against the 150-kDa neurotoxin neutralize its activity[62]. Antibodies may occasionally be formed against the non-toxin proteins in the botulinum neurotoxin complex, but these do not affect clinical responsiveness[62]. Within the botulinum toxin type A molecule, antibodies directed against the receptor-binding region in the heavy chain are neutralizing[61,63].

Despite the antigenic nature of botulinum neurotoxin proteins, antibody formation that interferes with the clinical responsiveness to botulinum toxin type A (BOTOX®) is infrequent[64–67]. This is probably because of the high potency of botulinum toxin type A, which produces clinical effects in extremely small quantities. However, frequent injections (i.e. more than every 3 months) or booster injections may increase the likelihood of an immune response against the neurotoxin[67]. Due to differences in manufacturing methods, different botulinum toxin preparations may show different antigenicity profiles even if they are based on the same serotype. The low rate of neutralizing antibody formation with botulinum toxin type A (BOTOX®, Allergan) has been confirmed in a recent study of 119 cervical dystonia patients[68]. None of these patients had detectable neutralizing antibodies in their serum after a mean of four treatments.

The finding of primary or secondary clinical non-responsiveness without evidence of neutralizing antibodies suggests that there may be other reasons for lack of response to botulinum neurotoxins. These reasons include patient perception; for example, subsequent injections may appear to have a less dramatic effect than the first[69], either because patients continue to experience some benefit from the previous injection or perhaps due to lack of memory about the severity of their condition prior to injection. The injections may not be directed into the optimal muscles or the muscles involved may have changed from the previous visit either due to progression of the disorder or neural adaptation[70,71]. These changes may require a modification of injection sites, dose, or both in order to maintain optimal treatment benefit.

Current developments

Possible mechanism(s) of action in pain

For many years it has been known that botulinum toxin type A reduces pain associated with cervical dystonia[72]. This observation led to additional study of the effects of botulinum toxin type A in pain associated with spasticity[73], myofascial pain[74], and certain headache disorders[75]. Investigations into the effects of botulinum toxin type A on migraine were prompted by reports of improvement in headaches following injection for facial lines[76,77].

Pain is transmitted to the central nervous system by two types of afferent nerves or primary nociceptive afferents: A delta fibers that mediate sharp, pricking pain and C fibers that mediate slow, long-lasting pain. The cell bodies of these neurons are located in the dorsal root ganglia, where they send out a single process that branches to innervate the periphery as free nerve endings (nociceptors – pain sensory organs) and the other to innervate the central nervous system, synapsing on neurons in the dorsal horn of the spinal cord. Pain sensations detected in the face and head are transmitted by trigeminal neurons (A delta and C fibers) whose cell bodies are located in the trigeminal ganglion and whose axons synapse in the brain stem. Type C fibers release substance P, somatostatin, and other neuropeptides from both central and peripheral terminals. These peptides mediate pain and inflammatory reactions.

The effects of botulinum toxin type A in migraine[78] and the lack of direct concordance between its effects on muscle relaxation and improvement in pain in neuromuscular conditions[79] suggest that pain relief may not be strictly secondary to the reduction of muscle contractions. This has led to an increase in research directed at identifying possible mechanisms by which botulinum toxin type A may act to reduce pain.

Botulinum toxin type A has been found to inhibit substance P release from cultured dorsal root ganglion neurons[80]. Substance P is a peptide neurotransmitter released by primary nociceptive afferents (C fibers). Additionally, recent results from our laboratory indicate that subcutaneous injection of botulinum toxin type A dose-dependently inhibits formalin-induced nociceptive behavior in rats (phase 2 but not phase 1), in the absence of any measurable effects on muscle weakness[81]. Additionally, botulinum toxin type A reduced formalin-evoked glutamate release in this model[81]. In another study, botulinum toxin type A has been found to reduce the stimulated but not basal release of calcitonin gene-related peptide (CGRP) from cultured trigeminal ganglia neurons[82]. CGRP is an inflammatory neuropeptide that is contained within dorsal root ganglia neurons and co-localized with substance P in most trigeminal and other sensory ganglia neurons. Current views of migraine pathophysiology emphasize the role of the trigeminovascular system, with trigeminal afferents thought to release CGRP, substance P, and possibly other neuropeptides that cause painful neurogenic inflammation of the meningeal vasculature[83,84]. Taken together, these results suggest a basis for non-cholinergic actions of botulinum toxin type A that may play a role in its analgesic effects.

Botulinum toxin type A inhibits the release of acetylcholine from both alpha and gamma motor neurons. Alpha motor neurons innervate extrafusal fibers of skeletal muscles and stimulate muscular contractions that lead to movement. Gamma motor neurons innervate the ends of intrafusal muscle fibers, which make up muscle spindles, and stimulate their contraction. Muscle spindles are proprioceptive organs situated among skeletal muscle fibers. Sensory fibers termed Ia afferents innervate the center of the intrafusal fibers. When the muscle spindle is stretched, the primary sensory ending sends impulses to the spinal cord.

Potential effects of botulinum toxin type A on pain may be relevant for dermatologists who encounter patients with neuropathic pain localized to facial regions such as post-herpetic neuralgia[85]. Intradermal injections of botulinum toxin type A have been reported to benefit such patients[86] although further study is needed (see Chapter 7).

Other current basic research findings

In order for botulinum neurotoxin preparations to be useful as therapeutics, the active neurotoxin molecule must remain at the site of injection. Uncontrolled diffusion leads to unwanted side effects through the weakening of nearby uninjected muscles or diffusion into the systemic circulation to induce more generalized or distant autonomic effects. Recent results suggest that the botulinum toxin type A 900-kDa complex may diffuse to a lesser extent than the free 150-kDa neurotoxin molecule[87], which suggests that the non-toxin proteins may play a role in the side-effect profiles of botulinum neurotoxin preparations.

The various botulinum neurotoxin serotypes are known to have different durations of action, with types A and C1 exhibiting the longest durations, types E and F much shorter durations, and type B an intermediate duration[88]. The longer duration of type A than other serotypes has been related to the persistence of the type A protease within the affected cell[88] and the prolonged turnover time of the type A cleavage product designated SNAP-25$_A$[89]. Recent results indicate that the protease domain of the type A light chain localizes in a punctate manner to the plasma membrane, in association with the cleaved product, SNAP-25$_A$ or SNAP-25(197)[90]. In contrast, the botulinum toxin type E light chain is localized to the cytoplasm. It has been hypothesized that localization of the type A protease to the plasma membrane and/or its interaction with the cleaved protein may partially protect it from degradation, thereby contributing to its extended duration of action compared with other serotypes[90]. In contrast, the cytoplasmic location of type E protease may make it more susceptible to degradation. This hypothesis is consistent with the much longer duration of type A than type E noted in humans and preclinical models[91,92].

Although much research has attempted to identify a protein binding site for botulinum toxin type A, polysialyated gangliosides remain the only well characterized acceptor/receptor candidates[93]. A recent study examined the binding of botulinum toxin type A to ganglioside GT1b using surface plasmon resonance, a technique that permits measurement of binding kinetics without the use of fluorescence or radiolabels[93]. This study found that the binding of botulinum toxin type A to GT1b in a phospholipid monolayer depended on ionic strength and proceeded at NaCl concentrations up to 150 mM. Binding did not follow a 1:1 model. Additional study indicated that the stability of the botulinum toxin type A–GT1b complex increased over time and that the conformation of botulinum toxin type A changed following incubation with GT1b. Using circular dichroism, a 25 per cent increase in alpha helix content and 23 per cent decrease in beta sheet content was observed over time[93].

In other research, Dong and colleagues reported that botulinum toxin type B binds to gangliosides as well as synaptotagmins I and II[26]. These molecules are thought to constitute co-receptors for botulinum toxin type B. However, botulinum toxin type A did not bind to synaptotagmins[26], although the possibility of another co-receptor protein for type A has not been ruled out. Yowler and Schengrund have hypothesized that the conformational change they observed following botulinum toxin type A binding to GT1b may permit subsequent binding to a protein co-receptor[93].

Summary

Botulinum toxin type A has a rich history of study that was first based on its identification as a toxin and later on its application as a potent medicine. Botulinum toxin type A and the six additional botulinum neurotoxin serotypes (B through G) share a similar molecular structure and basic mechanism of action. However, differences in the intracellular protein target or target site cleaved by the light chain of each serotype lead to variations in duration of action and possibly other effects. Evidence suggests that the clinical benefits of botulinum toxin type A may not only be due to its inhibition of acetylcholine release from motor efferent fibers, but also due to an indirect reduction in sensory feedback through the inhibition of acetylcholine release from gamma motor neurons. The onset and duration of botulinum toxin type A have been well characterized in many different disorders, with effects lasting longer in autonomic than neuromuscular conditions. Based on the available research, botulinum toxin type B appears to have a shorter duration of action than type A, as well as more autonomic side effects.

Basic and clinical research on botulinum neurotoxins is progressing rapidly, particularly in the area of pain. Evidence suggests that botulinum toxin type A inhibits release of neurotransmitters involved in the generation of pain, such as glutamate, substance P, and calcitonin gene-related peptide, which may form the basis for its beneficial effects in migraine and other painful conditions. Along with the frequent reports of potential novel uses of botulinum toxin, the developments in pain continue to make botulinum neurotoxin research a high priority.

References

1. Schantz EJ, Johnson EA. Botulinum toxin: the story of its development for the treatment of human disease. *Perspect Biol Med* 1997;40(3):317–27
2. Scott AB. Botulinum toxin injection into extraocular muscles as an alternative to strabismus surgery. *Ophthalmology* 1980;87(10):1044–9
3. Hatheway CL. Bacterial sources of clostridial neurotoxins. In: Simpson LL, ed. *Botulinum Neurotoxin and Tetanus Toxin*. San Diego: Academic Press, 1989: 3–24
4. Botox Prescribing Information, Allergan Inc., 2004
5. Myobloc Prescribing Information, Elan Pharmaceuticals, 2000
6. Dysport® Product Characteristics, Ipsen Ltd 2001. Available at: http://www.ipsen.com/staticfiles/Internet/Static_Files/Documents/Produits/Dysport_EN.pdf Accessed 9 September 2004
7. Markey AC. Dysport®. *Dermatol Clin* 2004:213–19
8. Rollnik JD, Matzke M, Wohlfarth K, Dengler R, Bigalke H. Low-dose treatment of cervical dystonia, blepharospasm and facial hemispasm with albumin-diluted botulinum toxin type A under EMG guidance. An open label study. *Eur Neurol* 2000;43(1):9–12
9. Mclellan K, Das RE, Ekong TA, Sesardic D. Therapeutic botulinum type A toxin: factors affecting potency. *Toxicon* 1996;34(9):975–85
10. Hatheway CL, Dang C. Immunogenicity of neurotoxins of *Clostridium botulinum*. In: Jankovic J, Hallett M, eds. *Therapy with Botulinum Toxin*. New York: Marcel Dekker 1994:25:93–107

11. Brin MF, Blitzer A. Botulinum toxin: dangerous terminology errors. *J R Soc Med* 1993;86:493–4

12. Brin MF, Aoki KR, Dressler D. Pharmacology of botulinum toxin therapy. In: Brin MF, Comella C, Jankovic J, eds. *Dystonia: Etiology, Clinical Features, and Treatment*. Philadelphia: Lippincott, Williams & Wilkins, 2004:93–112

13. Melling J, Hambleton P, Shone CC. *Clostridium botulinum* toxins: nature and preparation for clinical use. *Eye* 1988;2(Pt 1):16–23

14. Das Gupta BR, Sugiyama H. Role of a protease in natural activation of *Clostridium botulinum* neurotoxin. *Infect Immun* 1972;6(4):587–90

15. Sakaguchi G, Kozaki S, Ohishi I. Structure and function of botulinum toxins. In: Alouf JE, ed. *Bacterial Protein Toxins*. London: Academic Press, 1984:435–43

16. DasGupta BR, Sathyamoorthy V. Purification and amino acid composition of type A botulinum neurotoxin. *Toxicon* 1984;22:415–24

17. Setler PE. Pharmacology of botulinum toxin type B. *Eur J Neurol* 2001;8(Suppl 4):9–12

18. DasGupta BR, Sugiyama H. Molecular forms of neurotoxins in proteolytic *Clostridium botulinum* type B cultures. *Infect Immun* 1976;14:680–6

19. Duff JT, Wright GG, Yarinsky A. Activation of *Clostridium botulinum* type E toxin by trypsin. *J Bacteriol* 1956;72:455–60

20. Chen F, Kuziemko GM, Stevens RC. Biophysical characterization of the stability of the 150-kilodalton botulinum toxin, the nontoxic component, and the 900-kilodalton botulinum toxin complex species. *Infect Immun* 1998;66(6):2420–5

21. Lacy DB, Tepp W, Cohen AC *et al*. Crystal structure of botulinum neurotoxin type A and implications for toxicity. *Nat Struct Biol* 1998;5(10):898–902

22. Swaminathan S, Eswaramoorthy S. Structural analysis of the catalytic and binding sites of *Clostridium botulinum* neurotoxin B. *Nat Struct Biol* 2000;7(8):693–9

23. Simpson LL. Peripheral actions of the botulinum toxins. In: Simpson LL, ed. *Botulinum Neurotoxin and Tetanus Toxin*. San Diego, CA: Academic Press, 1989:153–78

24. Black JD, Dolly JO. Interaction of ^{125}I-labeled botulinum neurotoxins with nerve terminals: II. Autoradiographic evidence for its uptake into motor nerves by acceptor-mediated endocytosis. *J Cell Biol* 1986;103:535–44

25. Black JD, Dolly JO. Selective location of acceptors for botulinum neurotoxin A in the central and peripheral nervous systems. *Neuroscience* 1987;32:767–9

26. Dong M, Richards DA, Goodnough MC *et al*. Synaptotagmins I and II mediate entry of botulinum neurotoxin B into cells. *J Cell Biol* 2003;162:1293–303

27. Rummel A, Bade S, Alves J *et al*. Two carbohydrate binding sites in the H(CC)-domain of tetanus neurotoxin are required for toxicity. *J Mol Biol* 2003;326(3):835–47

28. Rummel A, Mahrhold S, Bigalke H *et al*. The HCC-domain of botulinum neurotoxins A and B exhibits a singular ganglioside binding site displaying serotype specific carbohydrate interaction. *Mol Microbiol* 2004;51(3):631–43

29. Pellizzari R, Rossetto O, Schiavo G *et al*. Tetanus and botulinum neurotoxins: mechanism of action and therapeutic uses. *Philos Trans R Soc Lond B Biol Sci* 1999;354(1381):259–68

30. Meunier FA, Herreros J, Schiavo G *et al*. Molecular mechanism of action of botulinal neurotoxins and the synaptic remodeling they induce in vivo at the skeletal neuromuscular junction. In: Massar EJ, ed. *Neurotoxicology Handbook*, Vol. 1. Totowa, NJ: Humana Press, 2001:307–49

31. Alderson K, Holds JB, Anderson RL. Botulinum-induced alteration of nerve-muscle interactions in the human orbicularis oculi following treatment for blepharospasm. *Neurology* 1991;41(11):1800–5

32. de Paiva A, Meunier FA, Molgo J *et al*. Functional repair of motor endplates after botulinum neurotoxin type A poisoning: biphasic switch of synaptic activity between nerve sprouts and their parent terminals. *Proc Natl Acad Sci USA* 1999;96:3200–5

33. Naumann M. Hypersecretory disorders. In: Moore P, Naumann M, eds. *Handbook of Botulinum Toxin Treatment,* 2nd ed. Malden, Mass: Blackwell Science, 2003:343–59

34. Filippi GM, Errico P, Santarelli R *et al.* Botulinum A toxin effects on rat jaw muscle spindles. *Acta Oto-Laryngol* 1983;113:400–4

35. Rosales RL, Arimura K, Takenaga S *et al.* Extrafusal and intrafusal muscle effects in experimental botulinum toxin-A injection. *Muscle Nerve* 1996;19:488–96

36. Simpson LL. The origin, structure, and pharmacological activity of botulinum toxin. *Pharmacol Rev* 1981;33(3):155–88

37. Burgen ASV, Dickens F, Zatman LJ. The action of botulinum toxin on the neuromuscular junction. *J Physiol* 1949;109:10–24

38. Lowe NJ, Yamauchi PS, Lask GP *et al.* Botulinum toxins types A and B for brow furrows: preliminary experiences with type B toxin dosing. *J Cosmet Laser Ther* 2002;4(1):15–18

39. Brashear A, Watts MW, Marchetti A *et al.* Duration of effect of botulinum toxin type A in adult patients with cervical dystonia: a retrospective chart review. *Clin Ther* 2000;22(12):1516–24

40. Dodel RC, Kirchner A, Koehne-Volland R *et al.* Costs of treating dystonias and hemifacial spasm with botulinum toxin A. *Pharmacoeconomics* 1997;12(6):695–706

41. Sloop RR, Cole BA, Escutin RO. Human response to botulinum toxin injection: type B compared with type A. *Neurology* 1997;49:189–94

42. Aoki KR. Botulinum neurotoxin serotypes A and B preparations have different safety margins in preclinical models of muscle weakening efficacy and systemic safety. *Toxicon* 2002;40(7):923–8

43. Hsiung GY, Das SK, Ranawaya R *et al.* Long-term efficacy of botulinum toxin A in treatment of various movement disorders over a 10-year period. *Mov Disord* 2002;17(6):1288–93

44. Defazio G, Abbruzzese G, Girlanda P *et al.* Botulinum toxin A treatment for primary hemifacial spasm: a 10-year multicenter study. *Arch Neurol* 2002;59:418–20

45. Dutton JJ, Buckley EG. Long-term results and complications of botulinum A toxin in the treatment of blepharospasm. *Ophthalmology* 1988;95(11):1529–34

46. Drummond GT, Hinz BJ. Botulinum toxin for blepharospasm and hemifacial spasm: stability of duration of effect and dosage over time. *Can J Ophthalmol* 2001;36(7):398–403

47. Tan EK, Jankovic J. Botulinum toxin A in patients with oromandibular dystonia: long-term follow-up. *Neurology* 1999;53(9):2102–7.

48. Hogikyan ND, Wodchis WP, Spak C *et al.* Longitudinal effects of botulinum toxin injections on voice-related quality of life (V-RQOL) for patients with adductory spasmodic dysphonia. *J Voice* 2001;15(4):576–86

49. Lagalla G, Danni M, Reiter F *et al.* Post-stroke spasticity management with repeated botulinum toxin injections in the upper limb. *Am J Phys Med Rehabil* 2000;79(4):377–84

50. Jankovic J, Schwartz KS. Longitudinal experience with botulinum toxin injections for treatment of blepharospasm and cervical dystonia. *Neurology* 1993;43(4):834–6

51. Garcia Ruiz PJ, Pascual Pascual I, Sanchez Bernardos V. Progressive response to botulinum A toxin in cerebral palsy. *Eur J Neurol* 2000;7(2):191–3

52. Giladi N. The mechanism of action of botulinum toxin type A in focal dystonia is most probably through its dual effect on efferent (motor) and afferent pathways at the injected site. *J Neurol Sci* 1997;152(2):132–5

53. Brin MF, Aoki KR. Botulinum toxin pharmacology. In: Mayer NH, ed. *Spasticity: Etiology, Evaluation, Management and the Role of Botulinum Toxin*. WE MOVE Worldwide Education and Awareness for Movement Disorders 2002:110–24

54. Naumann M, Lowe NJ. Botulinum toxin type A in treatment of bilateral primary axillary hyperhidrosis: randomised, parallel group, double blind, placebo controlled trial. *Br Med J* 2001;323(7313):596–9

55. Lowe NJ, Yamauchi PS, Lask GP et al. Efficacy and safety of botulinum toxin type A in the treatment of palmar hyperhidrosis: a double-blind, randomized, placebo-controlled study. Dermatol Surg 2002;28(9):822–7

56. Naumann M, Lowe NJ, Kumar CR et al. Botulinum toxin type A is a safe and effective treatment for axillary hyperhidrosis over 16 months: a prospective study. Arch Dermatol 2003;139(6):731–6

57. Dressler D, Adib Saberi F, Benecke R. Botulinum toxin type B for treatment of axillar hyperhidrosis. J Neurol 2002;249(12):1729–32

58. Dressler D, Benecke R. Autonomic side effects of botulinum toxin type B treatment of cervical dystonia and hyperhidrosis. Eur Neurol 2003;49(1):34–8

59. Leuchs J. Beitraege zur Kenntnis des Toxins und Antitoxins des Bacillus botulinus. Z Hyg Infektionsskr 1910;65:55–84

60. Burke GS. Notes on Bacillus botulinus. J Bacteriol 1919;4:555–65

61. Atassi MZ, Oshima M. Structure, activity, and immune (T and B cell) recognition of botulinum neurotoxins. Crit Rev Immunol 1999;19:219–60

62. Goschel H, Wohlfarth K, Frevert J et al. Botulinum A toxin therapy: neutralizing and nonneutralizing antibodies – therapeutic consequences. Exp Neurol 1997;147(1):96–102

63. Clayton MA, Clayton JM, Brown DR et al. Protective vaccination with a recombinant fragment of Clostridium botulinum neurotoxin serotype A expressed from a synthetic gene in Escherichia coli. Infect Immun 1995;63(7):2738–42

64. Jankovic J, Schwartz K. Response and immunoresistance to botulinum toxin injections. Neurology 1995;45(9):1743–6

65. Biglan AW, Gonnering R, Lockhart LB et al. Absence of antibody production in patients treated with botulinum A toxin. Am J Ophthalmol 1986;101(2):232–5

66. Gonnering RS. Negative antibody response to long-term treatment of facial spasm with botulinum toxin. Am J Ophthalmol 1988;105:313–15

67. Greene P, Fahn S, Diamond B. Development of resistance to botulinum toxin type A in patients with torticollis. Mov Disord 1994;9(2):213–17

68. Jankovic J, Vuong KD, Ahsan J. Comparison of efficacy and immunogenicity of original versus current botulinum toxin in cervical dystonia. Neurology 2003;60:1186–8

69. Brashear A, Bergan K, Wojcieszek J et al. Patients' perception of stopping or continuing treatment of cervical dystonia with botulinum toxin type A. Mov Disord 2000;15:150–3

70. Kessler KR, Benecke R. The EDB test – a clinical test for the detection of antibodies to botulinum toxin type A. Mov Disord 1997;12:95–9

71. Gelb DJ, Yoshimura DM, Olney RK et al. Change in pattern of muscle activity following botulinum toxin injections for torticollis. Ann Neurol 1991;29:370–6

72. Tsui JKC, Eisen A, Stoessl AJ et al. Double-blind study of botulinum toxin in spasmodic torticollis. Lancet 1986;2:245–7

73. Wissel J, Muller J, Dressnandt J et al. Management of spasticity associated pain with botulinum toxin A. J Pain Symptom Mgmt 2000;20(1):44–9

74. Foster L, Clapp L, Erickson M et al. Botulinum toxin A and chronic low back pain. A randomized, double-blind study. Neurology 2001;56:1290–3

75. Relja M, Telarovic S. Botulinum toxin in tension-type headache. J Neurol 2004;251(Suppl 1):I12–14

76. Binder W, Brin MF, Blitzer A et al. Botulinum toxin type A (BOTOX®-A) for migraine: an open label assessment. Mov Disord 1998;13:241

77. Binder WJ, Brin MF, Blitzer A et al. Botulinum toxin type A (BOTOX®) for treatment of migraine. Dis Mon 2001;48:323–35

78. Gobel H. Botulinum toxin in migraine prophylaxis. J Neurol 2004;251(Suppl 1):I8–11

79. Brin MF, Fahn S, Moskowitz C et al. Localized injections of botulinum toxin for the treatment of focal dystonia and hemifacial spasm. Mov Disord 1987;2:237–54

80. Welch MJ, Purkiss JR, Foster KA. Sensitivity of embryonic rat dorsal root ganglia neurons to *Clostridium botulinum* neurotoxins. *Toxicon* 2000;38:245–58

81. Cui M, Khanijou S, Rubino J *et al.* Subcutaneous administration of botulinum toxin A reduces formalin-induced pain. *Pain* 2004;107(1–2):125–33

82. Durham PL, Cady R, Cady R. Regulation of calcitonin gene-related peptide secretion from trigeminal nerve cells by botulinum toxin type A: implications for migraine therapy. *Headache* 2004;44(1):35–42

83. Buzzi MG, Bonamini M, Moskowitz MA. Neurogenic model of migraine. *Cephalalgia* 1995;15(4):277–80

84. Williamson DJ, Hargreaves RJ. Neurogenic inflammation in the context of migraine. *Microsc Res Tech* 2001;53(3):167–78

85. Argoff CE. A focused review on the use of botulinum toxins for neuropathic pain. *Clin J Pain* 2002;18(6 Suppl):S177–81

86. Kagan A. Case study of botulinum toxin type A for postherpetic neuralgia [letter]. *Am J Pain Mgmt* 2002;12(2):43–4

87. Tang-Liu DD, Aoki KR, Dolly JO *et al.* Intramuscular injection of ^{125}I-botulinum neurotoxin-complex versus ^{125}I-botulinum-free neurotoxin: time course of tissue distribution. *Toxicon* 2003;42(5):461–9

88. Foran PG, Mohammed N, Lisk GO *et al.* Evaluation of the therapeutic usefulness of botulinum neurotoxin B, C1, E, and F compared with the long lasting type A. Basis for distinct durations of inhibition of exocytosis in central neurons. *J Biol Chem* 2003;278(2):1363–71

89. O'Sullivan GA, Mohammed N, Foran PG, Lawrence GW, Oliver Dolly J. Rescue of exocytosis in botulinum toxin A-poisoned chromaffin cells by expression of cleavage-resistant SNAP-25. Identification of the minimal essential C-terminal residues. *J Biol Chem* 1999;274(52):36897–904

90. Fernandez-Salas E, Steward LE, Ho H *et al.* Plasma membrane localization signals in the light chain of botulinum neurotoxin. *Proc Natl Acad Sci USA* 2004;101(9):3208–13

91. Adler M, Keller JE, Sheridan RE, Deshpande SS. Persistence of botulinum neurotoxin A demonstrated by sequential administration of serotypes A and E in rat EDL muscle. *Toxicon* 2001:233–43

92. Eleopra R, Tugnoli V, Rossetto O *et al.* Different time courses of recovery after poisoning with botulinum neurotoxin serotypes A and E in humans. *Neurosci Lett* 1998;256(3):135–8

93. Yowler BC, Schengrund CL. Botulinum neurotoxin A changes conformation upon binding to ganglioside GT1b. *Biochemistry* 2004;43(30):9725–31

2 FACIAL ANATOMY AND THE USE OF BOTULINUM TOXIN

James M Spencer

Introduction

Botulinum toxin has the ability to block cholinergic nerve transmission to skeletal muscle and thus produce a temporary flaccid paralysis. This has enabled physicians to treat a number of medical problems characterized by hyperfunctional muscle. This has also enabled cosmetic physicians to soften or eliminate rhytides caused by hyperfunctional muscles. A thorough understanding of the muscular anatomy of the face is necessary for the judicious use of botulinum toxin (Appendix 4).

All cholinergic nerves have receptors for botulinum toxin, and thus are a potential target for the action of this protein. Normally, an action potential travels down the neuronal axon and reaches the distal portion at the neuromuscular junction. Within the distal end of the axon are preformed vesicles containing the neurotransmitter acetylcholine. In response to the action potential, the preformed vesicles dock and fuse with the terminal axonal membrane and release their contents out of the axon and into the synaptic cleft. In turn, the acetylcholine activates muscle contraction. A group of proteins known as the SNARE complex is responsible for fusing, docking, and release of acetylcholine from their vesicles. Botulinum toxin (BOTOX®) works by inactivating the SNARE complex. With time, new sprouts from the axon re-establish functional contact with the muscle. However, ultimately the original motor endplate regains function, and the sprouts regress. Thus the effects of BOTOX® are temporary.

For cosmetic use, the target of BOTOX® has principally been the muscles of facial expression. The muscles of the face can be divided into two groups: the muscles of facial expression, and the muscles of mastication[1]. The muscles of facial expression are somewhat unique in their arrangement and function. On the body, muscles typically have bony attachments via ligaments at either end and are responsible for movement of the body. Most of the muscles of facial expression are not attached to bone: rather they have soft tissue attachments. They tend not to move the body, but rather to move the skin and related structures to facilitate communication. Emotional states are communicated and understood by muscular action of the face. Raising or lowering the eyebrows can communicate surprise, anger, sadness, or tiredness. The muscles of facial expression are connected to the overlying skin through a series of fibrous septae and an intervening fascial layer known as the superficial muscular aponeurotic system (SMAS). Thus when the underlying muscle contracts, the overlying skin moves with it. The muscles of mastication, such as the masseter and temporalis, have bony attachments and function to move the jaw in a way similar to muscles elsewhere on the body[2].

With age, the muscles of the face tend to atrophy, resulting in sagging of the face. This sagging is addressed through surgical lifting procedures. However, with repeated contraction of the muscles, areas of the skin overlying the muscle can develop creases from repeated mechanical folding and pleating. As the muscle shortens during contraction, the overlying skin will be folded. This folding occurs perpendicular to the axis of muscle contraction. For example, the major muscle of the forehead is the frontalis (Figure 2.1). The fibers of the frontalis are vertically oriented, and thus contraction of this muscle shortens the forehead and pulls up the eyebrows. With repeated action over many years, the forehead can develop horizontal creases or rhytides. Many people in the course of normal activity overutilize a certain muscle: thus the muscle is hyperfunctional. The result will be permanent creases in the skin perpendicular to the long axis of the muscle. For example, habitual overuse of the corrugator muscles to pull the eyebrows down and in will result in vertical or oblique creases in the overlying skin. Normally, the muscles of facial expression communicate emotional states. However, a permanent crease sends an inappropriate message. A permanent glabellar crease communicates anger or worry when the person feels neither. Botulinum toxin can be used to temporarily weaken hyperfunctional muscles, and thus improve or eliminate the overlying skin crease.

In addition to animating the skin, the position of some important facial structures is partly determined by underlying muscle tension. At rest, our muscles are not completely flaccid, but rather maintain a resting tension that enables our body to maintain position. For example, contracture of the frontalis pulls the eyebrows up, but at rest normal muscle tension holds the eyebrows up at a normal position. If the function of the frontalis is completely lost, such as is seen with severing of the temporal branch of the 7th cranial nerve, the eyebrow will droop

Figure 2.1   Frontalis. This is the largest muscle of the upper face and a frequent site of botulinum toxin therapy

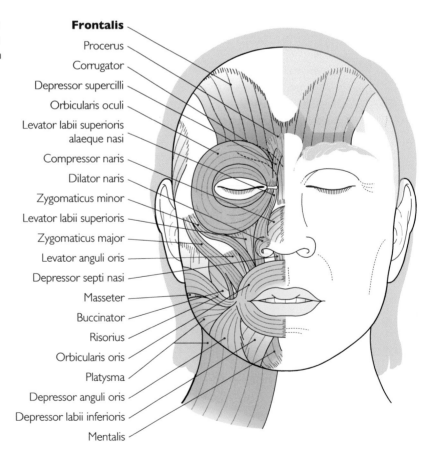

Frontalis
Procerus
Corrugator
Depressor supercilli
Orbicularis oculi
Levator labii superioris
alaeque nasi
Compressor naris
Dilator naris
Zygomaticus minor
Levator labii superioris
Zygomaticus major
Levator anguli oris
Depressor septi nasi
Masseter
Buccinator
Risorius
Orbicularis oris
Platysma
Depressor anguli oris
Depressor labii inferioris
Mentalis

downward (eyebrow ptosis) (Figure 2.2). Often, normal position results from the dynamic exchange of opposing muscle groups. Careful use of BOTOX® to alter such relationships can be used to alter the position of structures such as the eyebrows and corners of the mouth.

Upper face

The largest muscle of the upper face is the frontalis, and is a frequent site of BOTOX® therapy (Figure 2.1). The frontalis begins superiorly at the frontal scalp where the fibers originate from the galea aponeurotica, a fascial plane of the scalp that lies beneath the fat. The fibers of the frontalis extend vertically downward where they mesh with the skin and muscles at the eyebrow and glabella. The muscle actually has two halves, each separately innervated by the right and left temporal branches of the 7th cranial nerve. Thus in the superior aspect of the midline forehead there is no muscle, but rather a fascial band or aponiurosis separating the two halves of the frontalis[3].

The frontalis has one function: to raise the eyebrows. At rest, normal resting tension of the frontalis holds the eyebrows in a normal position. Evidence of the importance of unconscious normal resting tension is seen when the motor nerve supplying this muscle, the temporal branch of the 7th cranial nerve, is severed. Cutting this nerve produces not only complete hemiparalysis of the forehead, but with time ptosis of the eyebrow on the affected side (Figure 2.2). The resting position of the eyebrow is determined by the resting tension of the frontalis muscle pulling the eyebrow up, and the resting tension of the medial and lateral portions of the obicularis oculi muscle, which pull it down. By judicious use of this balance the eyebrow can be elevated: by weakening the downward pulling muscles, one now has unopposed upward

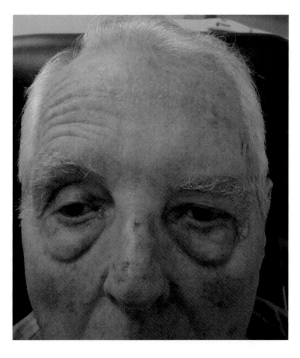

Figure 2.2 Brow ptosis resulting from cutting the temporal branch of the 7th cranial nerve

tension and the eyebrow will rise. This effect can be enhanced by selective use of BOTOX® within a single muscle. If the central portion of the frontalis is paralyzed while the lateral portions are not, the resting tension in the still functional lateral portions will increase, and thus the lateral aspect of the eyebrows will rise. This can be very helpful for patients with a lateral droop of their eyebrows.

With conscious effort, the vertically oriented frontalis will pull up the eyebrows. This is an important aspect of non-verbal emotional communication, but with repeated overuse, horizontal rhytides will develop. By weakening the middle and upper portions of the frontalis, these rhytides can be softened or eliminated. However, caution must be used to not paralyze too close to the eyebrows. If the portion immediately above the eyebrows is paralyzed, a brow ptosis may result. As a general principle, injections should always be at least 1 cm above the eyebrow, so functionality will remain to hold the eyebrows up.

The glabellar complex is composed of the paired corrugator supercilii and the single procerus (Figure 2.3). The corrugators roughly define a V, with the base at the nasal root. At its base, it is attached to the frontal bone. As the muscle travels up and laterally, it fans out and attaches to the skin. These muscles pull the eyebrows down and in. The procerus arises in the midline at the upper aspect of the nasal bone and travels vertically up between the corrugators

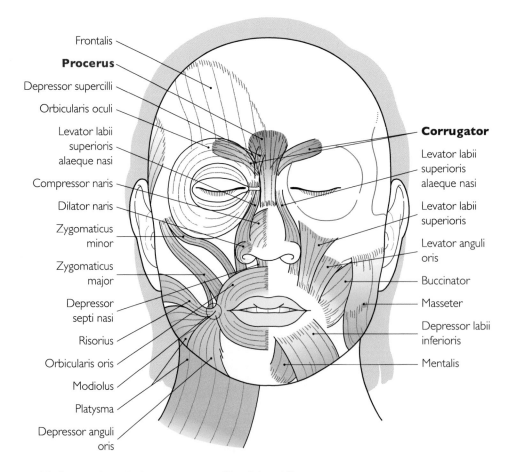

Figure 2.3   Glabellar complex; paired corrugator supercilii and the midline procerus

and attaches to the skin in the midline of the lower forehead. This muscle pulls the forehead down in this location. The fibers of the corrugators, procerus, and adjacent medial portion of the orbicularis oculi are often intertwined and fused in nature, and clean dissection of these structures is more a mental construct than a physical reality.

The orbicularis oculi is a circular muscle that functions to close the eyelids. It functions as a sphincter, encircling the globe, and upon contracture closes the eyelids (Figure 2.4). Around each eye, the orbicularis oculi arises from the medial canthal ligament, located just medial to the globe. The muscle fans out from the ligamentous attachment superiorly to about the level of the eyebrow where it inserts into the skin and frontalis, and inferiorly to the level of the lower orbital rim, to encircle the globe 360°. It is customarily divided into two portions: the palprebral portion which overlies the eyelids, and the orbital portion, which is outside the margins of the eyelids and over the bony orbital margin. It is the orbital portion that is a potential target for the use of BOTOX®. If the muscle were completely paralyzed, the patient would be unable to blink or close the eyelids. However, selective weakening of different portions of this muscle can produce cosmetic enhancement. Laterally, the fibers of this circular muscle travel vertically, and with

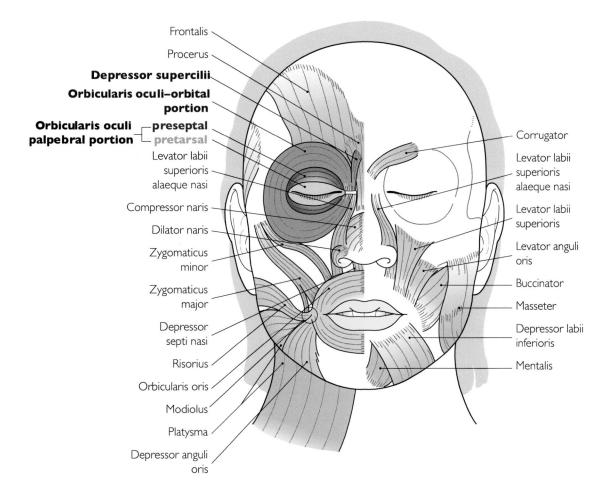

Figure 2.4   Orbicularis oculi. This muscle encircles the eye and functions as a sphincter. Note the fibers of this muscle are vertically oriented at the medial and lateral most aspects where they function as depressors of the eyebrow

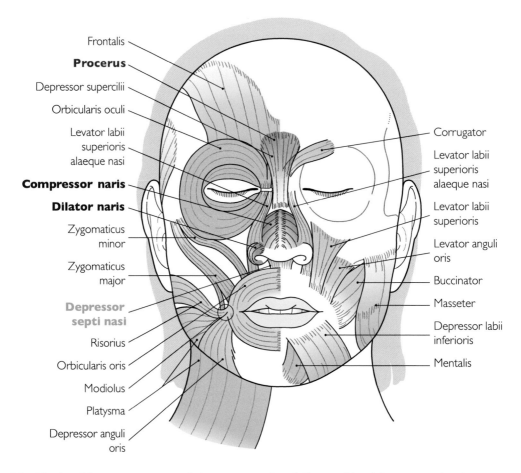

Figure 2.5   Muscles of the nose: procerus nasalis (compressor naris and dilator naris) and depressor septi nasi

contracture produce perpendicularly oriented 'crow's feet' rhytides. The application of BOTOX®
to the lateral portion of the orbicularis oculi muscle will treat crow's feet.

Treatment must be given outside the orbital rim (injection approximately 1 cm lateral to the
orbital rim) to avoid unwanted treatment of the muscles of ocular motion which are inside the
orbital rim. These same vertical fibers of the lateral orbicularis oculi also pull the lateral portion
of the eyebrow down, and thus treatment in this area can be used to raise the lateral eyebrows.
Similarly, the medial most portion of this muscle is also vertically oriented, and serves to pull the
medial eyebrow down. Since these medial vertical fibers are so closely associated with the
corrugator supercilii, treatment of the corrugators most likely provides some therapy of these
medial fibers as well. Some authors have identified a separate vertically oriented depressor in
this area just adjacent to the corrugators termed the depressor supercilii[4,5]. As mentioned
previously, in nature the fibers of the corrugators, procerus, and medial orbicularis oculi are
fused and intertwined, making clean and separate dissection of these muscles difficult at best. It
may be that in some patients, the medial vertically oriented portion of the orbicularis oculi is well
developed and gives the impression of a separate muscle.

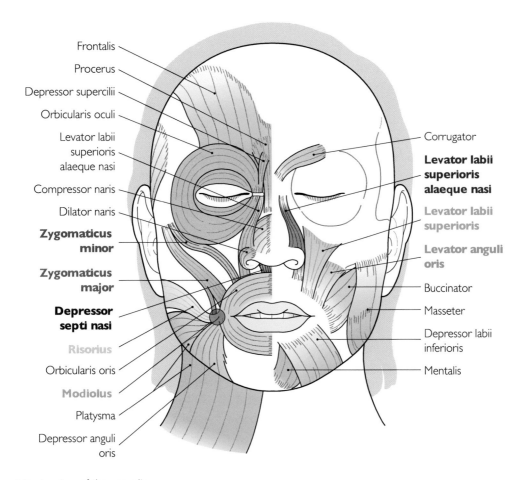

Figure 2.6   Levators of the upper lip

In the midline of the lower portion of the globe, the fibers of the orbicularis oculi are horizontally oriented and are vital for closing the eyelids. However, by selectively weakening this lower portion, it can help to soften creases seen with smiling at the outer half of the lower lid. Such creases can become quite prominent when the lateral vertical portion (crow's feet area) of the orbicularis oculi is paralyzed with BOTOX®. Furthermore, weakening the mid section of the lower lid palprebral portion of the orbicularis oculi has been shown to slightly relax the lower eyelid and thus 'opens' the eye, giving a larger, rounder eye[6].

The location of the orbicularis oculi in relationship to other structures is unique in the periocular region, and requires an adjustment of injection technique. In most areas of the body, the layers from outside to inside are: epidermis, dermis, fat, fascia, muscle, periosteum, bone. Thus, in most sites, one needs to pass the injection needle through skin, fat, and fascia to reach the muscle. However, the orbicularis oculi has a unique anatomy. The arrangement from outside to inside is: epidermis, dermis, muscle (orbicularis oculi), fascia (septum), fat. Thus the target muscle in the periocular area is just under the skin, and a very thin skin at that. Therefore, injections into the orbicularis oculi should be very superficial.

Mid face

The mid face contains few muscles amenable to therapy with BOTOX®, but some important muscles to avoid. The nose contains three main muscles: the procerus, which has already been discussed with the glabellar complex, the nasalis muscle, and the depressor septi muscle (Figure 2.5). The nasalis is shaped roughly like an upside-down horseshoe, with the upper part traveling transversely across the nasal dorsum (also known as the compressor naris), and two lower arms traveling vertically down the sides of the nose (also known as the dilator naris). Application of small amounts of BOTOX® to the lateral upper part of the nose may help soften 'bunny lines', which are oblique rhytides of the upper lateral nose seen in some patients with expression. The third nasal muscle, the depressor septi nasi, travels vertically up the columella from the upper lip, where it can pull the nasal tip down with smiling. It has been suggested that BOTOX® injection into to this location could elevate the nasal tip.

There are multiple levators of the upper lip, which generally originate from bony attachments and travel down to insert in the lip (Figure 2.6). In the midline is the depressor septi muscle, which attaches to the midline upper lip and runs up the columella of the nose. Extending laterally on both sides are a series of paired muscles required for the complex functions of the upper lip. Just lateral to the midline of the upper lip is the paired levator labii superioris alaque nasi, which inserts bilaterally to the medial portion of the upper lip and runs superiorly up along the side of the nose to originate from the skull at the level of the inner canthus. Moving laterally, the next muscle to insert in the upper lip is the levator labii superioris, which extends upward and attaches to bone at the level of the lower orbital rim in the mid pupillary line. Lateral to this is the zygomaticus minor and then the zygomaticus major. These muscles extend upward at an oblique angle from the upper lip and attach just below the lateral portion of the orbital rim. Paralysis of the upper poles of these muscles can be an unintended consequence of injecting too low in the lateral canthal area when treating crow's feet. The patient may note difficulty raising the lip to smile. Inserting into the lateral aspect of the upper lip is the levator anguli oris, which originates superiorly at the canine fossa. Lastly, the risorus muscle also inserts at the lateral portion of the upper lip and travels obliquely upward towards the ear. As several muscles come together to insert at the lateral commisure of the lips, this area is known as the modiolus, and can be thought of as a dense, fibromuscular interface that acts as a scaffold for the various muscles to pull on. The number of muscles in this area shows the complex functions performed by the mouth: eating, speaking, and emotional expression. As a general principle, none of the lip levators are targets for BOTOX® because of the importance of these functions, even though one could entertain the idea in order to soften the nasolabial folds.

Lower face

The muscles of the lower face are increasingly becoming targets for BOTOX® therapy. The major muscle of facial expression of the lower face is the orbicularis oris, a circular muscle that encircles the mouth and functions as a sphincter. The various levators and depressors of the lips insert into this muscle and the lip itself, and originate from bony attachments above and below respectively. Contracture of the upper, horizontally oriented fibers that travel along the upper lip is responsible for the vertical rhytides seen above the upper lip. However, complete paralysis of this portion of the orbicularis oris would interfere with eating and speaking and is to be avoided. However, very slight weakening of this upper portion, while still preserving overall function, can be used to soften upper lip vertical rhytides.

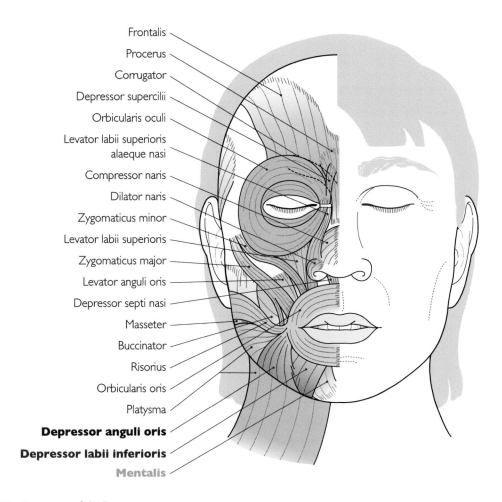

Frontalis
Procerus
Corrugator
Depressor supercilii
Orbicularis oculi
Levator labii superioris
alaeque nasi
Compressor naris
Dilator naris
Zygomaticus minor
Levator labii superioris
Zygomaticus major
Levator anguli oris
Depressor septi nasi
Masseter
Buccinator
Risorius
Orbicularis oris
Platysma
Depressor anguli oris
Depressor labii inferioris
Mentalis

Figure 2.7   Depressors of the lip

There are two depressors of the lips, the depressor anguli oris, and the depressor labii inferioris (Figure 2.7). These muscles insert superiorly into the lateral and medial orbicularis oris respectively, and originate inferiorly at the border of the mandible. The depressor anguli oris inserts at the corners of the mouth and travels down and slightly laterally to a bony origin at the border of the mandible. It is responsible for pulling down the corners of the mouth. If this muscle is weakened by injection at its lower mandibular head (so as not to affect the orbicularis oris), there is now an unopposed levator of the corner of the mouth. In this way, a subtle but noticeable elevation of the corners of the mouth can be achieved. It is important to avoid paralysis of the muscle just medial to this, the depressor labii inferioris. Lastly, the mentalis muscle inserts medially to the lower lip under the depressor labii muscle and travels straight down to attach at the midline of the chin. It is responsible for protrusion of the lower lip. It is also responsible in some patients for creation of the mental crease, a horizontal furrow under the lip on the upper portion of the chin. Injection of the mentalis muscle can soften the mental crease.

Neck

Botulinum toxin is used therapeutically in the neck for a variety of medical problems, but only one muscle in the neck is of cosmetic concern, the platysma. The platysma is a broad, thin muscle originating below the clavicle and extending upward to cover the entire anterior neck. Superiorly at the level of the mandible it meshes with the superficial fascia of the face, the SMAS. It is the most superficial muscle of the neck, and is thought to be responsible both for horizontal neck rhytides from repeated contracture, as well as vertically oriented platysmal bands, seen as the sheet-like muscle separates into cords with time. Multiple superficial injections of BOTOX® into this muscle can soften both of these cosmetic problems.

Nerves of the face

Use of BOTOX® is guided by a functional understanding of the muscles to be treated rather than the nerves that supply them. However, an understanding of the innervation of the face is important for a complete anatomic picture.

Innervation of the face is principally supplied by two nerves, the 5th cranial nerve and the 7th cranial nerve, which provide sensation and motor function respectively. The 5th cranial nerve is the trigeminal nerve and splits into three branches to provide cutaneous sensation of the face. The branches are termed V1, V2, and V3 and are arranged vertically, with V1 being superior, V2 in the middle, and V3 inferiorly. The first branch is the ophthalmic division, and innervates the upper one-third of the face. It originates in the semilunar ganglion and enters the orbit where it divides into the lacrimal branch to the upper lateral eyelid, a nasociliary branch to the glabella and nasal dorsum, and the larger frontal branch which supplies the forehead and periocular area. The frontal branch in turn gives rise to the supraorbital and supratrochlear branches. The supratrochlear branch exits at the level of the skull in the area of the corrugators while the supraorbital branch exits at the midline along the superior orbital rim, and thus both are a potential target for direct trauma from the needle used for BOTOX® injection. In the area of the glabellar complex where such trauma could theoretically occur, the supratrochlear nerve is deep to the muscle at the level of bone. Injection of BOTOX® in the middle of the superior orbital rim is not recommended, so damage to the supraorbital nerve can be avoided.

The maxillary division (V2) supplies sensation to the skin of the midface. This nerve also originates in the semilunar ganglia. This nerve gives rise to multiple branches that supply the sensation to the cheek and side of the face, the conjunctivae and the skin of the lower eyelid, the side of the nose and the nasal vestibule, and the mucosa and skin of the upper lip. The trunks and foramen of these nerves are not in locations where direct trauma from needle injection is likely.

The mandibular branch (V3) provides both a sensory and a motor function. The motor portion of the mandibular nerve provides function for the four muscles of mastication. Its main sensory branches supply the skin of the lower lip, chin, skin of the lateral cheek, lower mandibular region, lower gingival, and around the ear and temporal regions. Of note for injections of BOTOX®, the mental branch, which provides sensation to the lower lip and chin, exits the skull at the mental foramen, which is on the lower lateral aspect of the chin, and theoretically could be traumatized if the injection needle entered the foramen during injection of the depressor anguli oris.

Motor function of the face is provided by the 7th cranial nerve, the facial nerve. Although the action of BOTOX® is to block transmission from branches of this nerve to the muscles of facial expression, injection points are determined by the muscles themselves and not the course of the nerve. The facial nerve exits the skull at the stylomastoid foramen, which is located just below and medial to the auditory canal, under the parotid gland. The trunk typically divides into five branches, but there is significant anatomic variation. The temporal branch travels superiorly to innervate the orbicularis oculi, the frontalis, and the corrugator supercilii all targets of BOTOX® therapy. The zygomatic branch travels upwards towards the lateral canthus to further supply the orbicularis oculi. The buccal branch travels more medially to innervate the muscles of the mid face, and there may be significant anastomosis between the zygomatic and buccal branches. The mandibular branch travels down below the mandible, travels medially, and eventually crosses back up across the mandible (highly variable from person to person) to supply the orbicularis oris, the depressor anguli oris, and the mentalis. The cervical branch travels to the neck to supply the platysma.

Vascular supply

The consequence of intravascular injection of BOTOX® is ecchymosis or even a hematoma, but there is no systemic risk to the patient from intravascular injection with the amount used for cosmetic purposes. From primate data, it is estimated that the lethal dose of intravascular injection of BOTOX® would be in the range of 2800 units, or 28 vials of BOTOX®[7]. However, hitting a vessel may produce an unsightly ecchymosis, and the BOTOX® may not be delivered to the intended muscle and thus cannot do its job. Therefore, some knowledge of the location and course of the major vessels of the face is helpful.

The face receives arterial blood from various branches of the internal and external carotids. The majority of the skin and subcutaneous tissue of the face is supplied by branches of the external carotid artery, with the internal carotid supplying only the eyes, the upper two-thirds of the nose, and the central forehead via the ophthalmic branch.

The internal carotid enters the skull at the carotid canal, travels anteriomedially towards the cavernous sinus and ultimately towards the circle of Willis. From inside the skull it gives off the ophthalmic arteries, which in turn give rise to branches relevant to a discussion of BOTOX®. The ophthalmic artery travels anteriorly through the optic canal to enter the bony orbit. From here, they divide into several branches including the supraorbital and supratrochlear branches that exit the orbit through the foramen along the superior orbital rim. The supratrochlear branch emerges in the area of the corrugators deep to muscle with the supratrochlear branch of the 5th cranial nerve and travels superiorly with frequent branching as it goes. In the area of the corrugator complex this artery is vulnerable to needle puncture and bleeding from BOTOX® injection. The supraorbital branch exits the orbit in the midline of the superior orbital rim with the supraorbital branch of the 5th cranial nerve and travels superiorly deep to the frontalis muscle. Midline injection at the orbital rim with BOTOX® is ill advised, and thus the trunk of this branch and its accompanying nerve are not likely to be directly traumatized during injection.

The external carotid artery has multiple divisions that travel both superficially and deep to supply the head. However, there are a few points that merit special attention when injecting BOTOX®. As it travels up the lateral aspect of the neck, the external carotid gives off the facial artery. This branch travels medially and superiorly to cross the mandible and course across the cheek at a roughly 60° angle toward the nasal ala. At the level of the oral commissure it gives off two labial arteries that encircle the lips. The facial artery continues superiorly to the base of the nasal ala, where it anastomoses with the angular artery traveling down the junction of the cheek and lateral nose.

The external carotid itself continues up the lateral aspect of the neck to terminate into two branches below the dermis anteroinferior to the tragus of the ear. One of these is the superficial temporal artery that runs superiorly in front of the ear and up the lateral aspect of the temple and forehead. It runs superficially under the subcutaneous fat and fascia, above muscle, and thus is subject to trauma during cutaneous surgery or injections. The second branch of the terminus of the external carotid is the internal maxillary artery, which travels deep and is not relevant to BOTOX® injections.

Venous drainage of the face generally follows the arterial pattern. The veins of the face follow the pattern of arterial vessels, with flow in the opposite direction. The veins of the central forehead and glabellar region merit special mention. The supraorbital and supratrochlear veins run with the corresponding arteries and nerves, and drain into the bony orbits to terminate in the orbital veins. These in turn drain into the cavernous sinus, thus creating the potential portal for the spread of disease to intracranial structures. Despite this theoretic risk, infection has not been a reported problem with BOTOX® injections.

Botulinum toxin has rapidly become one of, if not the most, popular non-invasive cosmetic treatments currently available. Its cosmetic benefit derives from its ability to selectively relax or paralyze localized areas of facial muscle. A complete understanding of these muscles allows the physician to successfully utilize this medication.

Bibliography

1. Larrabee WF Jr, Makielski KH. *Surgical Anatomy of the Face*. New York: Raven Press, 1993
2. Williams P. *Gray's Anatomy*, 38th edn. New York: Churchill-Livingstone-Elsevier
3. Bentsianov B, Blitzer A. Facial anatomy. *Clin Dermatol* 2004;22(1):3–13
4. Daniel RK, Landon B. Endoscopic forehead lift; anatomic basis. *Aesthet Surg Jour* 1997;17:97–104
5. Cook Jr. BE, Lucarelli MJ, Lemke BN. Depressor supercilii muscle: anatomy, histology, and cosmetic implications. *Opthalmic Plast Reconstr Surg* 2001;17:404–11
6. Flynn TC, Carruthers J, Carruthers A. Botulinum A toxin treatment of the lower eyelids improves infraorbital rhytides and widens the eye. *Dermatol Surg* 2001;27:703–8
7. BOTOX® cosmetic (package insert). Irvine, CA: Allergan Inc., 2002

3 COSMETIC USES OF BOTULINUM TOXIN A IN THE UPPER FACE

Anthony V Benedetto

Introduction

Botulinum toxin (BTX) has taken the practice of medicine by surprise and with a furor. Rarely can one find such a simple protein that in its natural form is so deadly, but by purification and minor extraction techniques can be utilized for therapeutic purposes by both physicians and surgeons. The application of BTX in neuromuscular disorders has provided fortuitous relief for many tormented with incurable diseases, affording them an encouraging respite from their devastating afflictions. The countless possibilities for the use of BTX in medicine are on the verge of being discovered. From neurologists and physiatrists, to ophthalmologists and otolaryngologists, and now for gastroenterologists and even the cosmetic surgeons, BTX has proven to be a powerful adjunctive modality for a multitude of disorders.

Although this text is not the first concerning itself with the use of BTX, it is one of the few texts to address using BTX solely for dermatologic purposes. In the United States injecting BTX-A, specifically BOTOX® Cosmetic for any reason other than to diminish glabellar frown lines is considered off-label use and not FDA approved. Whether or not the FDA and other governmental regulatory agencies will ever approve every single indication for which BTX has proven to be efficacious, the fact remains that it is extremely reliable and non-toxic when administered as prescribed. Consequently, BTX is quickly becoming a part of the armamentarium of many physicians and surgeons worldwide.

In the subsequent four chapters any reference to BTX-A will denote explicitly BOTOX® Cosmetic unless stated otherwise. The dermatologic uses of BTX-A or BOTOX® Cosmetic in these chapters are presented in a systematic fashion, first by identifying the anatomical basis of different aesthetic changes acquired by men and women as they 'age' and 'wrinkle'. Next, normal functional anatomy is discussed to elucidate the reasons for these aesthetic changes so that a suitable plan of correction with BOTOX® Cosmetic can be initiated. Functional anatomy is emphasized because the only way to utilize any type of BTX properly is to have an in depth understanding of how to modify the normal movements of the mimetic muscles of the face. When injections of BOTOX® Cosmetic are appropriately performed, desirable and reproducible results without adverse sequelae are created. Various dilutions recommended for BOTOX® Cosmetic (henceforth identified simply as BOTOX®) also are presented so that precise dosing of the product can be applied to modify facial muscle movements, which in turn can improve a given esthetic problem. Emphasis is placed on what to do and what not to do when injecting BOTOX®. Outcomes and results of different injection techniques are discussed in order to avoid adverse sequelae and complications.

Some may criticize the 'cookbook' approach of these chapters. However, this systematic detailing of where, why and how much BOTOX® to inject is necessary to understand when treating a certain problem in a particular area of the body, and therefore was done intentionally. On the other hand, the reader must never lose sight of the fact that every single individual patient is different and should never be treated in an identical way without justification. This text strives to provide both the neophyte and experienced physician the rationale for why and how a patient should be treated with a particular amount of BOTOX® in one area or another for a distinct outcome. By explicitly presenting certain techniques and the reasons for their use, the reader also should understand that this is only the author's perception of a given esthetic problem and his approach to managing that problem, for that patient, who may or may not present again in the future in exactly the same way. Consequently, when a physician is preparing to treat a patient with BOTOX®, no matter if the patient is new or one who has been treated before, the physician should approach that patient as if he or she were receiving BOTOX® for the first time. The physician must comprehensively evaluate the patient's current esthetic problem prior to commencing with the injections of BOTOX® and not necessarily rely totally on past treatment dosing. The physician shoud be flexible and treat the patient's concerns and specific esthetic changes that are present at the time.

Clinical examples and solutions presented in the next few chapters are only paradigms of reasonably acceptable clinical outcomes. The reader therefore should be able to extrapolate for him or herself a preferred approach and injection technique when treating similar clinical problems, provided there is sound justification for such a manner of treatment.

In the not too distant future, we will be able to use new formulations of BTX-A in addition to new products of different serotypes of BTX. BTX-A of different formulations and brand names are currently in use in other parts of the world outside of the United States. Their equivalency to BOTOX® is still being measured and defined. It is extremely important to understand that the specific units and dosages of BTX-A indicated in this text, particularly in the next four chapters, are only for BOTOX® unless explicitly denoted otherwise. The same number of units of BOTOX® detailed in this text absolutely cannot be used to treat patients with BTX-A of another source or manufacturer, even if a ratio of equivalency is provided. Injectors of BOTOX® have quickly learned from their recently frustrating experience using BTX-B that comparative equivalencies are not easily extrapolated. Not only was it difficult to establish a conversion dosage for equating BTX-B with BTX-A, it also was found that a muscle in a particular area of the face or body did not respond equivalently with a fixed dose conversion ratio of BTX-B with BTX-A. The dose conversion ratio was even found to be different when similar or adjacent muscles in the same patient were treated. For example, if the average equivalency unit dose was found to be 150:1 (i.e. units of BTX-B to units of BTX-A) when treating the frontalis with BTX-B, then one would assume the same equivalency ratio would be applicable for treating any of the other mimetic muscles of the face. However, when BTX-B was used for another facial muscle, e.g. the orbicularis oculi or corruagator supercilii, the equivalency of BTX-B to BTX-A was not the same, but namely 125:1, or thereabouts. Diffussion characteristics and rates also seem to influence the inability to establish any type of fixed conversion ratio between BTX-B with BTX-A. Therefore the dose equivalent ratio for BTX-B could not be fixed, at least in the author's personal experience. This confounding of equivalencies using BOTOX® as the standard to which all other serotypes of BTX are measured will only become compounded when different formulations of BTX-A or other serotypes are administered, and the reasons for this are briefly touched upon in chapters 1, 8 and 9. Therefore, it appears that when using any other type of BTX other than BOTOX®, it is better to learn how to administer that particular type of BTX independently of any conversion ratios, as individual muscles may respond in a distinctly different manner with certain formulations and specific serotypes of BTX.

The understanding of the pharmacokinetics and pharmacodynamics of BTX is still only in its early phase, and the possibilities for future developments are boundless. It is intriguing to understand that all of this was started by the insight and convictions of two astute and courageous physicians, an ophthalmologist and a dermatologist. If it were not for the Carruthers' persistence in promoting their ingenious observations, many other perceptive and insightful physicians would not have had the opportunity or confidence to learn more about BTX and how to inject it. The challenge now being passed onto the reader is that with some basic knowledge of how to inject a few drops of BOTOX® safely and appropriately and treating patients with compassion and professionalism, additional innovative uses of BTX can be uncovered.

Horizontal forehead lines

Introduction: problem assessment and patient selection

The easiest area of the face to treat with injections of botulinum toxin (BTX) is the forehead[1]. Many individuals contract their frontalis constantly for various and sundry reasons, and, in so doing, the skin buckles, creating parallel grooves and elevations across their foreheads. On the other hand, the presence of horizontal forehead lines seems to be directly proportional to one's age or time spent in the sun. Older individuals generally have a number of forehead lines that become deeper with time. As one ages, the skin of the face, along with that of the rest of the body, typically becomes more inelastic and redundant. When this occurs in the upper face, a characteristic hooding of the brow over the upper eyelids also can result which commonly is observed in the sixth or seventh decade in those individuals so predisposed. For these individuals a properly functioning frontalis is essential, because it is this muscle that will keep the brow from drooping and producing a hood of skin that drapes over the upper eyelids, interfering with their forward and upward gaze.

Younger patients who have horizontal forehead lines commonly attempt to conceal their obtrusiveness by wearing their frontal hair with a fringe or in bangs (Figure 3.1).

Generally, the presence of horizontal forehead lines causes one to appear stressed, worried, tired, or old. Abruptly raising the eyebrows by acutely contracting the frontalis also can express an emotion of surprise or even fear: emotions that one usually may not want to express too readily or frequently (Figure 3.2). When done properly, injections of BOTOX® can diminish forehead wrinkling and replace one's negative expressions with those that are more positive.

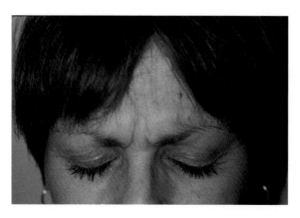

Figure 3.1 Patient before a BOTOX® treatment; note the fringe of hair concealing her forehead wrinkles. Bangs were separated for the photograph

Figure 3.2 Contracting the frontalis expresses surprise or even fear

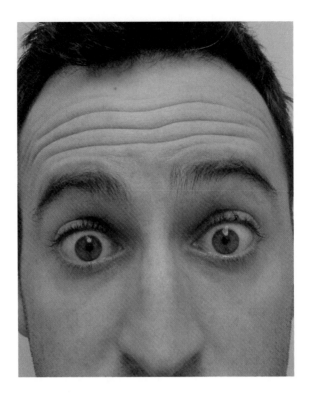

All too often it is the female rather than the male patient who is more concerned over the presence of forehead lines. Many of these women frequently are determined to eliminate any vestige of the appearance of a forehead wrinkle. A cautious and empathetic cosmetic physician will remind such patients that the absolute absence of a forehead wrinkle, especially at full contracture while expressing an emotion, may not be particularly appropriate for any reason, because it portrays an individual as too artificial and stone-like in appearance, and thus should not be desirable. Because of the various functions of the frontalis, its interaction with the depressor muscles of the glabella, and the potential risk of overtreatment causing brow ptosis, there are many who believe treating the frontalis with BOTOX® is not really as easy as one imagines[2].

Functional anatomy

The horizontal forehead lines are produced by the contraction of the muscle fibers of the frontalis, the only levator muscle of the upper third of the face (Figure 3.3). The function of the frontalis is to elevate the skin of the brow, the eyebrows, and the skin of the forehead, and to oppose the depressor action of the muscles of the glabella and brow. It also retracts the scalp.

The frontalis is a pair of quadrilaterally shaped, distinct muscles whose fibers are oriented vertically, producing the horizontal wrinkles of the forehead which are perpendicular to the direction of muscle contraction. The frontalis lies beneath a thick layer of sebaceous skin and subcutaneous tissue and has no attachment to bone. The frontalis originates from the epicranial, membranous galea aponeurotica superiorly and inserts at the level of the superciliary ridge (or arch) of the frontal bone into the subcutaneous tissue and skin of the brow. The fibers of the frontalis also interdigitate with the muscle fibers of the brow depressors, i.e. the procerus, corrugator supercilii, the depressor supercilii, and orbicularis oculi. In some patients there can be

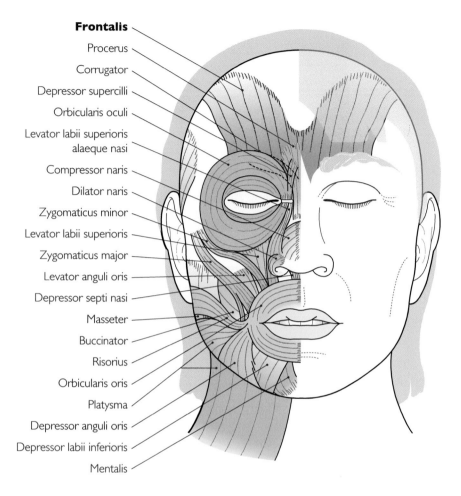

Frontalis
Procerus
Corrugator
Depressor supercilli
Orbicularis oculi
Levator labii superioris alaeque nasi
Compressor naris
Dilator naris
Zygomaticus minor
Levator labii superioris
Zygomaticus major
Levator anguli oris
Depressor septi nasi
Masseter
Buccinator
Risorius
Orbicularis oris
Platysma
Depressor anguli oris
Depressor labii inferioris
Mentalis

Figure 3.3   Frontalis, the only levator of the forehead

a downward extension of the membranous galea aponeurotica in the midline composed of little or no muscle fibers[3] (Figure 3.3). When present, injections of BOTOX® into this area are unnecessary. However, in some men and even women, there are well-developed muscle fibers in the center of the forehead. They can be detected by light palpation over the area while the patient actively raises and lowers the eyebrows. When functional muscle fibers of the frontalis can be detected in the center of the forehead, injections of BOTOX® in the midline of the forehead are needed to produce the desired effect (Figure 3.4). (see Appendix 4)

Dilution

Controlled, widespread diffusion of BOTOX® can be a desired effect when injecting BOTOX® in the forehead. To avoid brow ptosis, the muscle fibers of the frontalis must remain fully functional 1.5–2.5 cm above the brow (i.e. 3–4 cm above actual bony orbital margin). Then higher dilutions and larger volumes of BOTOX® can be injected into the upper forehead. Consequently, some injectors use from 1–2.5 ml of non-preserved saline to reconstitute a 100 U vial of BOTOX® when treating the forehead[4] (see Appendix 1).

Figure 3.4 Men and women who spend a lot of time outdoors have a well-developed frontalis

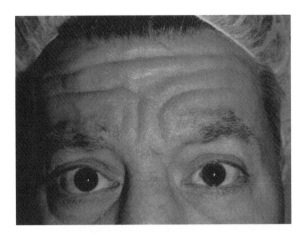

Figure 3.5 Typical injection sites in a woman with an average size forehead

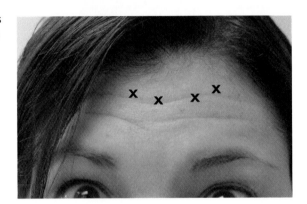

Dosing: how to correct the problem (what to do and what not to do)

A typical dose for injecting the forehead in women is approximately 8–12 U of BOTOX®.(see Appendix 1). This can be injected either subcutaneously or intramuscularly at four to six sites across the forehead with 2–4 U of BOTOX® placed in each site at intervals of 1.5–2 cm apart on either side of a deep crease[5,6] (Figure 3.5). For men, the typical dose is approximately 16–30 U of BOTOX® and occasionally higher. This can be injected at 4 to 12 or even more sites either subcutaneously or intramuscularly depending on the height and width of the forehead, with up to 4–5 U of BOTOX® placed in each site, depending on the strength of the frontalis[7] (Figure 3.6a,b). Some patients, either men or women, can have many rows of fine forehead wrinkles, whereas others can have one or two rows of deeply set folds and furrows. The number and dosage of the BOTOX® injections will depend on many factors, including the number and depth of the wrinkles, the size, shape and strength of the muscle and the height, width, and shape of the forehead[3,4]. More often than expected, and unbeknownst to the individual, a patient will present with asymmetrical eyebrows prior to their first treatment with BOTOX®. Patients must be made aware of their idiosyncratic differences and their anatomic particulars must be documented both in the patient's clinical chart and in their photographic record. Sometimes the eyebrows can be made symmetrically level with each other with carefully placed injections of BOTOX® (Figure 3.7a) and sometimes they cannot (Figure 3.7b).

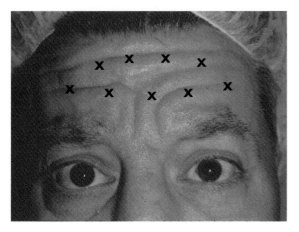

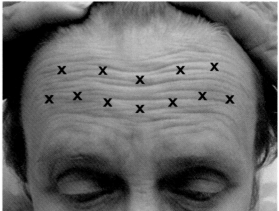

Figure 3.6a Typical injection sites in a man with an average size forehead. This patient had 3 U of BOTOX® injected at each site

Figure 3.6b Random pattern injections into a forehead that is high and wide with multiple parallel wrinkles. This patient had 2 U of BOTOX® injected at each site

The patient can be injected in an upright sitting position or even in a semireclined position. The pattern of injection across the forehead also can vary. One can randomly inject 2–4 U of BOTOX® subcutaneously or intramuscularly at any point on the forehead, that is at least 2–2½ finger breadths (i.e. 2–3 cm) above the margin of the bony orbit (Figures 3.6 and 3.7). One also can inject as much as 24 U of BOTOX® or more subcutaneously across the forehead in a horizontal plane parallel to the wrinkles present[3] (Figure 3.5). Another pattern that can be used is to inject 2–4 U of BOTOX® subcutaneously in a V configuration, whose arms diverge upward toward the lateral frontal hairline recession. This is accomplished by starting at a point in the midline approximately 2 cm above the medial aspect of the eyebrows, and injecting at three or four sites moving upwardly and laterally in a diagonal pattern, finishing toward the frontal

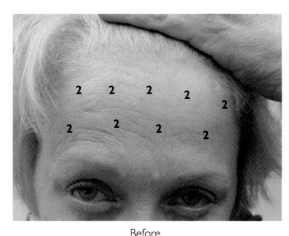

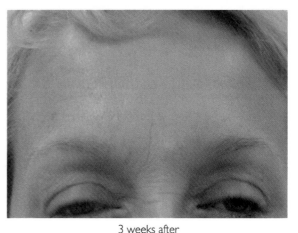

Before   3 weeks after
*Numbers indicate amount in units of BOTOX® injected

Figure 3.7a This 68-year-old patient with an average size forehead, and low set eyebrows, was unaware that her right eyebrow was higher than her left. After BOTOX® treatment they were symmetrical

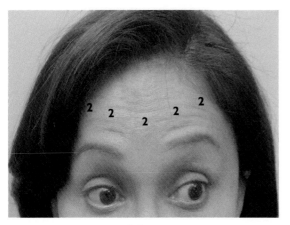 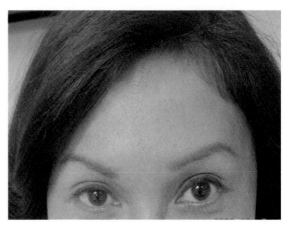

Before   I month after
*Numbers indicate amount in units of BOTOX® injected

Figure 3.7b This 36-year-old patient has a high and narrow forehead and multiple rows of forehead wrinkles. Note the left eyebrow is higher than the right before and after treatment with BOTOX®

hairline recession and 4–5 cm above the lateral side of the eyebrows, depending on the height of the forehead[2] (Figures 3.7b and 3.8). This pattern is best for women who have a relatively short rise to the height of their forehead. This pattern will keep BTX high above the eyebrows so they can form a peaked arch. Another technique is to inject subcutaneously approximately 2–4 U of BOTOX® at sites approximately 2 cm apart and across the entire forehead horizontally at a point midway between the brow and the hairline (Figure 3.5). This is advisable if the hairline is set low and if there are only one or two rows of horizontal wrinkles across the forehead (Figure 3.9).

If the width of the forehead is narrow, i.e. less than 12 cm between the superior temporal lines, then four or five injections subcutaneously of 2–4 U of BOTOX® at each injection site

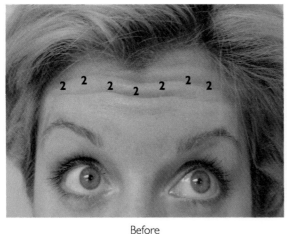 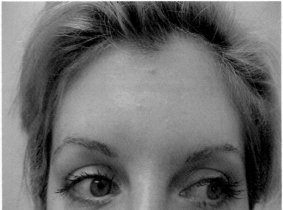

Before   I week after
*Numbers indicate amount in units of BOTOX® injected

Figure 3.8   This 40-year-old patient has a low and wide forehead with the right eyebrow higher than the left one before treatment with BOTOX®. Note the position of the right eyebrow one week after treatment with BOTOX®

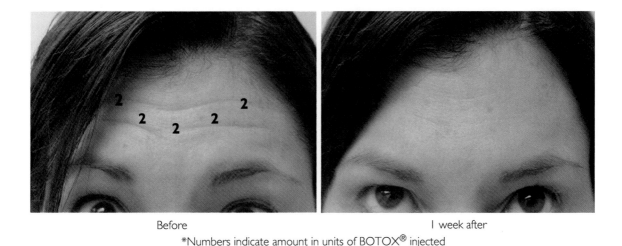

Before   1 week after

*Numbers indicate amount in units of BOTOX® injected

Figure 3.9   This 36-year-old patient has an average low and narrow forehead with the right eyebrow higher than the left

across the forehead are sufficient (Figures 3.7b and 3.9). One can feel the superior temporal line by first identifying the zygomatic process of the frontal bone, which is the superior portion of the upper lateral wall of the bony orbit (Figure 3.10). Its posterior edge continues upward, as a palpable protruding ridge up along the lateral edge of the frontal bone, and arches upward and backward, delineating the superior boundary of the temporal fossa. If an individual has a wider brow, i.e. more than 12 cm between the right and left superior temporal lines, then five, six, or possibly more injection sites across the forehead are probably necessary, with 2–4 U of BOTOX® injected at each site subcutaneously (Figures 3.7a and 3.11). The stronger the frontalis is, the more units of BOTOX® will be required to produce a desired effect.

Gentle massage upward and laterally at the injection sites for a few seconds helps to relieve the acute and transient pain of an injection and can help disperse the toxin locally. Prolonged or heavy-handed massage can disperse the liquid BTX beyond the intended area of injection, weakening adjacent muscles and producing unwanted results, e.g. brow ptosis.

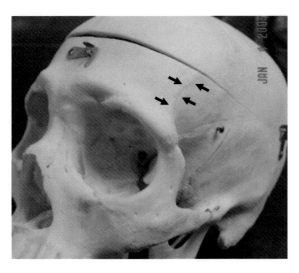

Figure 3.10 Anatomic photo of skull illustrating the location and extent of the superior temporal line

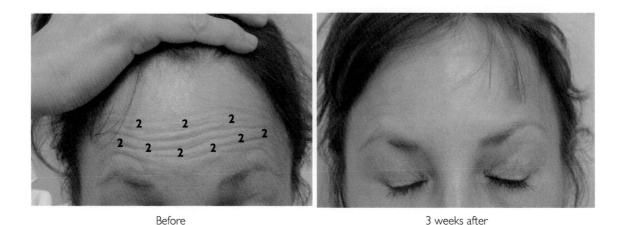

Before   3 weeks after
*Numbers indicate amount in units of BOTOX® injected

Figure 3.11 This 38-year-old patient has a high and wide forehead and an asymmetrically lower right eyebrow

Outcomes (results)

An adequate result when treating the frontalis is to completely eliminate the horizontal lines of the forehead when the patient is at rest, but to provide the ability for some movement and minimal wrinkling when the patient is animated or actively expressing an emotion (see Appendix 1). Ideally, weakening of the frontalis should last at least 3 full months when a sufficient dose of BOTOX® is injected. Frequently, after repeat treatments and occasionally after the first treatment session in some patients, the effects of BOTOX® weakening can last as long as 4 to 6 months after BOTOX® is injected[2]. Overgenerous intramuscular injections of the frontalis with high doses of BOTOX® will eliminate totally all movement of the muscle, even with forced contraction, creating a flat and motionless forehead. There usually is never a good cosmetic reason for such total paralysis of the frontalis or any other muscle of facial expression. In addition, the overall duration of results is usually not extended in any area when a higher dose than that adequate for the individual's problem is injected.

Often, especially with the initial treatment of forehead wrinkles, the effect of BOTOX® weakening may not occur symmetrically, and there may be wrinkling on one side of the forehead and not on the other, even at rest. It is imperative that the physician warn the patient of this before treatment and require the patient to return 2–3 weeks after a treatment session so that any minor asymmetries can be corrected. This is accomplished by injecting 1–2 U of BOTOX® in the vicinity of the persistent wrinkling. Remember, this should always be at least 2–2.5 cm above the brow, so as not to produce brow ptosis inadvertently. This is particularly important for those patients who have multiple rows of low-lying horizontal forehead lines. By allowing the lower fibers of the frontalis to remain active, there typically may be a wrinkle or two immediately above the eyebrow that might persist that cannot be reduced without causing brow ptosis. Most of the time, these narrow horizontal lines immediately adjacent to, if not within, the upper border of the eyebrow can be identified during the pretreatment physical examination and management planning (Figure 3.12a–d). When low lying horizontal forehead wrinkles occur, the patient should be made aware of their presence and given the option of other cosmetic procedures (e.g. fillers or resurfacing), before commencing with the injections of

BOTOX®. These minor horizontal forehead lines usually are the manifestation of excessively lax skin and the frontalis being recruited to elevate a weighty brow to prevent brow hooding. One runs the risk of brow ptosis if total reduction of these lower forehead lines is attempted. Consequently, the patient is better off totally ignoring these lines or, if they remain after treatment with BOTOX® and are obtrusively bothersome to the patient, having them treated with a soft tissue filler after the injection of BOTOX® has completely taken effect.

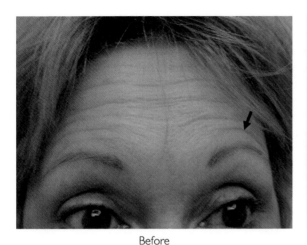

Before

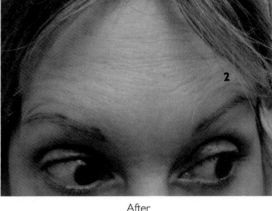

After

Figure 3.12a A 54-year-old patient with forehead wrinkles directly over the left eyebrow (arrow) observed with forced brow elevation before treatment

Figure 3.12b Same patient 2 weeks after initial treatment with BOTOX®. Note the left brow is now higher than the right brow with forced eyebrow elevation. An additional 2 U of BOTOX® were injected during this follow-up visit

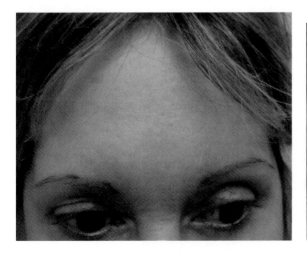

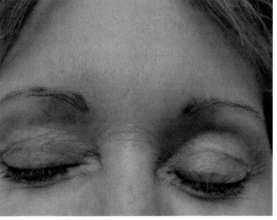

Figure 3.12c Same patient 5 weeks after the initial treatment with BOTOX® and 3 weeks after a touch-up of 2 U of BOTOX®. The left eyebrow remains slightly elevated laterally at rest with eyes wide open, but not with eyes closed

Figure 3.12d Same patient 5 weeks after the initial treatment with BOTOX® and 3 weeks after a touch-up of 2 U of BOTOX®. The left eyebrow remains slightly elevated laterally at rest with eyes wide open, but not with eyes closed

Complications (adverse sequelae) (see Appendix 5)

When treating the frontalis with BOTOX®, there does not appear to be a particular injection pattern or technique that might provide clinical results better than another. However, what does seem to be most important is avoiding brow ptosis[8–9]. This is best accomplished by remaining at least 2–3 cm above the supraorbital margin or 1.5–2.5 cm above the eyebrow when injecting the frontalis with BOTOX®. This will enable the muscle fibers of the frontalis to remain functional in the area directly above the brow so that the eyebrows will not droop and produce hooding over the upper eyelids (Figure 3.13a–c). In most patients, horizontal forehead lines are present in conjunction with glabellar frown lines. In these patients, it is imperative that the glabellar area is treated before or contemporaneously with the forehead; otherwise, because of the depressor action of the glabellar muscles, brow ptosis may be difficult to avoid. There is no antidote for brow ptosis, which can last as long as the BOTOX® injection is effective. Injections of low-dose,

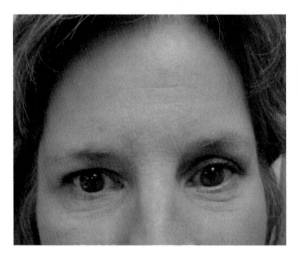

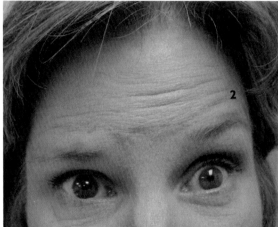

Figure 3.13a Unintentional ptosis of the right brow 3 weeks after a treatment of BOTOX®, in this 53-year-old, which lasted the entire 5 months of treatment efficacy

Figure 3.13b Same patient with an asymmetric left brow elevation found with forced raising of eyebrows. A touch-up of 2 U of BOTOX® was injected over the left eyebrow 3 weeks after the treatment of BOTOX®

Figure 3.13c Same patient 8 weeks after the initial BOTOX® treatment and 6 weeks after the touch-up

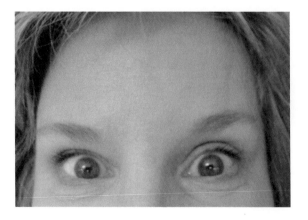

low-volume BOTOX® precisely placed in the superficial fibers of the upper, orbital portion of the orbicularis oculi may help to reduce the extent of brow ptosis (see below).

Clinical experience has indicated that when a more concentrated dose of BOTOX® is used (i.e. dilutions of 1 ml per 100 U vial of BOTOX®) there is minimal volume injected and migration of the BOTOX® is negligible, and the results also seem to last longer[9]. On the other hand, to prevent total paralysis of muscle movement, especially with the forced contraction of the frontalis, a different approach can be utilized when attempting to esthetically reduce horizontal forehead lines. Since there does not seem to be any agreement in the literature on which dilutions should be used when reconstituting a 100 U vial of BOTOX®, or which dosage regimens are most effective, one then can inject the forehead with the same number of units of BOTOX®, but with a more dilute solution[10,11]. Namely, a 100 U vial of BOTOX® can be reconstituted with 2–4 ml of saline when used solely for injecting the frontalis. This requires a greater volume to be injected. The toxin then can disperse over a wider area of the forehead, providing an effect that is less intensely paralyzing[4]. However, injecting large volumes of diluted BOTOX® possibly might limit the duration of its effectiveness[10,12]. As long as non-targeted muscle fibers (i.e. those of the lower frontalis) are not directly in the wake of the intended toxin diffusion, this may be a more forgiving alternative injection technique, especially for the neophyte injector.

Other more common adverse sequelae that occur with an injection of BOTOX® are related more to the actual injection rather than to the material injected. All of these adverse events are transient and generally do not last longer than 24–36 hours. They include local edema, erythema and pain at the injection and adjacent sites. For some patients, a dull and transient headache with or without general body malaise occurs after multiple injections of BOTOX® that can last beyond 24–72 hours. The occurrence of headache immediately after a BOTOX® injection seems paradoxical since BOTOX® injections are used to treat tension and migraine headaches by neurologists and many other medical specialists and subspecialists. Serious reactions, particularly immediate hypersensitivity such as anaphylaxis, urticaria, soft tissue edema, and dyspnea have been extremely rare. When they occur, appropriate medical treatment must be instituted immediately. (see Appendix 5)

Additional illustrations of injection techniques are shown in Figures 3.14 to 3.17.

Treatment implications when injecting the frontalis

1. Identify and document brow or forehead asymmetries prior to treatment with BOTOX®.
2. Inject the forehead subcutaneously or intramuscularly.
3. Weaken the frontalis; do not paralyze it.
4. The lower horizontal forehead lines may not be treatable if brow ptosis is to be avoided, especially in older patients.
5. Post-treatment forehead asymmetry can be corrected with a few units of BOTOX® given into the active fibers of the frontalis, 2–4 weeks after a treatment session.
6. Counteract brow ptosis and elevate the eyebrows by injecting the superficial fibers of the upper orbital portion of the orbicularis oculi with 1–2 units of low-volume BOTOX® injected into the medial and lateral aspects of the brow (see below). Otherwise, brow ptosis will remain as long as the current BOTOX® treatment is effective.
7. The frontalis is best treated after or in conjunction with glabellar frown lines.

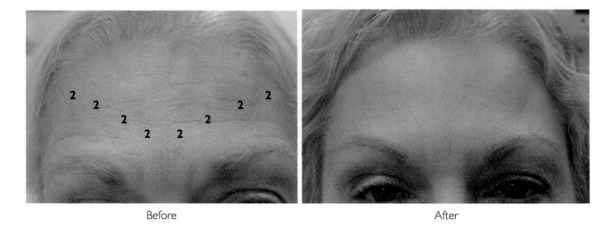

Figure 3.14a This 52-year-old has mild forehead wrinkling at rest before and 3 weeks after a BOTOX® treatment of only the forehead

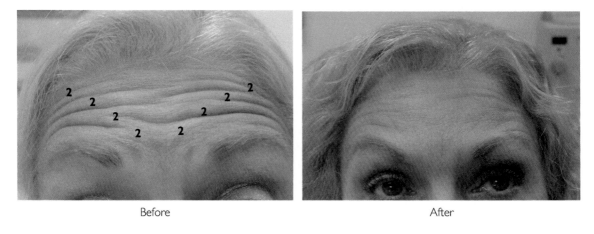

Figure 3.14b Same patient raising her eyebrows, before and 3 weeks after a BOTOX® treatment of only the forehead

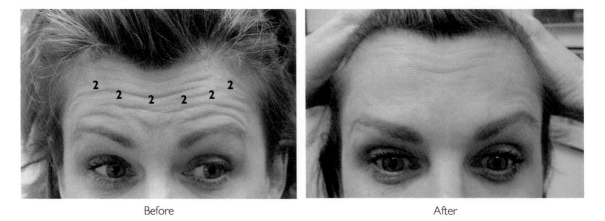

Figure 3.15 This 45-year-old patient is raising her eyebrows before and 3 weeks after BOTOX® treatment of only the forehead

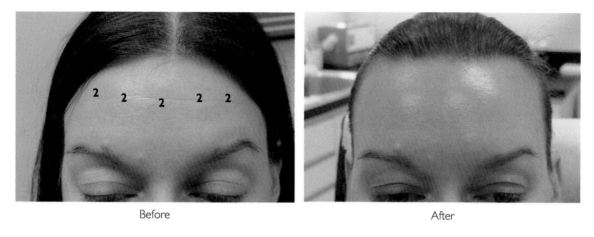

Before   After

Figure 3.16 This 35-year-old is shown at rest before and 2 weeks after a BOTOX® treatment of only the forehead

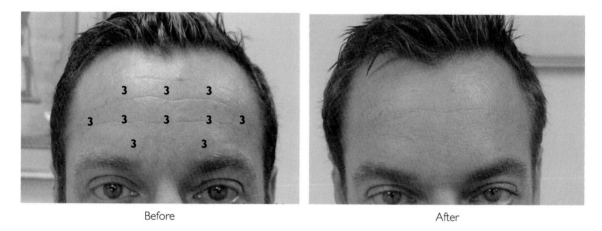

Before   After

Figure 3.17a This 40-year-old patient is shown at rest before and 3 months after a BOTOX® treatment of only the forehead

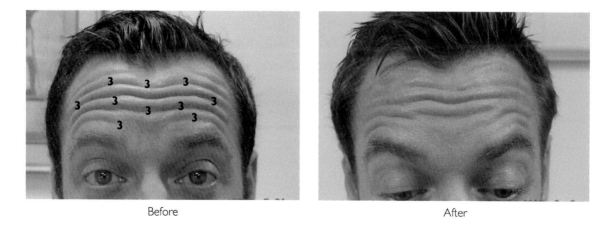

Before   After

Figure 3.17b Same patient raising his eyebrows before and 3 months after a BOTOX® treatment of only the forehead

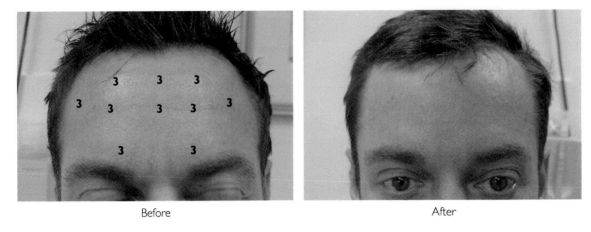

Before   After

Figure 3.17c   Same patient at rest before and one week after his fourth BOTOX® treatment of only the forehead

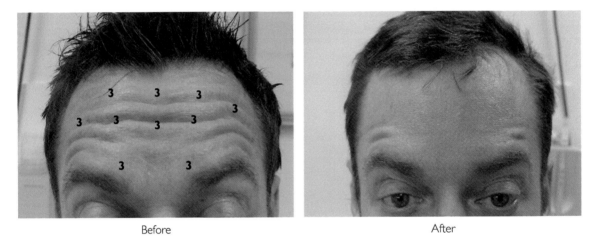

Before   After

Figure 3.17d   Same patient raising his eyebrows before and one week after his fourth BOTOX® treatment of only the forehead

Central brow (glabellar) frown lines

Introduction: problem assessment and patient selection

The area most frequently treated with BTX is the central brow or glabella and its frown lines[11–20]. The glabella is the smooth, flat, triangular elevation of the frontal bone superior to the nasal radix positioned between the two superciliary ridges or arches. The muscles of the 'glabellar complex' are the first and currently the only muscles of the face or body into which BOTOX® can be injected for cosmetic purposes that have been approved in the USA by the FDA. Treatment of all other muscles in any other part of the face or body with injections of BOTOX® for cosmetic reasons is done solely and explicitly in an off label manner.

There are four depressor muscles of the brow that cause the horizontal and vertical creases of the glabella. These muscles allow one to squint to protect the eyes from the elements (i.e.

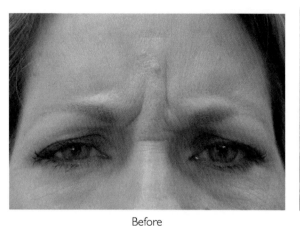

Before

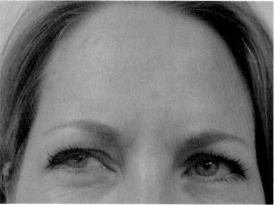

After

Figure 3.18a This 53-year-old patient, with unintentional frowning during intense concentration, is shown before a BOTOX® treatment

Figure 3.18b Same patient frowning 3 weeks after BOTOX® injections in the forehead and glabellar area

glaring light, gusts of air and wind, etc.), flying objects, and projectiles by lowering the eyebrows and adducting them medially. However, hyperkinetic depressor muscles can cause persistent, unintentional adduction and lowering of the medial aspect of the eyebrows, causing wrinkling between the eyes. For example, this central brow frowning during moments of intense concentration can be misinterpreted by others as a frown, which can express negative feelings of concern, tiredness, disappointment, frustration, anger, pain, and suffering, etc. (Figure 3.18a). Weakening the four depressors of the glabella with injections of BOTOX® can raise the eyebrows and virtually eliminate the frown lines of the central brow. This allows a person to appear more relaxed, conveying a positive sentiment when one ordinarily might be frowning and expressing a negative demeanor (Figure 3.18b). An elevated brow expresses a positive attitude, whereas a depressed brow expresses a negative one. In addition, low-set eyebrows may promote the formation of upper eyelid and lateral canthal hooding. In contrast, men in general prefer more horizontal eyebrows rather than arched or peaked eyebrows, which usually are more attractive in women. However, beware of women who pluck or have had permanent tattooing of their eyebrows, because the natural position of their brows may be deceptively displaced.

A detailed pretreatment assessment of how an individual's eyebrow position and shape conforms to the 'ideal brow' contour is key to producing acceptable results with injections of BOTOX®. The ideal contour of the female eyebrow is arched and positioned over the superciliary arch. The peak of the arch should be located just above the lateral limbus of the iris of the eye and sloping downward as far lateral as the lateral canthus, depending on the overall shape of a person's face and what is currently fashionable[21]. The tail of the eyebrow should lie on a horizontal plane 1–2 mm above the lowest point of its medial end. The overall silhouette of a female eyebrow should be that of the wing of a gull (Figure 3.19). The male eyebrow should have less of an arched contour and is positioned lower on the superciliary arch at about the level of the superior bony orbital margin (Figure 3.20). The pretreatment position and symmetry of

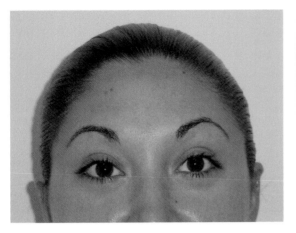

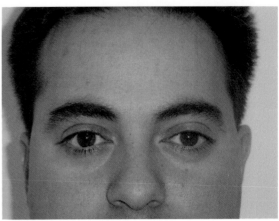

Figure 3.19 The ideal eyebrow of a woman outlines the wing of a gull

Figure 3.20 The ideal eyebrow of a man is less arched and lower set than a woman's

the eyebrows and eyelids will dictate the technique that will be needed to treat the glabellar frown lines. In women whose eyebrows are barely arched, strategically placed injections of BOTOX® can elevate them by allowing the lower fibers of the frontalis to raise the eyebrows unopposed by the decussating fibers of the corrugator supercilii and the superficial fibers of the orbital portion of the orbicularis oculi (Figure 3.21a,b).

Functional anatomy

Contracting any of the mimetic muscles of facial expression will cause wrinkling of the skin perpendicular to the direction of the muscle fibers. Therefore, the muscles that produce the vertical lines of the glabella because their fibers are oriented more or less horizontally are the

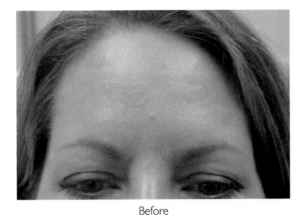

Before

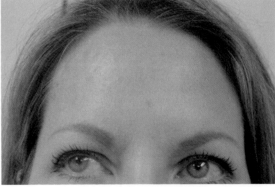

After

Figure 3.21a Arching an eyebrow with strategically placed BOTOX® injections in this 53-year-old patient with relatively flat arches

Figure 3.21b Arching an eyebrow with strategically placed BOTOX® injections in this 53-year-old patient 2 weeks after treatment

medial brow depressors, i.e. the corrugator supercilii and the medial fibers of the orbital portion of the orbicularis oculi. The corrugator supercilii is a small, narrow, deeply situated paired muscle that arises just inferior to the medial aspect of the superciliary arch approximately 4 mm lateral to the nasion (Figure 3.22). The nasion is the point of juncture of the nasofrontal with the internasal bony sutures[22]. Clinically it can be palpated as the center of the concavity at the nasal root. The corrugator extends laterally and upwardly through the palpebral and orbital fibers of the orbicularis oculi, inserting into the soft tissue and skin above the middle of the eyebrow in the vicinity of the supraorbital notch, overlying the inferior aspect of the superciliary arch[3,22]. It lies directly against the bone, and just beneath the interdigitating muscle fibers of the orbicularis oculi, procerus, depressor supercilii, and frontalis medially and beneath interdigitating fibers of the frontalis and orbicularis oculi laterally (Figure 3.22). Anatomic studies have demonstrated that the thickest portion of the belly of the corrugator is at or above a plane drawn through the middle of the eyebrow and approximately 1.6 cm from the nasion (i.e. the bony center of the nasal radix)[21–23]. (see Appendix 4)

The outer portion of the orbicularis oculi arises from the bony structures of the lateral nose and medial orbit, including the medial canthal ligament. Its fibers then run superiorly and

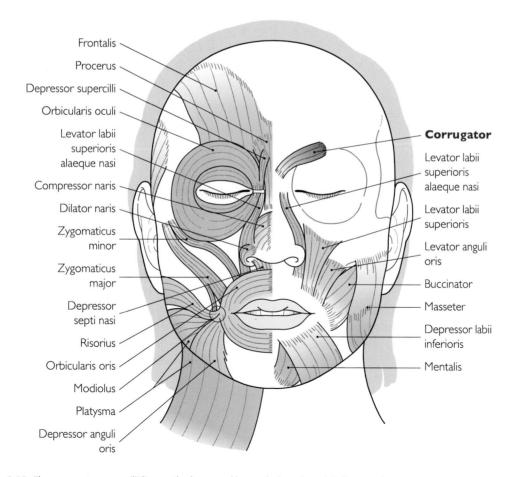

Figure 3.22 The corrugator supercilii lies on the bone and beneath the other glabellar muscles

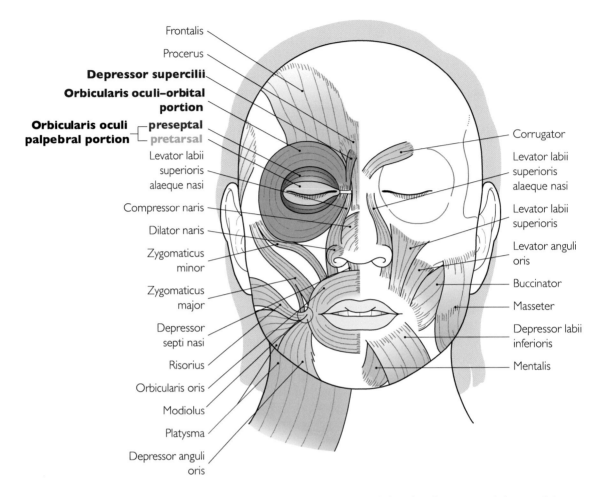

Figure 3.23 The orbicularis oculi has different subdivisions and interdigitates with the other depressors and elevator of the glabella

inferiorly, forming a wide sphincteric ring around the bony orbit that extends beyond the edges of the bony orbital rim and into the eyelids (Figure 3.23). The inner portion of the orbicularis oculi, identified as the palpebral portion of the muscle, is subdivided into preseptal and pretarsal portions (Figure 3.23). The medial aspect of the orbicularis oculi occasionally is referred to as the depressor supercilii by some authors. Contraction of the orbital portion of the orbicularis oculi approximates the upper with the lower eyelids, either voluntarily or involuntarily. (see Appendix 4)

The horizontal lines of the glabella and nasal root are produced by the contraction of the vertically oriented fibers of the procerus and the depressor supercilii, which are also medial brow depressors. The procerus is a thin, pyramidal muscle centrally located in the midline between the two eyebrows and lying 1–4 mm beneath the surface of the skin (Figure 3.24). The procerus arises from the fascia covering the nasal bridge and lower part of the nasal bone and the upper part of the upper lateral nasal cartilage and inserts superiorly into the skin and subcutaneous tissue at the nasal radix and lower part of the forehead between the two eyebrows. Contraction of the procerus pulls the medial aspect of the eyebrows downward, creating the horizontal

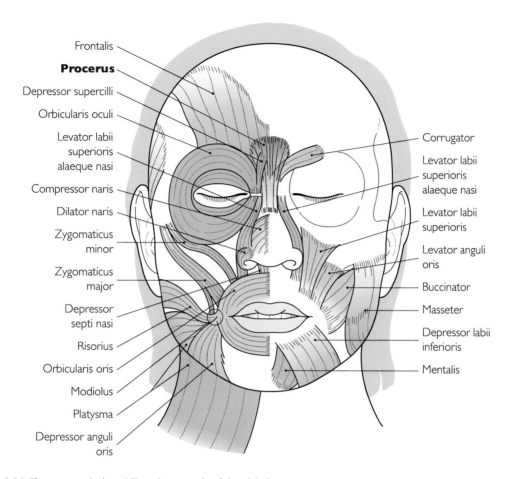

Frontalis
Procerus
Depressor supercilli
Orbicularis oculi
Levator labii superioris alaeque nasi
Compressor naris
Dilator naris
Zygomaticus minor
Zygomaticus major
Depressor septi nasi
Risorius
Orbicularis oris
Modiolus
Platysma
Depressor anguli oris

Corrugator
Levator labii superioris alaeque nasi
Levator labii superioris
Levator anguli oris
Buccinator
Masseter
Depressor labii inferioris
Mentalis

Figure 3.24 The procerus is the midline, deep muscle of the glabella

frown lines across the root of the nose. Anatomic studies have demonstrated that the procerus can be longer in women than in men[23,24]. The depressor supercilii is considered by many as a component part of the medial fibers of the orbital portion of the orbicularis oculi[21] (Figure 3.25). Yet others consider it a separate and distinct muscle from the orbicularis oculi and corrugator supercilii[25]. The depressor supercilii is a small muscle that has been found to originate directly from bone as one or two distinct muscle heads from the nasal process of the frontal bone and the frontal process of the maxilla, approximately 10 mm above the medial canthal tendon[25]. In cadaver dissections where the depressor supercilii originated as two separate heads, the angular vessels passed in between the two bundles of muscles[25]. In cadavers where there was only one head originating at the medial canthus, the angular vessels were found coursing anteriorly to the muscle. The depressor supercilii then passed vertically upward to insert into the undersurface of the skin at the medial aspect of the eyebrow, approximately 13–14 mm superior to the medial canthal tendon, which was superior in orientation to the medial aspect of the orbital portion of the orbicularis oculi[25]. Not only does it help move the eyebrow downward and close the eyelid, but it also participates in the functioning of the physiologic lacrimal pump by compressing the lacrimal sac (see below). (See Appendix 4)

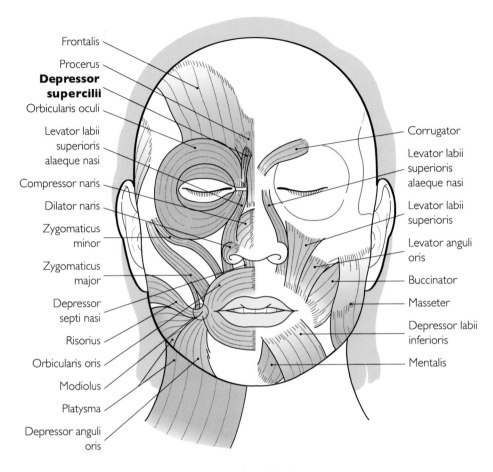

Frontalis
Procerus
Depressor supercilii
Orbicularis oculi
Levator labii superioris alaeque nasi
Compressor naris
Dilator naris
Zygomaticus minor
Zygomaticus major
Depressor septi nasi
Risorius
Orbicularis oris
Modiolus
Platysma
Depressor anguli oris

Corrugator
Levator labii superioris alaeque nasi
Levator labii superioris
Levator anguli oris
Buccinator
Masseter
Depressor labii inferioris
Mentalis

Figure 3.25 The depressor supercilii is the diminutive muscle of the glabella

Dilution

Different clinicians have their favorite pattern of injecting the glabella with varying doses of different concentrations of BOTOX®[18]. The manufacturer's package insert recommends reconstituting the 100 U vial of BOTOX® with 2.5 ml of unpreserved normal saline[26]. However, since the brow depressors decussate with each other and are in close proximity in a very small and confined area, it is extremely important to accurately inject precise amounts of BOTOX® in this area. Therefore, many seasoned and long time injectors of BOTOX® still dilute the 100 U vial of BOTOX® with only 1 ml of normal saline, and most have now switched to using preserved saline with 0.9% benzyl alcohol[27] (see Appendix 1). In this way, only minimal volumes of BOTOX® will be needed to produce the desired effects.

Dosing: how to correct the problem (what to do and what not to do)

The pretreatment evaluation should include examining the patient at rest and in full motion, lightly palpating the area with the palmar surface of the finger tips. This will help determine the location, size, and strength of the individual muscles of the glabella. A frequently used and standardized technique for treating the glabella is to inject BOTOX® into five different sites with doses that range anywhere from 4–10 U at each site (Figure 3.26)[14–20,26]. Electromyographic guidance in this area has not particularly improved treatment outcomes because these facial muscles are superficial and easily localized by topographical landmarks[19,22,23,28,29]. Patients who are hard to treat because they are less responsive to the effects of BOTOX® seem to be those who possess thick sebaceous skin with deep, intractable wrinkles whose furrows are difficult to pull apart with the fingers. Usually these turn out to be men and sometimes women who spend a lot of time outdoors. On the other hand, patients who possess thinner, less sebaceous skin with finer wrinkles and shallower skin folds that can be spread apart and reduced with the fingers ('glabellar spread test') seem to have better, longer-lasting results[20].

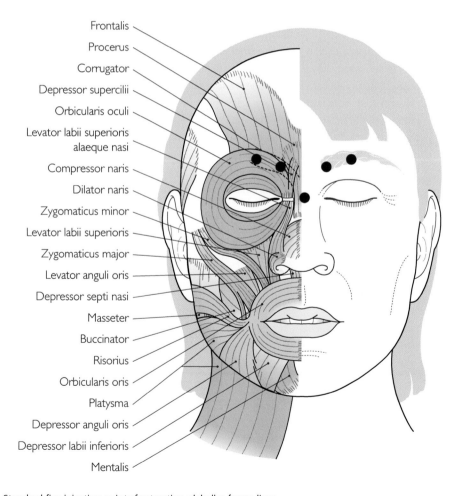

Figure 3.26 Standard five injection points for treating glabellar frown lines

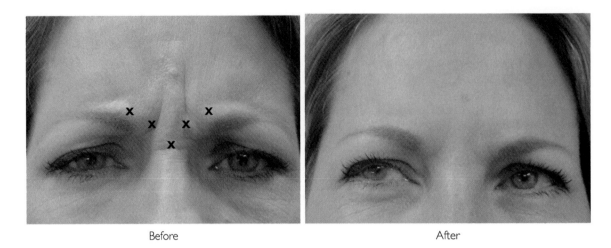

Before   After

Figure 3.27 Standard five injection points for treating glabellar frown lines in a female frowning

Generally, glabellar frown lines in women can be satisfactorily treated with a total dose of 25–40 U of BOTOX® injected into the standard five injection sites (Figure 3.27)[2,17,28-32]. Men, on the other hand, usually require a significantly higher dose of BOTOX® (40–80 U or even higher) injected at seven sites to produce a reasonable effect that lasts at least 3–4 months[2,31,33] (Figure 3.28). When glabellar lines are deeper, longer, or thicker on one side of the midline, that set of muscles (e.g. corrugator and medial aspect of the orbicularis oculi) should receive a slightly higher dose of BOTOX® than those on the contralateral side. The two injection points in addition to the standard five are those given over the midpupillary line, bilaterally, which usually are needed when treating men, so that the midbrow does not elevate and become more arched than is generally the case naturally (Figure 3.29a–d)[1]. Remember to remain at least 1–2 cm above the orbital rim at the midpupillary line to avoid blepharoptosis.

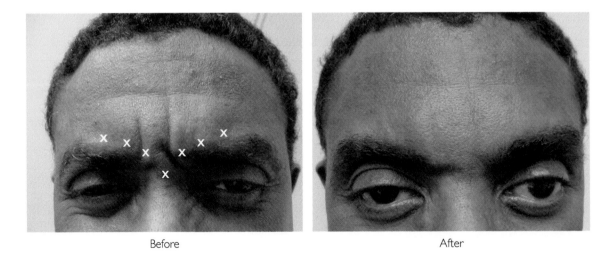

Before   After

Figure 3.28 Standard seven injection points for treating stronger glabellar muscles causing deeper furrows and frown lines in a male frowning

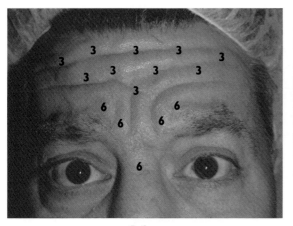

Before

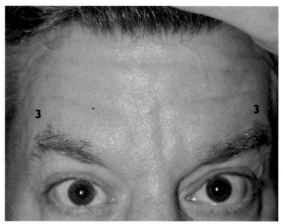

After

Figure 3.29a Typical injection points and number of units for a man who works outdoors and has strong depressors and levators of the brow and forehead causing very deep lines. Before treatment with BOTOX® injections

Figure 3.29b Same patient: an additional 6 U of BOTOX® were necessary to lower the lateral tail of the eyebrows in this man who usually has straight eyebrows. Two weeks after the initial BOTOX® treatment (note elevated lateral eyebrows and points where additional 3 U of BOTOX® were injected)

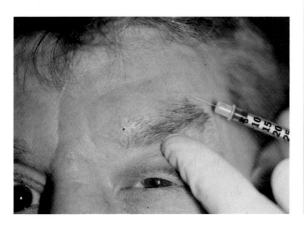

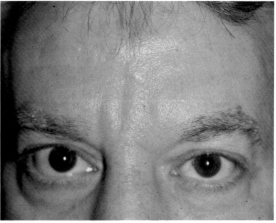

Figure 3.29c Injection of touch-up dose of 3 U of BOTOX® 2 weeks after initial BOTOX® treatment

Figure 3.29d Five weeks after the initial BOTOX® treatment and 3 weeks after a touch-up treatment with the patient frowning (note the flatter, less arched lateral eyebrows)

In order to treat the glabellar frown lines and produce optimal results with the least amount of complications, it is recommended that multiple injections of relatively concentrated doses and low volumes be used on both sides of the midline. With the patient sitting up or in the semireclined position gently palpate the medial aspect of the eyebrows as the patient squints and frowns. After locating the belly of the corrugator with the tips of the second and third fingers of the non-dominant hand, ask the patient to raise the eyebrows as high as possible, keeping the tip of your index finger positioned over the thickest part of the belly of the corrugator supercilii. Then 4–10 U of BOTOX® can be injected into the strongest portion of the

Figure 3.30 Technique of injecting the corrugator supercilii (note the position of the thumb and index finger of the non-dominant hand)

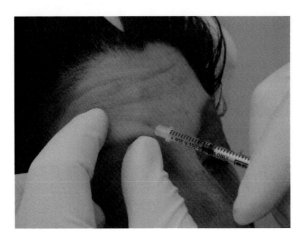

muscle, which is located approximately 12 mm lateral and 10 mm superior to the nasion or the center of the concavity at the nasal root[22].

Prior to inserting the needle, the index finger of the non-dominant hand should be advanced slightly cephalad and above the point of maximal muscle thickness. This usually is just above the eyebrow. The thumb now is placed at the lower margin of the supraorbital rim (or margin). The needle then is guided over the upper edge of the thumb, between it and the index finger, and inserted into the skin at a 60–90° angle until penetration into the corrugator supercilii can be felt[22,31]. Entry into the corrugator is usually discerned when, after passing through the dermis and subcutaneous tissue, an abrupt release of resistance is felt as the needle penetrates fascia and muscle fibers of the corrugator. At this point, the needle may or may not impinge onto bone. If it does, the patient will sense sharp pain. The needle should then be withdrawn gently enough to move away from the bone, but not enough to exit the belly of the corrugator. The bore of the needle tip should be pointed upward and away from the globe, as it is slowly advanced into the belly of the corrugator supercilii in an oblique direction, slightly upward and lateral. Always remain deep within the muscles and medial to the supraorbital notch and approximately 1.5–2.0 cm superior to the bony supraorbital margin (Figure 3.30). Refrain from striking the frontal bone with the needle tip, so as not to inflict any additional pain upon the patient, which occurs when periosteum is pierced. However, this may not be avoidable when first learning how to find the deeply seated corrugators and effectively inject them at the proper depth. Placing the non-dominant thumb and index finger on the brow just above and below the eyebrow prior to injecting BOTOX® serves many purposes. It prevents injecting BOTOX® too low and close to the orbital rim. By applying direct pressure inferior to the border of the supraorbital rim, Binder et al. felt that they were able to reduce migration of BOTOX® behind the orbital septum[22,31]. This maneuver also assists in identifying the location and direction of the corrugator supercilii, because it can be felt by light palpation. It is important to inject slowly to avoid dispersing the BOTOX® to surrounding, non-targeted muscles.

The medial orbital portion of the orbicularis oculi is injected with another 4–10 U of BOTOX® at a point just above the medial end of the eyebrow. The level of the needle tip is directed away from the orbit and perpendicular to the skin surface and advanced slightly upward toward the hair line, always avoiding contact with the frontal bone and remaining 1–1.5 cm above the medial aspect of the superorbital margin (Figure 3.31)[32, 33]. Because the

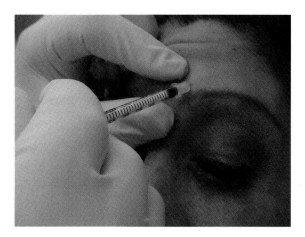

Figure 3.31 Technique of injecting the medial aspect of the orbicularis oculi and depressor supercilii (note the position of the index finger and the thumb of the non-dominant hand)

fibers of the orbicularis oculi are closely adherent to the overlying skin, injections can be given subcutaneously at this site, which also should affect the depressor supercilii. A pleasing vertically upward lift to the medial brow can be accomplished by this technique, if fibers of the frontalis are not affected[34,35]. Gentle massage in an upward and lateral direction for a few seconds immediately after the injection helps relieve the acute pain of injection the patient might experience, and can disperse the toxin into the areas intended for treatment. Heavy-handed massage will definitely disperse the BOTOX® beyond the area and into muscle fibers not intended for the treatment, i.e. into the fibers of the lower frontalis, which can produce brow ptosis. When present, do not forget to identify, photograph, and indicate to the patient prior to any BOTOX® injection any variation in the anatomy that might cause the patient's eyebrows to be asymmetric. Documentation of the conversation and the patient's response is absolutely necessary and must always be completed prior to initiating treatment with BOTOX®.

Next, an injection of approximately 4–10 U of BOTOX® is given between the eyebrows at the nasal root into the belly of the procerus and into the interdigitating fibers of the depressor supercilii. The dose needed for this injection of BOTOX® will depend on the overall muscle strength and depth of the horizontal glabellar wrinkles that are present[23]. The strength of the procerus can be determined by gently palpating the glabellar area while the patient repeatedly squints and frowns. Glabellar wrinkles tend to be deeply fixed in the skin, especially the horizontal ones. Those that are more resistant to treatment with BTX commonly are found in men and women who spend a lot of time outdoors, because their glabellar muscles are significantly hypertrophied from frequent squinting. Intramuscular instead of subcutaneous injections of BOTOX® into the procerus can be done. This can be accomplished by grasping the soft tissue of the root of the nose between the thumb and the index finger of the non-dominant hand, elevating skin and muscle before placing the needle between the two fingers and injecting into one or two sites in the center of the nasal radix (Figure 3.32). The site of injection should be anywhere from 1–3 mm above or below the center of the horizontal plane that intersects both medial canthi. The weaker muscle fibers of the procerus are injected with at least 4 U of BOTOX®, while the stronger ones can be injected with up to 10 U and possibly more. The depressor supercilii already will have been partially treated by the injections given at the medial aspect of the eyebrows when the medial portion of the orbicularis oculi is treated. Likewise, when the procerus is injected some diffusion of the BOTOX® into the interdigitating fibers of the

Figure 3.32 Technique of injecting the procerus (note the position of the index finger and the thumb of the non-dominant hand)

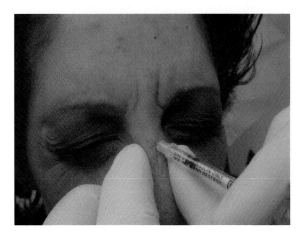

depressor supercilii will occur, particularly when gentle massage upward and laterally toward the procerus is performed immediately after injection (see Appendix 1).

Outcomes (results)

There can be a noticeably high arching of the eyebrows, approximately 2–3 mm, caused by the levator action of the frontalis in those patients whose glabellar depressors have been substantially weakened, but the interdigitating muscle fibers of the frontalis immediately above the brow have not[34–36]. Accentuated high arching eyebrows may be attractive in most women, but usually are not in men. In order to avoid a high arching brow in men, an additional 4–6 U of BOTOX® can be injected subcutaneously 1–1.5 cm above the supraorbital margin at the midpupillary line (Figures 3.28, 3.29)[8,13]. There also can be an increase in the distance between the eyebrows and an elevation of the medial aspect of the eyebrows when glabellar frown lines are treated with BOTOX® because of the dynamic relationship between the brow depressors and levator[30,34–36].

On the other hand, to enhance and elevate the arching of the lateral eyebrow, especially in women, 2–4 U of BOTOX® can be injected subcutaneously into the lateral depressor, i.e. the lateral orbital portion of the orbicularis oculi, at a point of maximal contraction which usually is in the vicinity where the lateral aspect of the superciliary arch meets the lower aspect of the superior temporal line (Figure 3.33a). Depending on the idiosyncratic anatomy of the patient being treated, this point can be just above or below the hairs of the lateral aspect of the eyebrows (Figure 3.33b). One or multiple (usually no more than three) injections of 2–4 U of BOTOX® can be given at points of maximal muscle contraction (higher doses can be used for a lesser number of injections). Injecting BOTOX® in this area reduces the depressor action of the vertical muscle fibers of the orbicularis oculi at the lateral aspect of the brow, and allows the muscle fibers of the lateral aspect of the frontalis to elevate the lateral eyebrow[34–38] (Figure 3.34a, b and c). Approximately 2 U to no more than 8 U of BOTOX® should be injected into one and usually no more than three injection sites, starting from the lateral aspect of the eyebrow and finishing at a point just lateral to the midpupillary line in patients with a strong orbicularis oculi who warrant such an injection (Figure 3.35). Ordinarily, one to three injections of 2–3 U of BOTOX® placed into the lateral aspect of the brow and upper eyelid will suffice to produce an esthetically pleasing lateral brow lift (Figures 3.35 and 3.36). With the bore of the needle

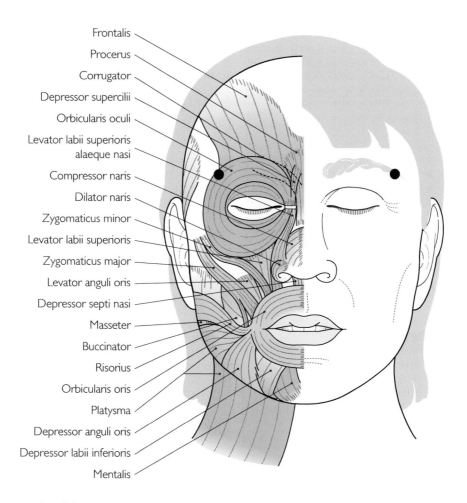

Frontalis
Procerus
Corrugator
Depressor supercilii
Orbicularis oculi
Levator labii superioris alaeque nasi
Compressor naris
Dilator naris
Zygomaticus minor
Levator labii superioris
Zygomaticus major
Levator anguli oris
Depressor septi nasi
Masseter
Buccinator
Risorius
Orbicularis oris
Platysma
Depressor anguli oris
Depressor labii inferioris
Mentalis

Figure 3.33a Location of the main injection point when attempting to elevate the lateral aspect of the eyebrow

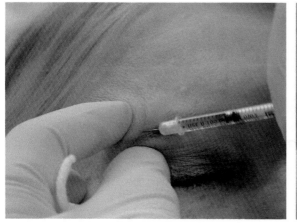
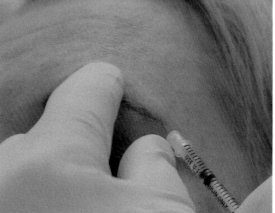

Figure 3.33b Injection point for a lateral lift. The exact location on the skin in relationship to an individual's eyebrow may vary according to the person's anatomy

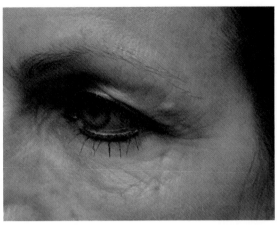
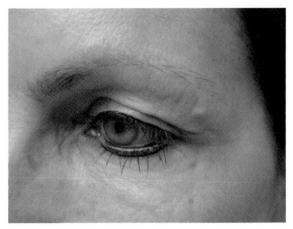

| Before | 3 weeks after |

Figure 3.34a This 49-year-old patient is shown before and 3 weeks after BOTOX® was injected into the lateral aspect of the orbicularis oculi (note muscle fibers of the lower lateral frontalis raising the tail of the eyebrow and diminished lateral hooding of the lateral aspect of the upper eyelid)

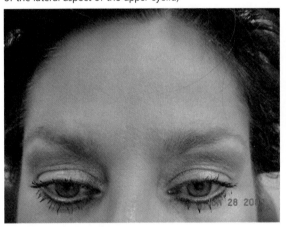
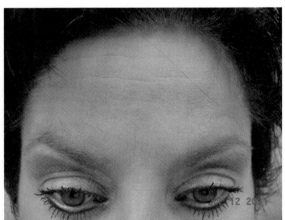

| Before | 3 weeks after |

Figure 3.34b This 56-year-old patient is shown before and 3 weeks after BOTOX® was injected into the lateral aspect of the orbicularis oculi (note muscle fibers of the lower lateral frontalis raising the tail of the eyebrow)

pointing upward and away from the orbit, BOTOX® must be injected slowly and subcutaneously into each lateral brow (Figure 3.33b). This technique might help reduce the risk of the BTX dispersing beyond the intended area and producing adverse sequelae, i.e. brow and eyelid ptosis, ectropion, diplopia, and xerophthalmia or dry eye. (see Appendix 5)

High lateral eyebrows convey an expression of surprise, happiness, or approval. Depressed, or low positioned lateral eyebrows convey an expression of sadness, fatigue, anxiety, disdain and disapproval. Lateral brow elevation is best appreciated as a decrease in hooding of the lateral aspect of the upper eyelid[34–40] (Figure 3.34 and 3.36). Elevating the eyebrows at their medial, central, or lateral aspects can be unpredictable when first attempted, but usually reproducible when the proper technique is used and appropriate specific clinical records and sequential

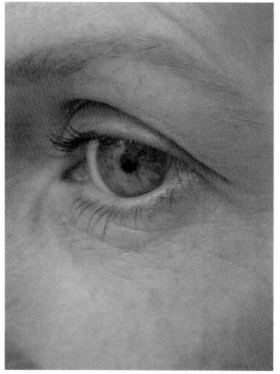
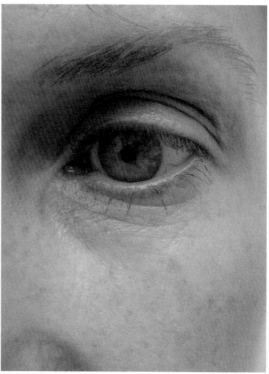

Before   2 weeks after

Figure 3.34c   This 45-year-old patient is shown before and 2 weeks after BOTOX® was injected into the lateral aspect of the orbicularis oculi (note the reduction in the lateral brow hooding)

photographs are kept[36–40]. (see Appendix 3) With the proper technique the complication rate is low and the results may be subtle at best. Each patient's clinical record must include diagrammatic as well as photographic documentation along with their written or typed progress notes if reproducible results are desired and expected. The preference of lifting the eyebrows for one patient or another, i.e. the medial, central, or lateral aspect, will depend on current fashion standards, the patient's overall physiognomy and idiosyncratic anatomy, and whether or not the physician is capable of injecting BOTOX® with a reproducible technique.

Ordinarily, one can expect the effect of a BOTOX® treatment of glabellar frown lines to last at least 3–4 months, with progressively longer-lasting results with each subsequent treatment session. Patients who are treated for the very first time with BOTOX® may experience some asymmetry and therefore should return for an evaluation and possible touch-up treatment within 2–3 weeks. Ordinarily, the effects of a BOTOX® treatment last longer with each sequential treatment. Therefore, after the first 1–2 years of treatment sessions regularly scheduled every 3–5 months, the patient may prefer to return for their next retreatment on an as-need basis (see Appendix 2).

Complications (adverse sequelae) (see Appendix 5)

Ptosis of the upper eyelid is the most significant complication seen when injecting BOTOX® in and around the glabella[16,17] (Figure 3.37). It is felt by some that blepharoptosis is caused by the

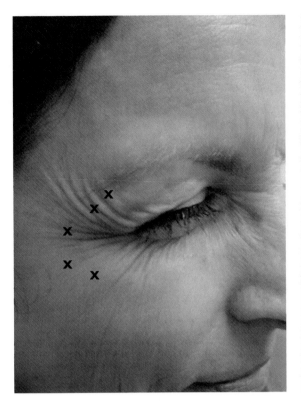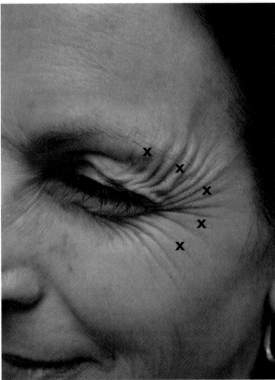

Figure 3.35 This 49-year-old patient with many wrinkles of the upper lid and lateral eye is shown before a treatment of BOTOX®. (X marks where 1 to 3 U of BOTOX® can be injected subcutaneously in the lateral aspect of the upper eyelid)

migration of injected BOTOX® through the orbital septum, weakening the levator palpebrae superioris. This is found to occur more frequently when BOTOX® is injected close to the bony supraorbital margin at the midpupillary line. Only at this point do some of the muscle fibers of the levator palpebrae superioris insert inferiorly to the bony attachment of the orbital septum, allowing for easy diffusion and access of BOTOX® into the fibers of the upper eyelid levator, and producing ptosis of the upper eyelid. Blepharoptosis, when it occurs, is seen as a 1–2 mm or more drop in the upper eyelid, obscuring the upper border of the iris (Figure 3.37). Ptosis can appear up to 7–10 days after a BOTOX® injection and can last 2–4 weeks or even longer[8,11,16,17]. Blepharoptosis seems to occur more frequently when large volumes of highly diluted BOTOX® are injected into the glabellar complex.

An antidote for blepharoptosis is apraclonidine 0.5% eye drops (Iopidine®, Alcon Laboratories, Inc., Fort Worth, TX, USA). The ocular instillation of Iopidine®, an alpha-2-adrenergic agonist with mild alpha-1 activity, causes Mueller's muscle (a non-striated sympathomimetic levator muscle of the upper eyelid) to contract, temporarily raising the upper eyelid approximately 1–2 mm. One or two drops should be instilled into the affected eye. If ptosis persists after 15–20 minutes, intraocular instillation of an additional one or two drops may be required before the affected eyelid will elevate. This procedure can be repeated three to four times a day. It is advisable to use apraclondine eyedrops only when absolutely necessary,

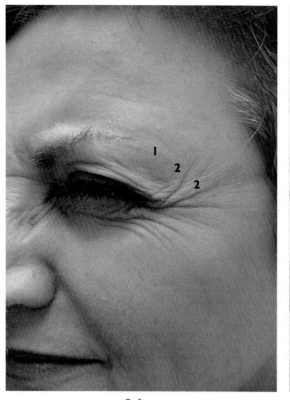 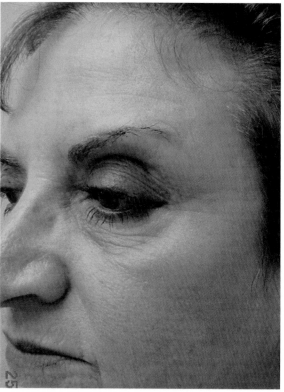

Before   After

Figure 3.36 This 68-year-old patient is shown before and 3 weeks after BOTOX® was injected into the lateral aspect of the orbicularis oculi (note the elevation of the hooding of the lateral aspect of the upper eyelid). The numbers indicate the amount of BOTOX® units injected

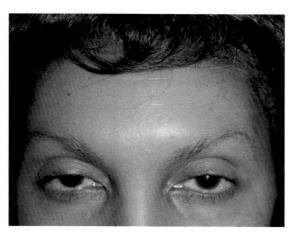

Figure 3.37 Brow and eyelid ptosis in this 67-year-old patient. Note a drop of 2 mm of the right brow and the upper eyelid that occurred approximately 10 days after BOTOX® was used to treat forehead and glabellar wrinkles. Patient is actively blinking

because approximately 20% of patients can develop a contact conjunctivitis with frequent use. The mydriatic and vasoconstrictor phenylephrine (Neo-Synephrine® HCl, 2.5% ophthalmic solution, Sanofi Pharmaceuticals, Inc., New York, NY USA or Myfrin™ 2.5%, Alcon Laboratories,

Inc., Fort Worth, TX, USA) is an alpha-1 agonist that also can be used when Iopidine® is not available[33]. However, there are more potential side effects associated with its use than with Iopidine®. Specifically, even when only the 2.5% ophthalmic solution is used, phenylephrine can acutely exacerbate narrow angle glaucoma, cardiac arrhythmias, and hypertension. Because it also is a mydriatic, even one drop of Neo-Synephrine® will prevent the patient from accommodating as usual and visual acuity can be compromised. Naphazoline (Naphcon®, Alcon Laboratories, Inc., Fort Worth, TX, USA) is another ophthalmic solution that can be used to stimulate Mueller's muscle to contract, temporarily lifting a ptotic upper eyelid.

Blepharoptosis also can be induced secondarily when the lower fibers of the frontalis are weakened, producing a drop in the height of the brow. The weight of the ptotic brow then impinges upon the upper eyelid and causes it to droop. This seems to occur more frequently in older patients who possess dermatochalasis of the skin of the eyelids and brow. In order to compensate for a heavy, lax brow, they unconsciously use the lower fibers of their frontalis to lift the soft tissue of the brow, which also maintains their upper eyelids in a raised position[22]. When this compensatory action of the frontalis is weakened by BOTOX®, a secondary blepharoptosis is created.

Overzealous treatments of BOTOX® in the area of the lateral canthus that are either forcibly injected or given with high doses of high volume BOTOX® can result in brow ptosis, ectropion, diplopia, xerophthalmia, or lagophthalmos and even superficial punctate keratosis because of corneal exposure. Brow ptosis is caused by the diffusion of BOTOX® into the lower fibers of the frontalis when BOTOX® is injected rapidly, or the area is massaged vigorously (Figure 3.13). Patients can cause brow ptosis if they manipulate the injected area excessively, enough to disperse the BOTOX® beyond the targeted area. Injecting large volumes of low concentrations of BOTOX® also increases the risk of dispersion beyond the targeted muscle. Ectropion occurs when the muscular sling of the lateral orbicularis is inadvertently weakened. This is generally seen as excessive rounding of the contour of the lateral canthus. Diplopia occurs when the lateral rectus or other extraocular muscles are weakened because BOTOX® has diffused through the orbital septum. Xerophthalmia or dry eye will occur if BOTOX® is injected too deeply in the upper lateral aspect of the periocular area and affects the secretion of the lacrimal glands. Lagophthalmos results when there is a loss of the normal sphincteric function of the orbicularis oculi, and the upper eyelid does not close and approximate firmly against the lower eyelid. Loss of the sphincteric functions of the orbicularis oculi either with involuntary blinking or with voluntary forced eye closure can occur when BOTOX® diffuses onto the palpebral portion of the orbicularis oculi, causing undue eyelid weakness.

Incomplete eyelid closure or lagophthalmos has been seen more frequently in patients treated for strabismus when extraocular muscles are treated with substantial doses of BOTOX® than when patients are treated for cosmetic reasons, especially if minimal volume BOTOX® is injected[47]. On the other hand, patients who have an attenuated orbital septum because of age or other reasons may be more prone to this adverse sequela. If the incomplete eyelid approximation is present for extended periods of time, exposure of the cornea can result in symptomatic dry eyes or exposure keratitis. There is no antidote for lagophthalmos, which can remain as long as the effects of the BOTOX® are present, or it can remit sooner. So protecting the patient from developing secondary dry eyes is extremely important, because excessive corneal exposure will lead to desiccation of the cornea and superficial punctate keratosis. Immediate consultation with an ophthalmologist at the first sign of lagophthalmos will prevent any additional, unintended eye injury.

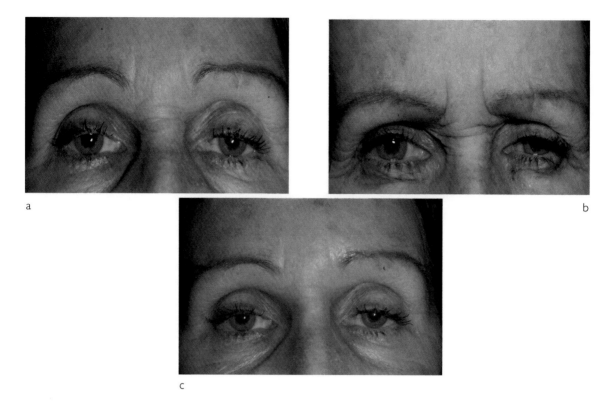

Figure 3.38 This 70-year-old with compensatory brow lifting and an undetected left eyelid droop at rest (a) and frowning (b) before BOTOX®. Blepharoptosis (c) is seen at rest one month after BOTOX®. The patient and treating physician assumed the blepharoptosis was caused by BOTOX® until the before and after treatment pictures were compared which then prompted the diagnosis of 'pseudoblepharoptosis'

Asymmetry is a minor adverse sequela that sometimes is unavoidable, particularly when a patient is treated for the first time with BOTOX® (Figure 3.38). There are three types of asymmetry that can be corrected with injections of BOTOX®; iatrogenic; idiosyncratic; and incidental or acquired. An example of incidental or acquired asymmetry is Bell's or facial (7th cranial) nerve palsy, or when one side of the face acquires a weakness because of an illness (e.g. cerebral vascular accident), or an accidental or traumatic injury. Idiosyncratic asymmetry occurs when a person is born with the inability to control or move a facial muscle to its fullest extent, while its counterpart muscle on the contralateral side of the face is unaffected. This can result, for example, in a crooked, asymmetric smile (see Chapter 5), or one eyebrow or eyelid higher than the other (see above).

Many of those individuals who possess, unbeknownst to them, a lower lying asymmetric brow on one side, commonly will also possess a lower lying upper eyelid on the same side. With age, compensatory brow lifting will lift the brows to maintain unobstructed vision. When these patients are treated with injections of BOTOX® to such a degree that the lower fibers of the frontalis are weakened, the patient's compensatory brow lifting is interrupted. With a drop in brow height comes a drop in upper eyelid height, and those patients who already have an asymmetrically lower upper eyelid on one side now appear to have blepharoptosis or pseudoblepharoptosis (Figure 3.38). When the patient first realizes that one upper eyelid is lower than the other, blame on the injector and the product is a foregone conclusion[41]. However, the astute and conscientious physician will evaluate the patient carefully and document his or her findings with pretreatment photographs. This will enable the physician to discuss the true problem with the patient and graphically demonstrate its presence prior to embarking on a perilous path to treatment failure. So instead of the physician being led to believe that the patient developed blepharoptosis because of his or her poor injection technique, the physician will be able to identify that the patient always has had an idiosyncratic subclinical upper eyelid asymmetry that can be unmasked and even exaggerated with injections of BOTOX®. This manifestation of pseudoblepharoptosis frequently occurs in patients over the age of 65–70 years who are treated for glabellar frown lines with injections of BOTOX®.

The best way to avoid additional difficulties with patient rapport and confidence is to keep carefully documented written and photographic clinical notes (see Appendix 3). Discuss the physical findings with the patient and point out existing iodiosyncratic asymmetries, anatomical differences, and potential outcomes prior to treatment. Informing the patient of such findings before any treatment commences always is considered by the patient an accurate diagnosis of a unique situation. Explaining the circumstances and reasons for a particularly poor outcome after treatment always is considered by the patient an excuse for an improperly executed therapeutic procedure.

Iatrogenic asymmetry arises when an injection of BOTOX® causes one side of the face to become weaker than the other. There are many reasons for this. The primary reason for one side of the face to become weaker than the other after an injection of BOTOX® is when the stronger side is not injected with the equivalent dose of BOTOX® as the contralateral side. This could be the result of the BOTOX® not diffusing completely through all the muscle fibers. Another reason could be that some of the fibers might have been physically resistant to the BOTOX®, because those particular fibers were idiosyncratically thicker or stronger than the rest of the area and may have required a higher dose of BOTOX®. Another possibility is that the injection was not given precisely symmetrically or in the thickest and strongest part of the muscle, causing a particular section of muscle to retain most or some of its strength. Iatrogenic asymmetry is probably the easiest to rectify. Generally with a few additional units of BOTOX® injected into the appropriate area, iatrogenic asymmetry can be easily and expeditiously ameliorated (Figure 3.39a,b).

Other untoward sequelae of more limited significance and duration can occur. These are the same adverse sequelae as those experienced with any type of subcutaneous or intramuscular injection. They include ecchymoses, edema, and erythema at the injection sites (Figure 3.40), headache, and flu-like malaise. Rarely, if ever, do any of these side effects last beyond the day of the treatment, except for ecchymoses, which can last up to 10 days or more. Also, for the first time recipient of a periocular BOTOX® treatment, the presence of periocular edema lasting a few hours to days may occur. This could be attributed to lymph stasis, possibly produced by a non-detectable attenuation of the sphincteric pumping action of the orbicularis oculi, reducing the efficiency of lymph fluid clearance from the surrounding soft tissue.

For some women, habitual scowling is the result of spending a lot of time outdoors, or suffering from constant and persistent headaches, or being plagued with poor vision and refusing to wear corrective lenses, among many other things. Incessant contraction of the corrugator supercilii, manifested by habitual scowling, causes the medial end of the eyebrows to approach the midline. Many of these women will pluck and shorten the transverse length of their eyebrows by removing eyebrow hair from the medial end of their brow. This will widen the

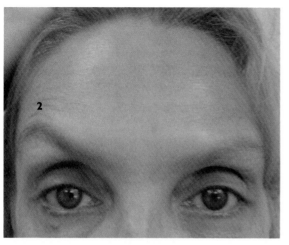

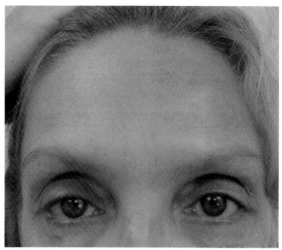

Before

After

Figure 3.39a This 42-year-old patient is seen at rest with a higher right eyebrow 2 weeks after BOTOX® injections of the glabella and forehead and just before an additional 2 U of BOTOX® were given

Figure 3.39b Same patient at rest 3 weeks after the additional 2 U of BOTOX® were given and 5 weeks after her initial treatment with BOTOX®. Notice the relative asymmetry of both eyebrows

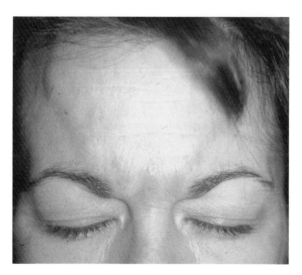

Figure 3.40 Patient 5 to 10 minutes after a BOTOX® treatment for forehead, glabellar and lateral canthal wrinkles. Note the erythema and edema in the pattern of the injections

glabellar interbrow space, so they do not look like they are habitually scowling, when they actually are. After injections of BOTOX® are given to reduce the number and extent of glabellar frown lines, the corrugators are no longer contracting repeatedly and adducting the eyebrows toward each other, narrowing the interbrow glabellar space. In fact, the transverse width of the glabella returns to normal because the corrugators are in a more relaxed state at rest. However, those women who have plucked the medial portion of their eyebrows to visually widen a scowling brow before BOTOX®, now complain after BOTOX® that they look practically hyperteloric because their eyebrows are now widely separated, when in fact it is only that the medial aspects of their eyebrows have been excessively plucked. Such an adverse sequela is difficult to predict, but warning prospective patients who pluck their eyebrows of such a side effect will prevent further disappointment on the part of the patient and additional frustration on the part of the physician. Also, beware of the patients who color in the shape of their eyebrows, because the shape that is chosen that day may not necessarily correspond to the natural anatomical position of that person's brow. Injections of BOTOX® may return the area to its natural anatomic position, which paradoxically may appear to be distorting the glabellar area, when in reality it is not. Patients with permanent eyebrow tattooing may present similar challenges and treatment disappointments.

Figures 3.41–3.48 are some examples of different patients treated with BOTOX® for glabellar frown lines. Some had simultaneous treatment of their forehead frown lines.

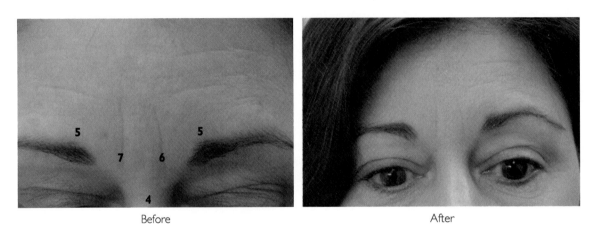

Before　　　　　　　　　　　　　　　After

Figure 3.41a This 56-year-old patient is shown at rest before and one month after a BOTOX® treatment for forehead and frown lines. Note the different dosages for areas of stronger muscle contraction

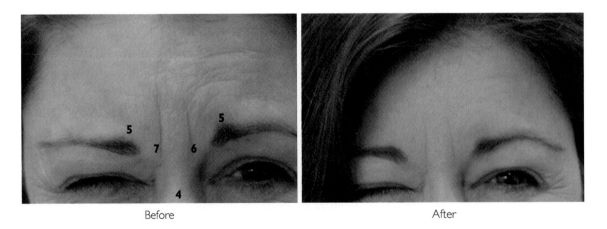

Before　　　　　　　　　　　　　　　After

Figure 3.41b Same patient frowning before and one month after BOTOX® treatment for forehead and frown lines. Note the different dosages for areas of stronger muscle contraction

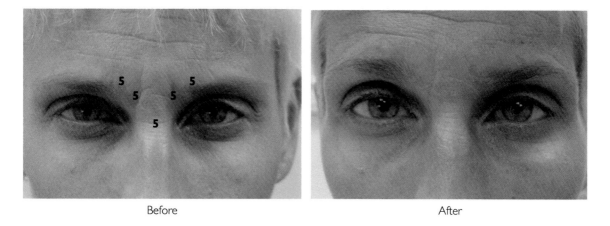

Before   After

Figure 3.42 This 43-year-old patient is shown at rest before and 2 weeks after a BOTOX® treatment of frown lines only

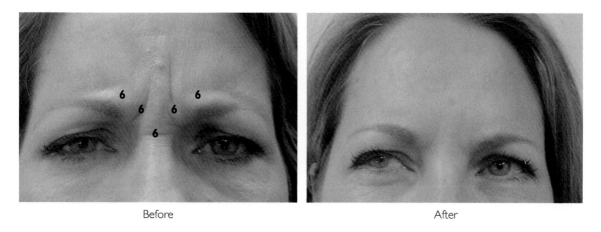

Before   After

Figure 3.43 This 53-year-old patient is shown frowning before and 3 weeks after a BOTOX® treatment of glabellar frown lines only

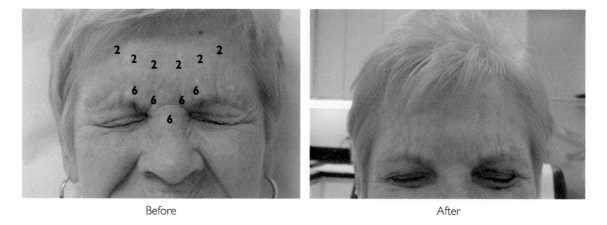

Before   After

Figure 3.44 This 66-year-old patient is shown frowning before and 4 weeks after a BOTOX® treatment of forehead and glabellar frown lines

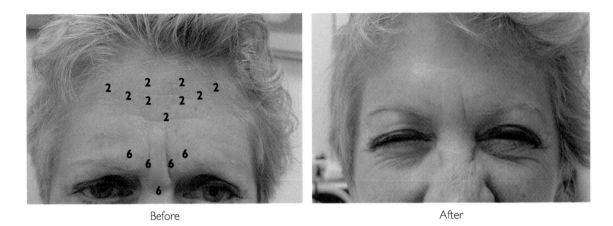

Before   After

Figure 3.45 This 57-year-old patient is shown at rest before and frowning 2 weeks after a BOTOX® treatment of forehead and glabellar frown lines

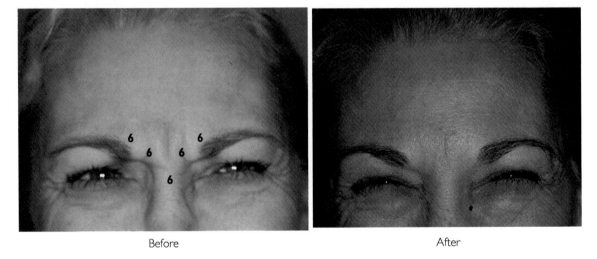

Before   After

Figure 3.46 This 52-year-old patient is shown before and 3 weeks after a BOTOX® treatment of glabellar frown lines only

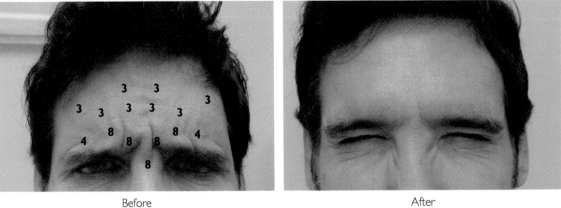

Before   After

Figure 3.47 This 48-year-old patient is shown frowning before and 3 weeks after a BOTOX® treatment of forehead and glabellar frown lines

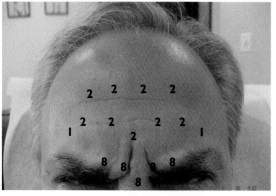
Before

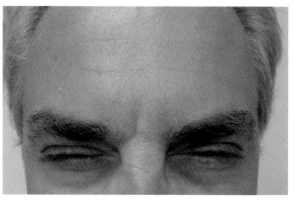
After

Figure 3.48 This 56-year-old patient is shown frowning before and 2 weeks after a BOTOX® treatment of forehead and frown lines

Treatment implications when injecting the glabella

1. Precise amounts of accurately placed injections of minimal volume BOTOX® reduce the incidence of brow and eyelid ptosis.
2. Men may need higher doses of BOTOX® than women for comparable results.
3. Women prefer arched eyebrows; men prefer straight, non-arched eyebrows.
4. BOTOX® injections should remain medial to the midpupillary line and 1.5–2.0 cm above the supraorbital margin, placed deeply into the corrugator supercilii.
5. Blepharoptosis can be transiently reversed with alpha-adrenergic agonist eye drops, but brow ptosis cannot be reduced and remits only when the effects of BOTOX® diminish.
6. Patients with inelastic, redundant skin of the brow develop brow ptosis and secondary blepharoptosis easily with injections of BOTOX®.
7. Pre-existing asymmetry of the brow and eyelids should be discussed with the patient before treatment, and might be corrected by accurately injecting appropriate doses of BOTOX® on the affected side.

Periocular lines – Lateral canthal lines

Introduction: problem assessment and patient selection

One of the first signs of aging is the wrinkles that radiate away from the lateral canthus outwardly and laterally which are sometimes referred to as "crow's feet" (Figure 3.49). Depending on a person's skin type, history of sun exposure, and muscle strength, crow's feet can appear in someone as young as 20 years of age. The natural thinness and abundance of the skin in the lateral periorbital area make this area prone to wrinkling. These lateral canthal lines initially appear only during animation, they soon accentuate while smiling, laughing, or squinting and become increasingly noticeable with time. Their presence causes one to appear perpetually tired and fatigued and even older than one's current age. For a woman, crow's feet

Figure 3.49 Crow's feet accentuated by squinting in a person who is 68 years old

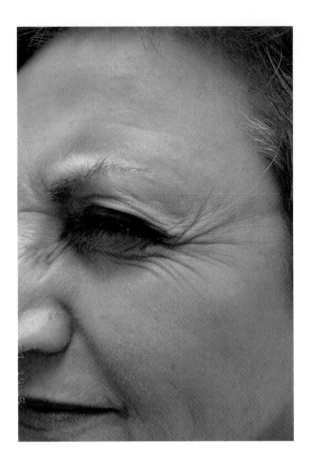

are the bane to her appearance, especially when make-up accumulates in the depths of the creases. For men, crow's feet are a sign of hard work and fun in the sun.

Functional anatomy

Lateral canthal wrinkles are caused by the contraction of the lateral side of the orbital portion of the orbicularis oculi and therefore are referred to as dynamic wrinkles. They are the result of infolding and pleating of the overlying skin, which radiate away from the lateral canthus (Figure 3.49). These wrinkles are perpendicular to the direction of the lateral muscle fibers of the orbital portion of the orbicularis oculi, which run mostly in a vertical direction around the lateral canthus (Figure 3.50). These types of wrinkles can be diminished by injections of BOTOX® [42,43]. In some patients, however, age and photodamage are the major contributing factors that produce lateral canthal wrinkles. These types of wrinkles are always present whether a person is actively animating or not and therefore are referred to as static wrinkles. When the bulk of crow's feet are produced by static wrinkles, then injections of BOTOX® will be less effective. Only a resurfacing procedure or a soft tissue filler might help modify static wrinkling of the lateral canthus. When the bulk of crow's feet are produced by the hyperactivity of the lateral orbital portion of the orbicularis oculi, then injections of BOTOX® can play a significant role in diminishing the wrinkling (Figure 3.51a,b).

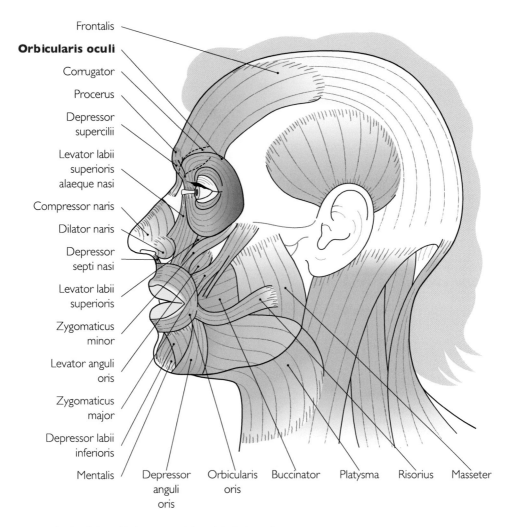

Figure 3.50 Lateral side of the orbital portion of the orbicularis oculi

The orbicularis oculi is divided into three parts, the orbital, palpebral, and lacrimal portions. The orbital part is the outermost portion of the muscle that forms a complete ellipse around the bony orbit (Figure 3.52). In its superior aspect it interdigitates with the muscle fibers of the frontalis, corrugator supercilii, depressor supercilii, and the procerus. It inserts into the soft tissue of the brow, anterior temple (superficial temporalis fascia), cheeks, and medial and lateral canthal tendons. Contraction of the orbital portion of the orbicularis oculi approximates the upper with the lower eyelids, as with forced, volitional eyelid closure, and depresses the medial and lateral aspects of the eyebrow. Certain medial fibers of the orbital portion of the orbicularis oculi have been referred to by some as the depressor supercilii. However, the depressor supercilii in recent anatomic studies has been identified as a distinct and separate pair of muscles, which insert into the undersurface of the skin at the medial aspect of the eyebrows. They pull the eyebrows downward when they contract[24,25]. (see Appendix 4)

The fibers of the palpebral part of the orbicularis oculi are subdivided into preseptal and pretarsal portions (Figure 3.53). The pretarsal portion courses over the eyelids and the preseptal

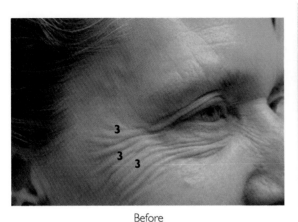

Before

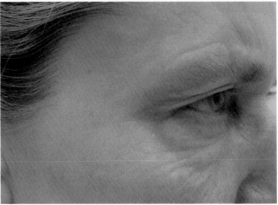

After

Figure 3.51a Squinting produces a myriad of lateral orbital wrinkles in this 64-year-old before a treatment of BOTOX® into her crow's feet

Figure 3.51b Same patient squinting 3 weeks after BOTOX® injections

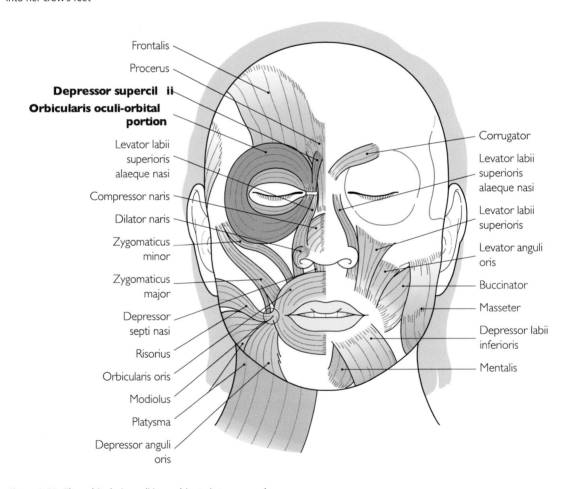

Figure 3.52 The orbicularis oculi is a sphincteric type muscle

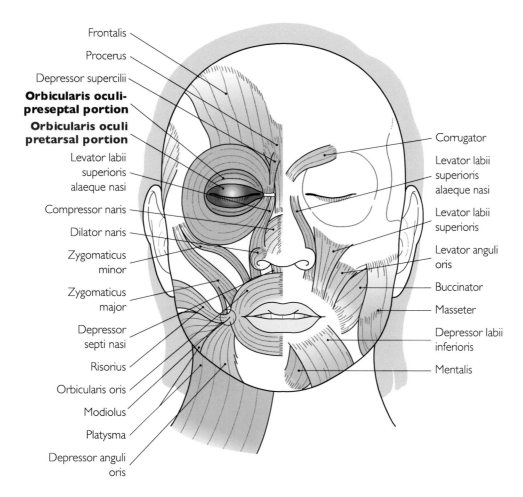

Frontalis

Procerus

Depressor supercilii

**Orbicularis oculi-
preseptal portion**

**Orbicularis oculi
pretarsal portion**

Levator labii
superioris
alaeque nasi

Compressor naris

Dilator naris

Zygomaticus
minor

Zygomaticus
major

Depressor
septi nasi

Risorius

Orbicularis oris

Modiolus

Platysma

Depressor anguli
oris

Corrugator

Levator labii
superioris
alaeque nasi

Levator labii
superioris

Levator anguli
oris

Buccinator

Masseter

Depressor labii
inferioris

Mentalis

Figure 3.53 Orbicularis oculi: the palpebral orbicularis oculi is divided into the preseptal and pretarsal portions

portion lies superficial to the orbital septum. The preseptal fibers arise from the bifurcation of the medial palpebral ligament, while the upper and lower pretarsal fibers traverse laterally to join and form the lateral palpebral raphe.

Contraction of the palpebral part of the orbicularis oculi provides the sphincteric action of the eyelids and gently closes them involuntarily, as occurs with blinking or sleep. The palpebral portion of the orbicularis oculi should not be treated with BOTOX®, because it can cause loss of the voluntary and involuntary functions of eyelid closure.

The lacrimal part of the orbicularis oculi is located posterior to the medial palpebral ligament and lacrimal sac (Figure 3.54). Its fibers arise from the posterior lacrimal crest and travel posteriorly to the lacrimal sac and insert onto the upper and lower tarsal plates medial to the lacrimal punctum. Contraction of the lacrimal portion of the orbicularis oculi draws the eyelids posteriorly against the globe, compressing the lacrimal sac and facilitating the lacrimal pump (see p 107) by creating negative back pressure within the canalicular system, and allowing tears to flow into the nasolacrimal duct.

Because crow's feet are enhanced during smiling or laughing, the contraction of the risorius and zygomaticus major et minor also contributes to the formation of these lateral canthal

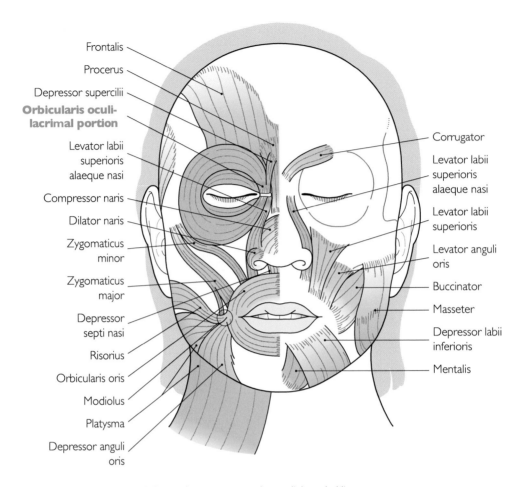

Frontalis
Procerus
Depressor supercilii
**Orbicularis oculi-
lacrimal portion**
Levator labii
superioris
alaeque nasi
Compressor naris
Dilator naris
Zygomaticus
minor
Zygomaticus
major
Depressor
septi nasi
Risorius
Orbicularis oris
Modiolus
Platysma
Depressor anguli
oris

Corrugator
Levator labii
superioris
alaeque nasi
Levator labii
superioris
Levator anguli
oris
Buccinator
Masseter
Depressor labii
inferioris
Mentalis

Figure 3.54 Orbicularis oculi: third subdivision lies posterior to the medial canthal ligament

rhytides. The zygomaticus major originates anterior to the zygomatic temporal suture deep to the orbicularis oculi and travels diagonally toward the corner of the mouth (Figure 3.55). It decussates with the modiolus and inserts into the skin and mucosa of the corners of the mouth. The zygomaticus major moves the angle of the mouth superiorly, laterally, and posteriorly when a person laughs, smiles, or chews.

The zygomaticus minor originates from the zygomatic bone posterior to the zygomaticomaxillary suture, just anterior to the origin of the zygomaticus major, travels downward and forward and inserts into the lateral aspect of the upper lip (Figure 3.56). The zygomaticus minor helps to create and elevate the nasolabial fold and to elevate the lateral aspect of the upper lip, producing the expression of disdain.

The risorius is bandlike, usually poorly developed, and lies at the upper border of the facial platysma (Figure 3.57). It does not originate from bone, but from the connective tissue overlying the parotid gland and the fascia of the masseter. The risorius travels horizontally across the face, superficially to the platysma, decussates with the modiolus, and inserts into the skin of the oral commissure. The risorius at times can be indistinguishable from the platysma. The risorius can stretch the lower lip and displace the skin of the cheek posteriorly when laughing or smiling,

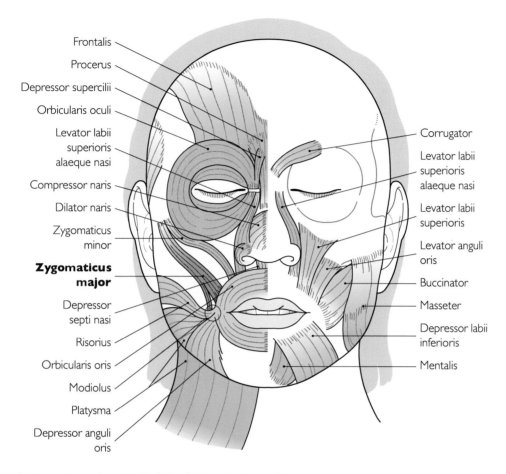

Figure 3.55 Zygomaticus major assists in lifting the lateral oral commissure

producing dimples in some individuals. Along with the platysma, the risorius can move the oral commissures in downward, upward, and lateral directions.

Consequently, when a person laughs, smiles, or grins they contract the risorius and zygomaticus major et minor, which also can accentuate the lower aspect of their crow's feet (Figures 3.36 and 3.51a). (See Appendix 4).

Dilution

When injecting BOTOX® in the periocular area, it is imperative that minimal volumes be accurately placed. This will necessitate diluting a 100 U vial of BOTOX® with only 1 ml of normal saline (see Appendix 1).

Dosing: how to correct the problem (what to do and what not to do)

When one performs injections of BOTOX® or any other pharmaceutical in the periocular area, both the patient and the physician should remain unencumbered, comfortable, and without

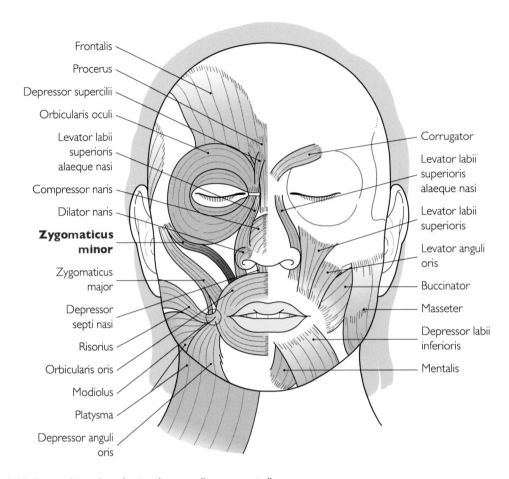

Frontalis
Procerus
Depressor supercilii
Orbicularis oculi
Levator labii
superioris
alaeque nasi
Compressor naris
Dilator naris
**Zygomaticus
minor**
Zygomaticus
major
Depressor
septi nasi
Risorius
Orbicularis oris
Modiolus
Platysma
Depressor anguli
oris

Corrugator
Levator labii
superioris
alaeque nasi
Levator labii
superioris
Levator anguli
oris
Buccinator
Masseter
Depressor labii
inferioris
Mentalis

Figure 3.56 Zygomaticus minor elevates the upper lip more centrally

distractions. The patient should be in a sitting or semireclined position, approachable from both the left and right sides. When injecting BOTOX® in the lateral canthal area, one should stand on the opposite side of the area to be treated with the patient facing toward the injector. This will allow the physician to approach the area to be treated with the tip of the needle pointed lateral to and away from the patient's eye. Stretching the skin over the area to be injected with the non-dominant hand enables the physician to visualize most of the blood vessels that lie just beneath the surface of the skin in this area (Figure 3.58).

Since the skin of the periorbital area is thin, the tip of the needle should be inserted no more deeply than 2–3 mm below the skin surface. This will allow the BOTOX® to diffuse slowly and evenly into the underlying muscle fibers. While injecting BOTOX® into the lateral canthus, it is important to remain at least 1–1.5 cm lateral to the lateral bony orbital rim. Approximately 2–4 U of BOTOX® can be injected into each of two to four sites subcutaneously at the lateral orbital area 1.0–1.5 cm apart from each other for a total of 4–16 U of BOTOX® on each side (Figure 3.51a,b). Men may need slightly higher dosing, approximately 10–20 U per side for comparable results[2].

Because there can be variable patterning of the lateral canthal lines from one person to the next, BOTOX® treatments should be individualized for each patient. Generally, the lateral canthal lines can be identified as upper eyelid creases, lateral canthal creases, or lower eyelid or malar

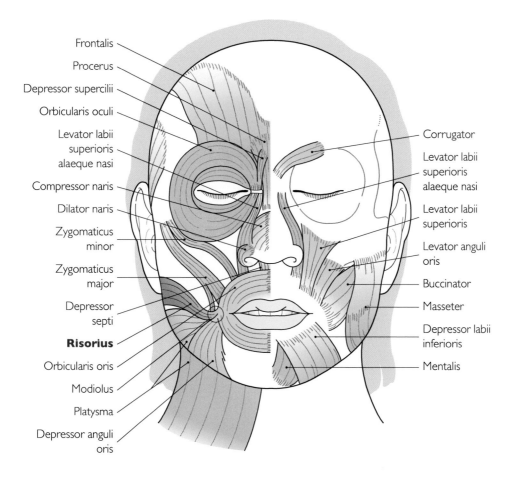

Frontalis

Procerus

Depressor supercilii

Orbicularis oculi

Levator labii superioris alaeque nasi

Compressor naris

Dilator naris

Zygomaticus minor

Zygomaticus major

Depressor septi

Risorius

Orbicularis oris

Modiolus

Platysma

Depressor anguli oris

Corrugator

Levator labii superioris alaeque nasi

Levator labii superioris

Levator anguli oris

Buccinator

Masseter

Depressor labii inferioris

Mentalis

Figure 3.57 Risorius is the muscle of laughter

creases (Figure 3.59a). Characteristically, a patient can possess any one or multiple patterns of creases that can even be different from the left to right side of the face (Figure 3.59b). In addition, a person may have a certain percentage of either static or dynamic wrinkles, but only the dynamic ones are reducible by injections of BOTOX®. The number of injection sites and the

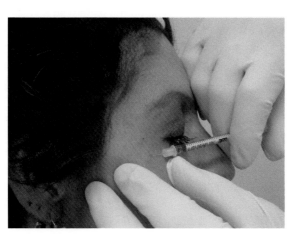

Figure 3.58 Technique of injecting the crow's feet or lateral orbicularis oculi. Note the injector stands on the opposite side, pointing and inserting the needle away from the lateral canthus and globe. Stretching the skin with the non-dominant hand assists in visualizing superficial periocular vasculature

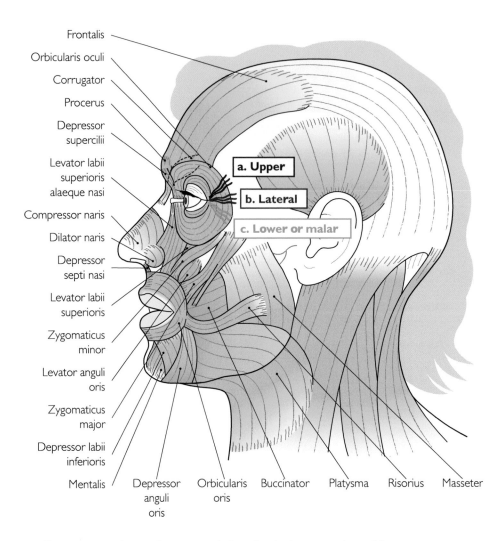

Figure 3.59a Different patterns of crow's feet: a, upper b, lateral and c, lower or malar eyelid creases

amount of BOTOX® injected will depend on the patterning and severity of the lateral canthal wrinkling as well as the thickness of the skin and the presence or absence of blood vessels[36,43–47,49]. Men, generally, will be satisfied with less of a reduction in wrinkling of the lateral canthi, especially with active movements such as smiling and laughing.

In order to avoid puncturing any one of the many superficial vessels found in and around the lateral canthus, the total dose of BOTOX® can be injected subcutaneously at one or two sites as a single or double bolus, producing one or two wheals on the surface of the skin. The wheals of BOTOX® are then gently massaged laterally and away from the orbital fossa in an upward and downward direction. By carefully kneading a bolus of BOTOX® around the lateral canthus, the injected BOTOX® is dispersed subcutaneously and over the muscle fibers of the lateral orbicularis oculi. This maneuver can prevent post-injection ecchymoses if none of the many periocular vessels found at the lateral canthus are punctured. The bolus of BOTOX® is always injected 1–1.5 cm lateral to the lateral bony orbital margin.

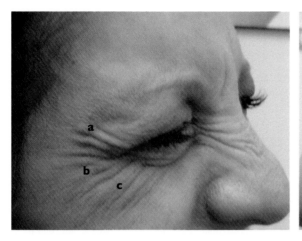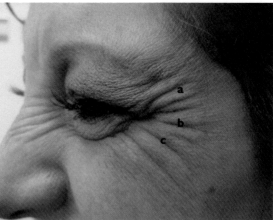

Figure 3.59b Different patterns of crow's feet: a, upper b, lateral and c, lower or malar eyelid creases of the left and right side of a 49-year-old patient squinting before a treatment of BOTOX®

When treating crow's feet, especially at the level of the lower eyelid and lateral malar prominence, it is extremely important to inject BOTOX® in the subcutaneous plane, where the superficial muscle fibers of the orbicularis oculi can be found.

The duration of effect of BOTOX® treatments of the lateral canthus usually are somewhat shorter than that seen in other areas of the face. At least 3 months and sometimes up to 4 months of diminished crow's feet can be obtained with proper dosing and accurate placement of the injections. For some patients the duration of effect is extended with subsequent treatments of BOTOX®[43]. (see Appendix 2).

Outcome (results)

If the treated crow's feet are dynamic and the result of the contraction of the orbicularis oculi, there will be a significant improvement to the area (Figures 3.60 and 3.61). However, if the crow's feet are mostly static and the result of photodamage and chronological aging, then the improvement will be disappointing, especially if the patient was not warned of this prior to treatment. It is important always to assess and discuss a particular problem and its solution in detail with the patient before commencing a course of treatment. It is also in the best interest of both patient and physician to document the pretreatment consultation both in writing and with photographs (see Appendix 3). The documentation should include any remarks the patient may have voiced during the interview. All too often, memory of a physician's concerns and predictions are easily forgotten by patients.

Most of the time, the best way to diminish lateral canthal static wrinkling is by some form of ablative resurfacing, whether by laser ablation, dermabrasion, or chemical peeling. The different types of non-ablative facial rejuvenation techniques still have not been able to eliminate completely the deep and dense solar elastosis that creates the pronounced crow's feet in the manner in which many patients over 50 years of age would like. In such cases, oftentimes a treatment regimen of BOTOX® injections and ablative resurfacing, and even injections of a soft tissue filler and daily applications of topical retinoids, alpha-hydroxy acids, or similar type products, is the only way many patients will be able to realize the kind of facial improvement

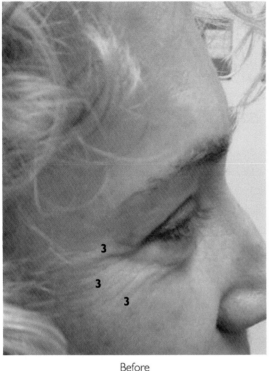
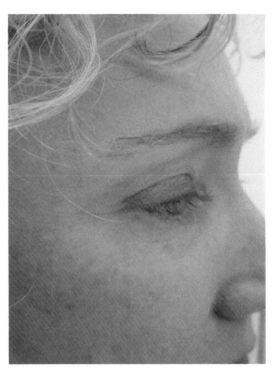

Before   6 weeks after

Figure 3.60 This 46-year-old patient is shown at rest and 6 weeks after treatment with BOTOX®

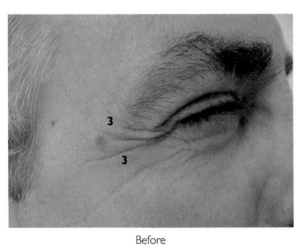
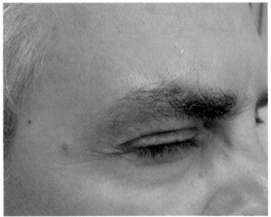

Before   2 weeks after

Figure 3.61 This 56-year-old man is shown squinting before and 2 weeks after a treatment with BOTOX®

they are seeking[30,49] (Figure 3.62). Maintenance of such improvements then can be accomplished regularly, albeit infrequently throughout the year, with non-ablative laser, intense pulsed light, or similar types of superficial facial rejuvenation treatments.

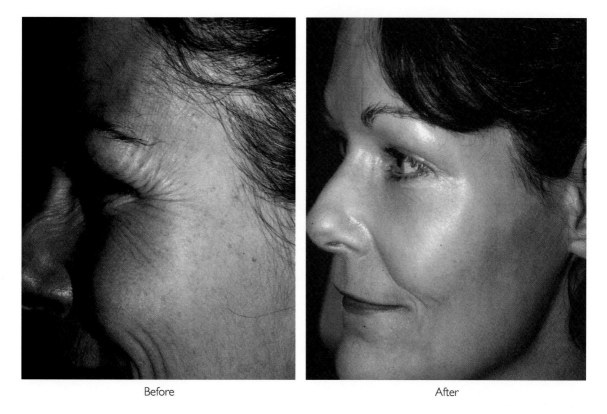

Before   After

Figure 3.62 Patient's crow's feet before a treatment with BOTOX® and 2½ months after BOTOX® and 2 months after full face CO_2 laser resurfacing

When the orbicularis oculi is exceptionally hyperfunctional, causing deep and elongated crow's feet that are recalcitrant and resist improvement with injections of BOTOX® placed in the usual sites, additional injections placed posteriorly toward the lateral limits of the orbicularis oculi in the temporal area can be beneficial[50] (Figure 3.63a–d).

Be cautious when treating the lower malar type of lateral canthal lines, because the majority of these lines may be produced by a hyperkinetic zygomaticus major. If the patient possesses redundant skin around the lateral canthus, then injecting BOTOX® into the lower crow's feet area can create additional skin folding over the lateral malar prominence and exacerbate diagonal wrinkling of the mid and lateral cheeks. The propensity for this may be identified prior to treating the patient with BOTOX® by having the patient smile repeatedly. If their lower lateral canthal lines are continuous with diagonal wrinkles of the mid and lateral cheeks, caution must be taken when injecting the lower malar crow's feet (Figure 3.64). Soft tissue fillers or resurfacing may be the best way to rid the patient of these types of rhytids. Treating the zygomaticus major with BOTOX® can easily result in an asymmetric smile and upper lip incompetence (see below) (see Appendix 1).

Complications (adverse sequelae) (see Appendix 5)

BOTOX® should be injected subdermally and not any more medially to an imaginary vertical line that passes through the lateral canthus, nor below the level of the superior margin of the

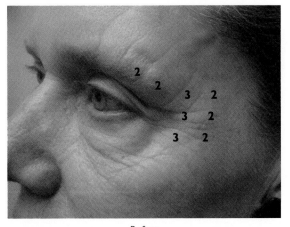

Before

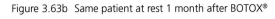

After

Figure 3.63a A 64-year-old patient at rest with deep, extensive and recalcitrant crow's feet before BOTOX®

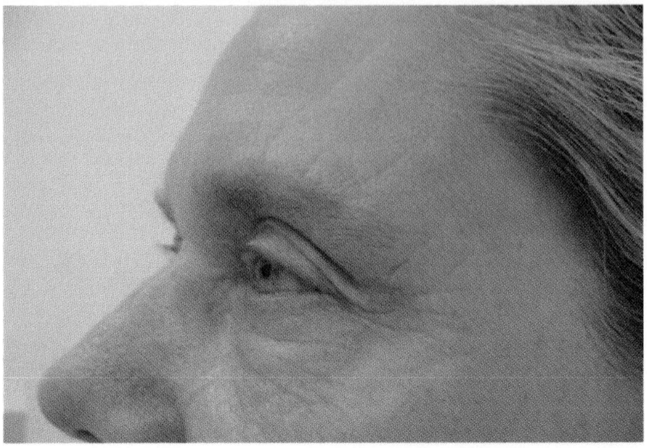

Figure 3.63b Same patient at rest 1 month after BOTOX®

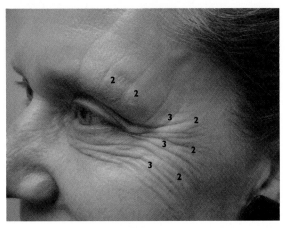

Before

After

Figure 3.63c Same patient squinting before BOTOX®

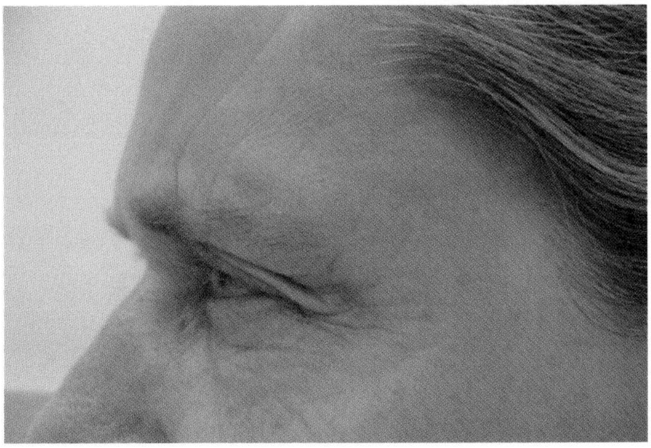

Figure 3.63d Same patient squinting 1 month after BOTOX®

Figure 3.64 Lower crow's feet extend down the mid and lateral cheeks in this smiling 42-year-old patient

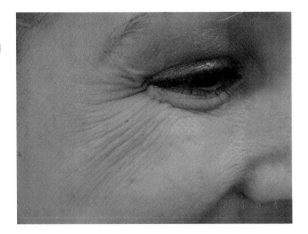

zygomatic arch. Otherwise, the muscle fibers of some of the levators of the lateral upper lip and corners of the mouth will be affected by the diffusion of the BOTOX®, and result in lateral upper lip ptosis and possibly oral sphincter incompetence[40,47]. This can occur because the zygomaticus major et minor originate at or near the lateral aspect of the superior margin of the zygomatic arch. If the zygomaticus major is injected with BOTOX®, the lateral edge of the upper lip will be weakened, causing a drooping of the affected side of the upper oral commissure, an asymmetric smile, and possible drooling and incontinence of food and liquid. If BOTOX® is injected or even diffuses more medially and inferiorly to the superior margin of the zygomatic arch, then the central and deep lip levators (levator labii superioris, levator labii superioris alaeque nasi, and levator anguli oris) can be affected, causing a more profound interference with upper lip competence and basic sphincteric functions, including speaking and eating.

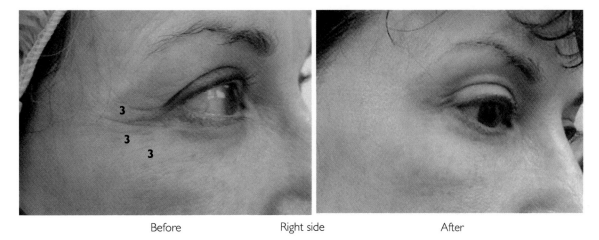

Before   Right side   After

Figure 3.65a This 56-year-old patient is shown at rest before and 3 weeks after a BOTOX® treatment. Note the difference in pattern between the left and right crow's feet

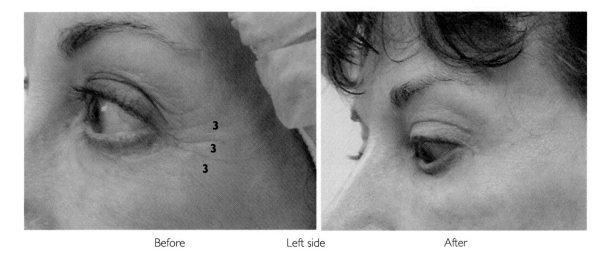

Before   Left side   After

Figure 3.65b Same patient at rest before and 3 weeks after a BOTOX® treatment. Note the difference in pattern between the left and right crow's feet

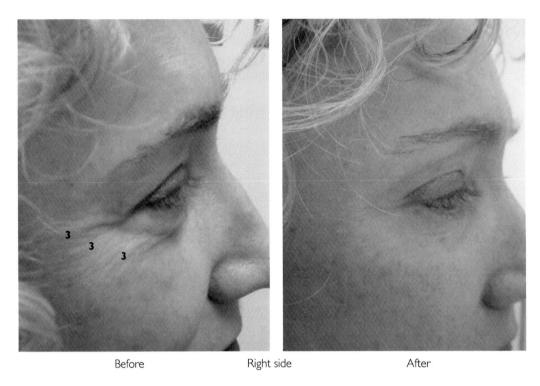

Before   Right side   After

Figure 3.66a   This 54-year-old patient is shown at rest before and 2 weeks after a BOTOX® treatment. Note the difference in the pattern of wrinkles between the left and right crow's feet

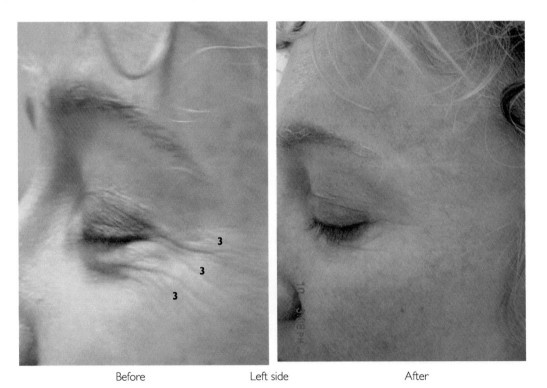

Before   Left side   After

Figure 3.66b   Same patient at rest before and 2 weeks after a BOTOX® treatment. Note the difference in the pattern of wrinkles between the left and right crow's feet

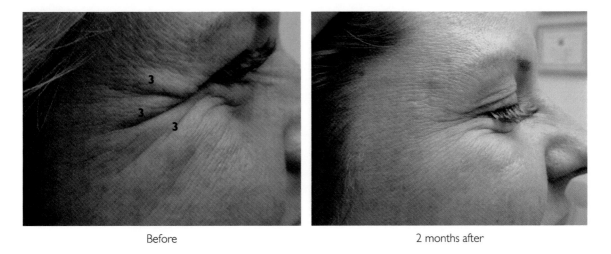

Before   2 months after

Figure 3.67a This 37-year-old patient is shown squinting before and 2 months after a BOTOX® treatment. Note the difference in the pattern of wrinkles between the left and right crow's feet

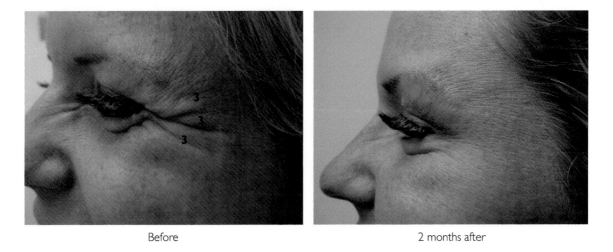

Before   2 months after

Figure 3.67b Same patient squinting before and 2 months after a BOTOX® treatment. Note the difference in the pattern of wrinkles between the left and right crow's feet

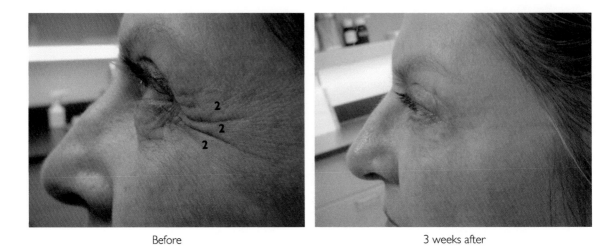

Before   3 weeks after

Figure 3.68a   This 58-year-old patient is shown at rest before and 3 weeks after a BOTOX® treatment.

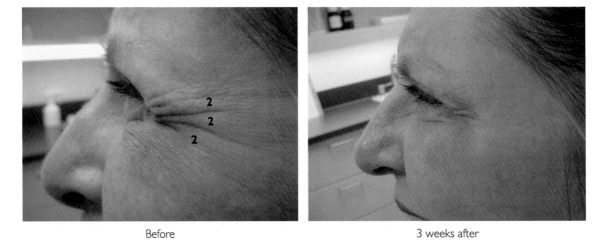

Before   3 weeks after

Figure 3.68b   Same patient squinting before and 3 weeks after a BOTOX® treatment.

Injecting small volumes of concentrated BOTOX® far enough (i.e. 1.0–1.5 cm) away from the lateral side wall of the bony orbit will prevent the unintended migration of BOTOX® medially and into the superior or inferior, or both, palpebral portion of the orbicularis oculi. If this occurs, weakening of the lateral canthal tendon occurs, producing lower eyelid ectropion which manifests as rounding of the lateral canthus. Rounding can lead to secondary complications of possible prolonged corneal exposure, secondary dry eye, and eventually corneal damage (superficial punctuate keratitis). If any of the extraocular muscles are inadvertently weakened by BOTOX®, diplopia will result. Because of their position within the orbit the lateral and inferior rectus or inferior oblique are especially disposed to accidental diffusion of injected BTX. If any of these serious complications does occur, immediate consultation with an ophthalmologist is imperative[47].

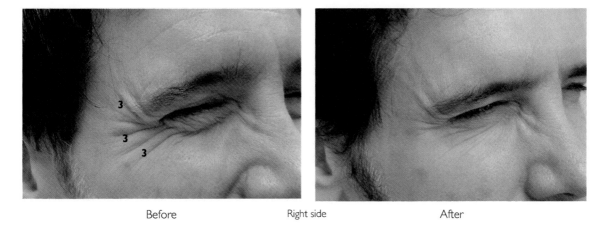

Before   Right side   After

Figure 3.69a This 48-year-old patient is shown squinting before and 3 weeks after a BOTOX® treatment. Note the difference in pattern between the left and right crow's feet

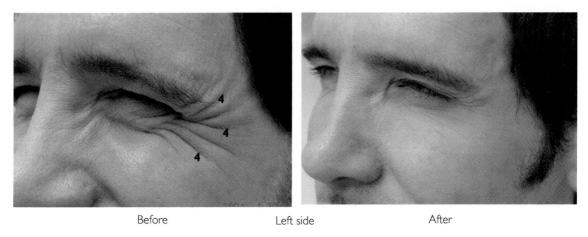

Before   Left side   After

Figure 3.69b Same patient squinting before and 3 weeks after a BOTOX® treatment. Note the difference in pattern between the left and right crow's feet

Loss of the sphincteric function of the orbicularis oculi with either involuntary blinking or voluntary forced eye closure can occur when BOTOX® diffuses onto the palpebral portion of the orbicularis oculi. Lagophthalmos has been seen more frequently in patients treated for strabismus than when they are treated for cosmetic reasons, especially if minimal volume BOTOX® is injected. On the other hand, patients who have an attenuated orbital septum because of age or other reasons may be more prone to this adverse sequela. There is no antidote for lagophthalmos, which will resolve when the effects of the BOTOX® remit. So protecting the patient from developing secondary dry eyes is extremely important. Consultation with an ophthalmologist will prevent any additional, unintended eye injury. Figures 3.65–3.70 are some examples of different patients treated with BOTOX® for crow's feet.

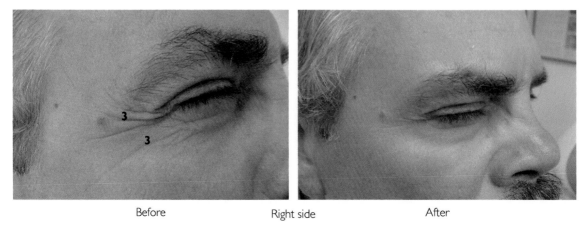

Before   Right side   After

Figure 3.70a This 56-year-old patient is shown squinting before and 2 weeks after a BOTOX® treatment. Note the difference in the pattern between the right and left crow's feet

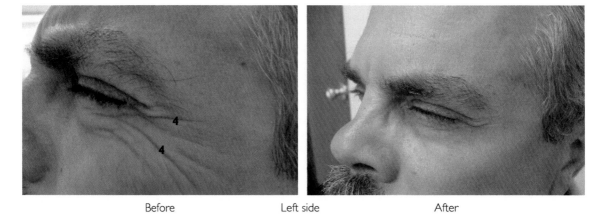

Before   Left side   After

Figure 3.70b Same patient squinting before and 2 weeks after a BOTOX® treatment. Note the difference in the pattern between the right and left crow's feet

Treatment implications when injecting the lateral orbicularis oculi (crow's feet)

1. Older patients will have varying degrees of improvement, depending on the amount of photoaging, redundant skin, and static wrinkling present.
2. Injecting the lateral canthus can produce upper lip asymmetry and cheek ptosis. Inject well above the superior margin of the zygoma and remain 1.0–1.5 cm lateral to the lateral canthus.
3. All periocular injections of BOTOX® should be placed in the lower dermis or subcutaneously, and not any more deeply.
4. Inject 1–1.5 cm lateral to the lateral canthus (bony orbital rim) to avoid diplopia.
5. Post-treatment ecchymoses can last over one week, fallaciously suggesting a substandard injection technique by an incompetent injector.
6. Upper lateral canthal injections of the orbicularis oculi also can be used to produce a lateral eyebrow lift when used in conjunction with BOTOX® injections of the glabellar and forehead muscles.
7. Accurately placed and precisely dosed low-volume BOTOX® injections are essential in order to avoid untoward sequelae in the periocular area.

Lower eyelids

Introduction: problem assessment and patient selection

Along with crow's feet, many people have additional folds and creases of the lower eyelids, which give them the appearance of being tired, sleep deprived, or even older than their current age. These 'festoons' or 'jelly rolls' are produced by hyperkinetic palpebral (preseptal and pretarsal) orbicularis oculi (Figure 3.71a,b). They also help create the appearance of dark, baggy eyes that women and even men alike would prefer not to have. Likewise, a tired, disinterested, downtrodden, and unambitious demeanor is projected when the palpebral aperture is narrowed because of a hyperfunctional pretarsal orbicularis oculi. Various facial movements, primarily smiling or laughing, also will narrow momentarily the palpebral aperture.

Functional anatomy

The orbicularis oculi helps protect the eyes from bright light and fast flying projectiles and, when contracted abruptly, causes one to shut the eyes completely or partially, i.e. to squint. Those working outdoors or in a brightly lit environment maintain their orbicularis oculi in a constant hyperkinetic state, causing the muscle fibers of the orbicularis oculi to hypertrophy. In younger patients, hypertrophic palpebral orbicularis oculi can be observed as producing additional periocular folds, and are sometimes referred to as 'jelly rolls', especially in the vicinity of the lower eyelid (Figure 3.71b). These lower eyelid folds can be diminished by BOTOX® (Figure 3.72a–d). In older patients, however, the skin of the eyelids becomes thin and less elastic and the orbital septum attenuates, making it less effective. Because of a weakening of this anatomical bulwark, the inferior periorbital fat bulges from behind the preseptal orbicularis oculi and creates characteristic suborbital 'festoons' (Figure 3.73a,b). BOTOX® injections of the already weakened and incompetent preseptal orbicularis oculi invariably will enlarge this type of suborbital festooning, and therefore should not be performed[48].

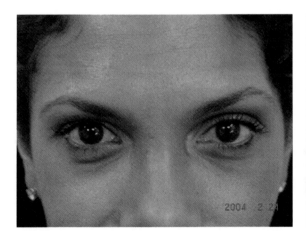

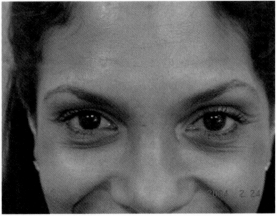

Figure 3.71a Early festoons and wrinkles of the lower eyelid in this 42 year old patient at rest

Figure 3.71b Same patient with periocular wrinkles exaggerated when she smiles. She also complained of dark circles under her eyes

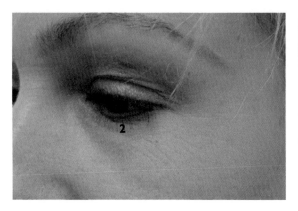

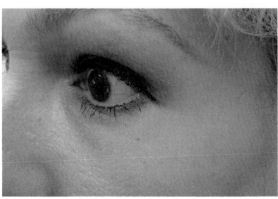

Figure 3.72a Left lower eyelid of a 42-year-old woman at rest and before BOTOX®

Figure 3.72b Same patient at rest 3 weeks after BOTOX®

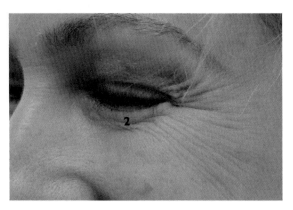

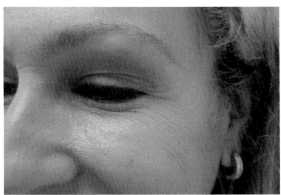

Figure 3.72c Same patient smiling before BOTOX®

Figure 3.72d Same patient smiling 3 weeks after BOTOX®

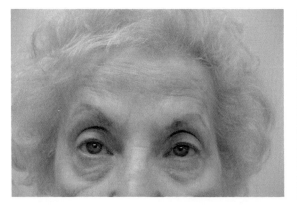

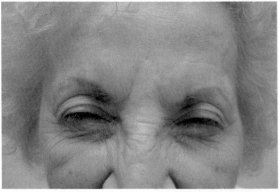

Figure 3.73a This 75-year-old woman has thinning of the preseptal orbicularis oculi which is seen as festoons of the lower eyelids

Figure 3.73b Same patient squinting causes the orbital and palpebral portions of the orbicularis oculi to contract. Injections of BOTOX® in the lower eyelid will make the orbicularis oculi incompetent at rest and intensify her festooning and wrinkles with squinting. Therefore, BOTOX® injections in the lower eyelids should not be performed in this patient

A major function of the palpebral portion of the orbicularis oculi is its sphincteric action that aids in the maintenance of corneal moisture. It accomplishes this with each blink of the eye, which distributes over the anterior surface of the globe the drops of tears that are secreted from the main and accessory lacrimal glands (Figure 3.74). Opening and shutting the eyes activates the so-called lacrimal pump, shunting the secreted tears through the canalicular system into the lacrimal sac and down the nasolacrimal duct, where they are then released into the nasal cavity from the inferior meatus under the inferior nasal turbinate. As the secreted tears flow from the upper lateral aspect of the orbit, they collect in the lower medial corner of the orbit to form the lacrimal lake. With the eyelids open, the lacrimal portion of the orbicularis oculi compresses the lacrimal sac and positions the patulous punctum in direct contact with the globe and the lacrimal lake. This allows the tears to flow into and through the patent canaliculi. Contracting the superficial fibers of the pretarsal orbicularis oculi shuts the eyelids and distributes the tears over the anterior surface of the globe from a superior lateral to an inferior medial direction. Opening the eyes again causes the deep fibers of the pretarsal orbicularis oculi to contract, shutting down the upper and lower canalicular system. Contemporaneously, the deep fibers of the preseptal orbicularis oculi pull on the lateral walls of the lacrimal sac, enlarging its lumen and contributing to the negative pressure gradient within the nasolacrimal canalicular system, which causes the tears to be aspirated into the lacrimal sac (Figure 3.74). Upon re-opening the eyelids, the positive pressure within the canalicular system is recreated and the lacrimal sac collapses, propelling the tears into the nasolacrimal duct, then through the inferior

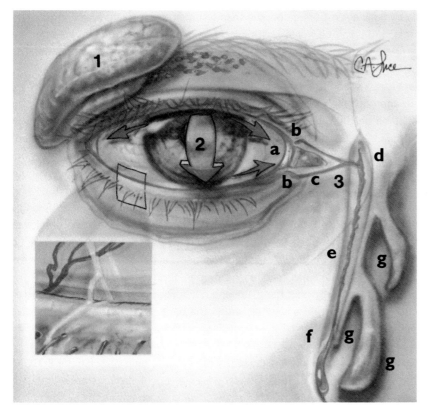

Figure 3.74 Tears are produced by main and accessory lacrimal glands (1). The distribution of these tears over the surface of the eye is achieved by movements of the eyelids performing a 'squeegee' action (2) of the marginal tear bead shown here in optical cross-section by a slit lamp beam (inset). The passage of tears into the nose occurs via the lacrimal drainage system (3) (Reproduced with permission from Zide B, Jelks G (eds) 1985 *Surgical Anatomy*, p.34. Philadelphia: Lippincott)

a. Lacrimal late
b. Puncta
c. Canaliculi
d. Lacrimal sac
e. Nasolacrimal duct
f. Inferior meatus
g. Turbinates

meatus and into the nasal cavity. Simultaneously, the puncta and canaliculi reopen to collect more tears from the lacrimal lake and the cycle recreates itself with each opening and shuting of the eyelids.

Dilution

When treating the periocular area with BOTOX® it is imperative to be precise with dosing and accurate with injecting minimal volumes of the BTX. Therefore, a 100 U vial of BOTOX® should be reconstituted with only 1 ml of normal saline. (see Appendix 1).

Dosing: how to correct the problem (what to do and what not to do)

Appropriate candidates for BOTOX® treatment of the lower eyelids are those who have normal eyelid elasticity, determined by a normal snap test, and who have not had any previous lower eyelid surgery, including blepharoplasty or some form of resurfacing, either by laser or chemical peeling. To perform a lower eyelid snap test, grasp the skin of the lower eyelid between the thumb and index finger. Gently pull the lid away from the globe and then release it. If the eyelid recoils immediately back against the globe, the snap test indicates that the eyelid's elasticity is ostensibly normal, and it can be treated with injections of BOTOX®. If the recoil is sluggish, indicating insufficient elasticity of eyelid skin, then the patient's lower eyelids should not be injected with BOTOX®, because the probability of post-injection ectropion is high.

If the patient is in a sitting or a semireclined position for the injection, it will be easier for the physician to approach the patient with a needle head-on toward the eye. The physician injector should stand on the side of the lower eyelid to be treated, and the patient should gaze directly forward. As the injector approaches the patient with the needle, the patient should be asked to gaze directly upward and to take a deep breath without moving. Contemporaneously, the physician pulls the lower eyelid skin inferiorly with the non-dominant hand and inserts the needle tip through the skin at a point 2–3 mm from the lower lid margin at the midpupillary line. The needle tip should be advanced at about a 45° angle and approximately 2–3 mm deep through the skin, but remaining at the depth of the lower dermis and no deeper than the subcutaneous layer (Figure 3.75a,b). Even with the needle tip advanced 2–3 mm into the skin, it should maintain its superficial position. When the tip of the needle is through the skin and has reached its proper depth, an injection of 2 U (i.e. 0.02 ml) of BOTOX® will remain within the tissue and not leak or track out along the path of the needle puncture, provided there is no air within the barrel of the syringe. The injector should observe the rise of a wheal of fluid, which should reassure the physician that an adequate dose of BOTOX® has been delivered as intended (Figure 3.75b). Delicate massage of the injected area directed laterally will distract the patient and help disperse the BOTOX® safely along the superficial fibers of the pretarsal orbicularis oculi. When this technique is

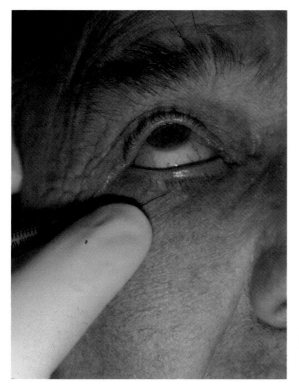

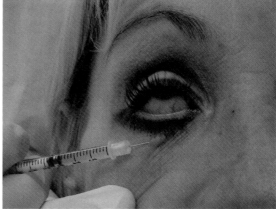

Figure 3.75a Technique of injecting the lower eyelid with BOTOX®. Note the index finger of the non-dominant hand pulling down on the skin of the lower eyelid making it taut. The needle tip is inserted at a 45° angle, 2–3 mm from the lid margin and approximately 2–3 mm deep within the deep dermal to subcutaneous layer

Figure 3.75b The appearance of a wheal indicates that the bolus of BOTOX® has been delivered successfully

executed in a calm and expeditious manner, the patient will not cower away from the needle pointed directly at his or her eye, and s/he may even compliment the physician on the painless fashion and ease with which the treatment was executed. An additional 1–2 U of BOTOX® can be injected intradermally or subcutaneously and approximately 2–3 mm below the lid margin, at a point halfway from the lateral canthus and the midpupillary line[52,53]. For most patients this second injection in the lower eyelid is superfluous and not necessary. It may even lead to a lateral lower lid ectropion and other annoying adverse sequelae (see Appendix 2).

Outcomes (results)

It was discovered serendipitously that an injection of 1–2 U of BOTOX® subcutaneously in the pretarsal portion of the orbicularis oculi of the lower eyelid at the midpupillary line, approximately 2–3 mm below the lid margin, can improve the rolls of festooning redundant skin that occur on and just inferior to the lower eyelid[51] (Figures 3.71 and 3.72). Lower eyelid

TABLE 3.1   IPA – INCREASE IN PALPEBRAL APERTURE AT REST AND AT FULL SMILE

	Pretarsal area treated alone			Pretarsal area treated together with crow's feet		
BOTOX® units	2 U	4 U	8 U	2 U	4 U	8 U
IPA at rest (mm)	0.5	1.75	1.95	1.75	2.2	1.5
IPA at full smile (mm)	1.3	2.5	4.5	2.9	2.9	4.0

Adapted from Flynn TC, Carruthers J, Carruthers A. Botulinum A toxin treatment of the lower eyelids improves infraorbital rhytides and widens the eye. *Dermatol Surg* 2001;27:703–8

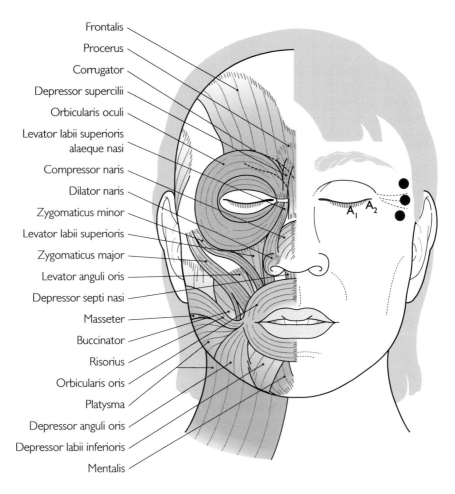

Frontalis
Procerus
Corrugator
Depressor supercilii
Orbicularis oculi
Levator labii superioris alaeque nasi
Compressor naris
Dilator naris
Zygomaticus minor
Levator labii superioris
Zygomaticus major
Levator anguli oris
Depressor septi nasi
Masseter
Buccinator
Risorius
Orbicularis oris
Platysma
Depressor anguli oris
Depressor labii inferioris
Mentalis

Figure 3.76 When treating the lower eyelid folds and festoons, depending on the depth of the folds, one (A₁) injection at the midpupillary line or a second (A₂) injection midway between A₁ and the lateral canthus can be performed, depending on the strength of the palpebral orbicularis oculi. Additional injections (●) of BOTOX® may be needed to treat crow's feet, the dosage of which will depend on the strength of the lateral orbicularis oculi

pretarsal injections of BOTOX® also were found to produce a desirable relaxation of the palpebral aperture both at rest and during smiling, laughing, and various other facial movements, especially when they were applied in conjunction with BOTOX® treatments of lateral canthal rhytides (crow's feet). The increase in palpebral aperture was dependent on the amount of units injected pretarsally and whether simultaneous treatment of crow's feet was performed. For those patients who were treated with only 2 U of BOTOX® injected at only one site in the lower lid pretarsal midpupillary line, the average increase in palpebral aperture (IPA) was approximately 0.5 mm at rest and 1.3 mm at full smile (Figure 3.76). When combined with a fixed dose of 12 U of BOTOX® given in three separate doses 1.5 mm apart at the lateral canthus to treat concomitant crow's feet, the average IPA was approximately 1.75 mm at rest and 2.9 mm at full smile (Table 3.1). When 4 U of BOTOX® were injected pretarsally into the lower eyelid at two separate sites, equally positioned from the lateral canthus and the midpupillary line (Figure 3.76), the average IPA was approximately 1.75 mm at rest and 2.5 mm at full smile. When 2 U of BOTOX® were injected pretarsally into the lower eyelid at two separate sites (total of 4 U) equally positioned, one at the midpupillary line (Figure 3.76 A$_1$), the other midway from the midpupillary line and the lateral canthus (Figure 3.76 A$_2$) in conjunction with treating the crow's feet with 4 U of BOTOX® injected in the lateral canthus at three sites each equally spaced (total of 12 U), the average IPA at rest was approximately 2.2 mm and 2.9 mm at full smile. When 8 U of BOTOX® were injected pretarsally in the lower eyelid at two separate sites in the same manner that the 4 U of BOTOX® were given (Figure 3.76 A$_1$, A$_2$), the average IPA was approximately 1.95 mm at rest and approximately 4.5 mm in full smile. When the 8 U of BOTOX® were injected pretarsally into the lower eyelid at the two separate sites as above (A$_1$ and A$_2$ in Figure 3.76) and in conjunction with treating the crow's feet with 12 U of BOTOX® injected in three equal (4 U) doses in the lateral canthus (Figure 3.76), the average IPA was approximately 1.5 mm at rest and 4.0 mm at full smile. Interestingly, there appeared to be a synergistic effect to the response of the lower pretarsal orbicularis oculi when the lateral orbital orbicularis oculi was simultaneously treated during the same session. This technique of injecting the pretarsal orbicularis oculi produces an 'open-eyed look' that gives the patient the appearance of one who is vibrantly active and cheerfully youthful (Figure 3.77).

In most cases, the second intermediary injection of BOTOX® between the lateral canthus and midpupillary line is not necessary (Figure 3.76 A$_2$). It may even increase the chance for lateral canthal rounding and lower eyelid ectropion. This technique of injecting the lower eyelids with BOTOX® also has been surprisingly popular among Asian patients who desire a more rounded, Western eyelid aperature[49,52,53].

Figures 3.78–3.82 are some examples of different patients treated with BOTOX® for folds and creases of the lower lids.

Complications (adverse sequelae) (see Appendix 5)

Rounding of the lateral canthus can be produced by the weakening of either the upper or lower, or both, pretarsal orbicularis oculi. Injecting at least 1.0–1.5 cm lateral to the lateral canthus can help avoid such an unwanted outcome. The second intermediate injection of the lower pretarsal orbicularis oculi (Figure 3.76 A$_2$) also has been found to cause rounding of the lateral canthus and ectropion of the adjacent lateral aspect of the lower lid margin, especially when a full treatment of BOTOX® is injected into the adjacent upper and lower crow's feet area (Figure 3.83). Therefore, unless the patient has recalcitrant lower eyelid festoons that wrap around the lateral canthus and

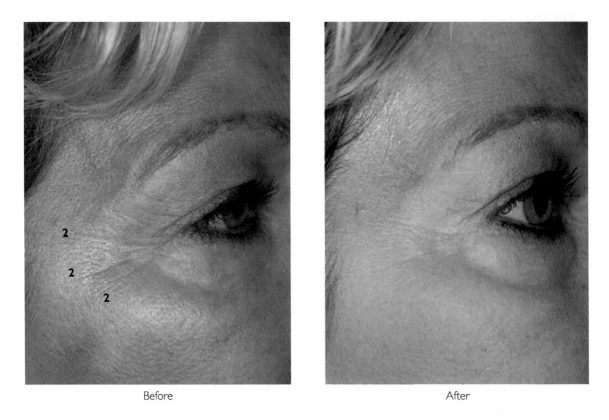

| Before | After |

Figure 3.77 This 56-year-old patient seen at rest before and after 2 U of BOTOX® were injected into the lower eyelid at the midpupillary line 2–3 mm from the lid margin and 6 U of BOTOX® for crow's feet. Note the wide eyed open look

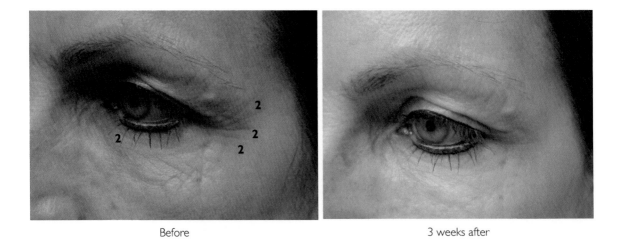

| Before | 3 weeks after |

Figure 3.78 This 49-year-old patient is shown at rest and forward gazing before and 3 weeks after a BOTOX® of the lower lid. Note the wide eyed open look

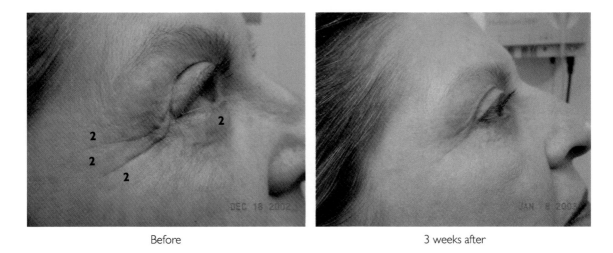

Before   3 weeks after

Figure 3.79a, b This 58-year-old patient is shown at rest and forward gazing before and 3 weeks after a BOTOX® treatment of the lower lid and crow's feet. Note the reduction of the lower lid festoons

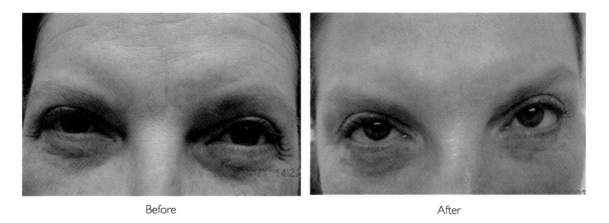

Before   After

Figure 3.80 The same patient is shown at rest and forward gazing before and 3 weeks after a BOTOX® treatment of the lower lid and crow's feet. Note the reduction of the lower lid festoons

are continuous with deep and resistant lateral canthal lines, this second (Figure 3.76 A_2), intermediate, lateral pretarsal injection of BOTOX® should be withheld, and only the central pretarsal injection of the lower eyelid at the midpupillary line should be given (Figure 3.76 A_1).

It is imperative that the pretarsal injections be placed into the deep dermis, barely reaching the subcutaneous tissue, and nowhere near the bony malar prominence, since most of the upper lip levators originate along the superior margin of the zygomatic arch (Figure 3.84). Otherwise, upper lip ptosis, asymmetry, and even sphincter incompetence of the upper lip can result, because the levators of the lateral aspect of the upper lip (zygomaticus major and levator anguli oris) and even the levators of the central aspect of the upper lip (levator labii superioris, zygomaticus minor and levator labii superioris alaeque nasi) can be weakened by diffusion of the BOTOX®.

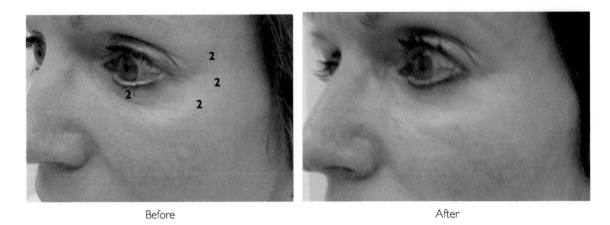

Before

After

Figure 3.81a This 50-year-old patient is shown at rest and forward gazing before and 3 weeks after a BOTOX® injection of the lower lid. Note the wide eyed open look

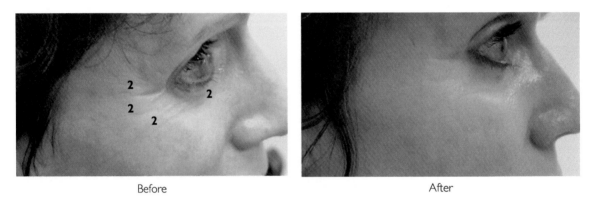

Before

After

Figure 3.81b Same patient at rest and forward gazing before and 3 weeks after a BOTOX® of the lower lid. Note the wide eyed open look

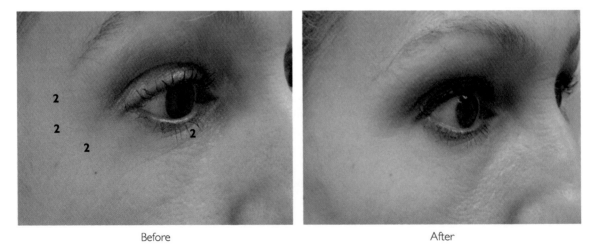

Before

After

Figure 3.82 This 42-year-old patient is shown at rest and forward gazing before and 3 weeks after a BOTOX® injection of the lower lid. Note the wide eyed open look

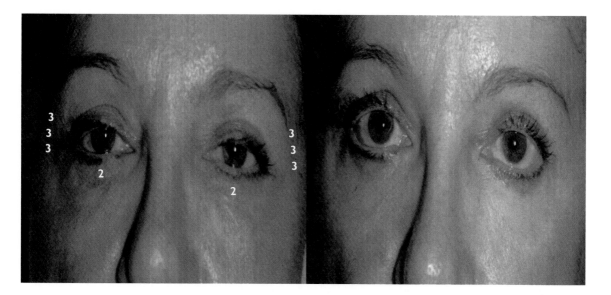

Figure 3.83 2 U of BOTOX® were injected into each lower eyelid at the mid pupillary line 2 mm from the lid margin along with 9 U of BOTOX® into the lateral canthus of this 55-year-old woman who is 8 years post-blepharoplasty. Although she had a normal Snap test her previous blopharoplasty may have contributed to this patient's asymptomatic lateral canthal rounding and lower eyelid ectropion. Note the scleral show and unnatural and unattractive rounding of the lateral canthi

Injecting BOTOX® medial to the midpupillary line of the lower eyelid runs the risk of weakening the voluntary and involuntary sphincteric function of the palpebral orbicularis oculi which would compromise forced eyelid closure and the blink reflex. This in turn could either diminish the action of the lacrimal pump and cause temporary epiphora[23,49] or even result in xerophthalmia or dry eyes because of supervening lagophthalmos and corneal exposure. This can occur more readily in older patients who have attenuated muscular strength and a thinned orbital septum.

Post-injection ecchymoses are more commonly produced whenever thin eyelid skin is injected (Figure 3.85). The use of small insulin syringes and fine 30-gauge needles, a slow injection technique, pre- and post-treatment icing, and gentle massage and point pressure all may help to prevent or limit the extent of post-injection ecchymoses, which otherwise should resolve in a few (approximately 10–15) days.

Pseudoherniation of the infraorbital fat pad can be enhanced when BOTOX® is injected into the inferior palpebral orbicularis oculi in patients who have festooning caused by protruding periorbital fat in inelastic, incompetent lower eyelids. A worsening of pseudoherniation by BOTOX® is easy to produce, particularly in older patients or in patients who have had a blepharoplasty or other type of lower eyelid surgery in the past, because the sling-like support of their preseptal orbicularis oculi is weak and ineffective (Figure 3.73). Injections of BOTOX® in the inferior palpebral, inferolateral canthal, and high malar areas of patients with lax lower eyelid skin can compromise further the integral strength of the orbicularis oculi, accentuating the infraorbital festoons, instead of reducing them[40]. Lower eyelid injections of BOTOX® in such individuals should not be performed[48].

In their dose-defining studies, Flynn et al. found no substantial adverse events in the patients treated with 2 U of BOTOX® injected at one site pretarsally in the lower eyelid (Figure 3.76). In

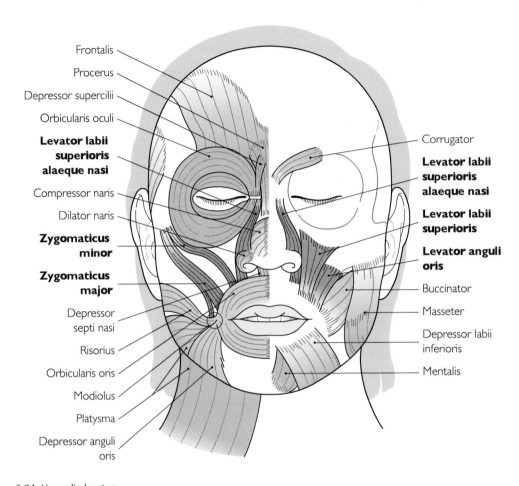

Frontalis
Procerus
Depressor supercilii
Orbicularis oculi
Levator labii superioris alaeque nasi
Compressor naris
Dilator naris
Zygomaticus minor
Zygomaticus major
Depressor septi nasi
Risorius
Orbicularis oris
Modiolus
Platysma
Depressor anguli oris

Corrugator
Levator labii superioris alaeque nasi
Levator labii superioris
Levator anguli oris
Buccinator
Masseter
Depressor labii inferioris
Mentalis

Figure 3.84 Upper lip levators

Figure 3.85 Two days after 2 U of BOTOX® were injected in both lower eyelids for the first time in this 53-year-old woman. The ecchymosis in the right eyelid lasted for about 10 days

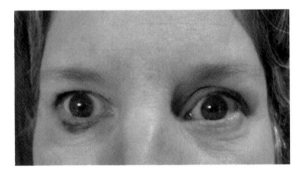

those patients who had 4 U of BOTOX® injected pretarsally in two divided doses of 2 U each (Figure 3.76 A$_1$, A$_2$), less than half of them suffered from 'dry eyes' and one patient could not wear her contact lenses[52,53]. There were additional, temporary adverse events that were more of an annoyance than a serious complication and they occurred after 8 U of BOTOX® were injected pretarsally in two divided doses of 4 U each into the lower eyelid (Figure 3.76 A$_1$, A$_2$). They included transient lower eyelid edema, which gave the patient an increasing sense of lower eyelid fullness, persistently 'dropped bags' and a sensation of puffy lower eyelids, which became worse toward the end of the day[52]. Also, there were patients who developed photophobia, and who were unable to go outdoors in bright light because they had difficulty with squinting and could not protect their eyes from sunlight. Still others were bothered by incomplete sphincteric eyelid closure, which caused stinging of their eyes when they washed their faces with or without soap. All of these annoyances remitted within 3 months from the time the 8 U of BOTOX® were injected into the two sites in the mid and lateral aspects of the pretarsal portion of their lower eyelids.

Treatment implications when injecting the lower eyelids

1. Lower eyelid injections of BOTOX® produce a 'wide-eyed', actively youthful appearance.
2. Inject only 1–2 U and no more than 3 U of BOTOX® into the lower dermis or the upper subcutaneous tissue in the pretarsal midpupillary line.
3. Pretarsal injections of BOTOX® at the intermediate point between the lateral canthus and the midpupillary line increases the risk for lower eyelid ectropion, rounded lateral canthus, and various other adverse sequelae.
4. Pretarsal injections of BOTOX® in the lower eyelid medial to the midpupillary line may cause epiphora by weakening the blink reflex, or dry eyes by creating persistent lagophthalmos and corneal exposure.
5. Injections of BOTOX® lower than 2–3 mm from the lower eyelid margin can result in lip asymmetry and cheek ptosis.
6. Low-volume, highly concentrated injections of BOTOX® are best when injecting the superficial fibers of the lower pretarsal portion of the orbicularis oculi.
7. Anyone who has had other periocular cosmetic procedures and who has a sluggish snap test should not be treated with BOTOX® injections in the lower pretarsal orbicularis oculi.

References

1. Benedetto AV. The cosmetic uses of botulinum toxin type A. *Int J Dermatol* 1999;38:641–55
2. Carruthers J, Fagien S, Matarasso, SV et al. Consensus recommendations on the use of botulinum toxin type A in facial aesthetics. Supplement to *Plastic Reconstr Surg* 2004;114:1S–18S
3. Wieder JM, Moy RL. Understanding botulinum toxin. Surgical anatomy of the frown, forehead, and periocular region. *Dermatol Surg* 1998;24:1172–4
4. Hsu TS, Dover JS, Arndt KA. Effect of volume and concentration on the diffusion of botulinum exotoxin A. *Arch Dermatol* 2004;140:1351–4
5. Carruthers A, Carruthers J, Cohen J. A prospective, double-blind, randomized, parallel-group, dose-ranging study of botulinum toxin type A in female subjects with horizontal forehead rhytides. *Dematol Surg* 2003;29:461–7
6. Flynn TC, Clark RE. Botulinum toxin type B (Myobloc) versus botulinum toxin type A (Botox) frontalis study: rate of onset and radius of diffusion. *Dermatol Surg* 2003;29:519–22,
7. Le Louarn C. Botulinum toxin A and facial lines: the variable concentration. *Aesthetic Plast Surg* 2001;25:73–84
8. Carruthers A, Carruthers J. Clinical indications and injection technique for the cosmetic use of botulinum A exotoxin. *Dermatol Surg* 1998;24:1189–94

9. Klein AW. Complications and adverse reactions with the use of botulinum toxin. *Dis Mon* 2002;48;336–56

10. Klein AW. Dilution and storage of botulinum toxin. *Dermatol Surg* 1998;24:1179–80

11. Carruthers A, Carruthers J. Botulinum toxin type A: history and current cosmetic use in the upper face. *Semin Cutan Med Surg* 2001;20:71–84

12. Fulton JE. Botulinum toxin. The Newport Beach experience. *Dermatol Surg* 1998;24:1219–24

13. Carruthers A, Carruthers J. The treatment of glabellar furrow with botulinum A exotoxin. *J Dermatol Surg Oncol* 1990;16:83

14. Carruthers JD, Carruthers JA. Treatment of glabellar frown lines with C. botulinum-A exotoxin. *J Dermatol Surg Oncol* 1992;18:17–21

15. Blitzer A, Brin MF, Keen MS, Aviv JE. Botulinum toxin for the treatment of hyperfunctional lines of the face. *Arch Otolaryngol Head Neck Surg* 1993;119:1018–22

16. Carruthers JD, Lowe NJ, Menter MA, Gibson J, Eadie N for the Botox Galbellar Lines II Study Group. Double-blind, placebo-controlled study of the safety and efficacy of botulinum toxin type A for patients with glabellar lines. *Plast Reconstr Surg* 2003;112:1089–98

17. Carruthers JA, Lowe NJ, Meneter Ma *et al.* A muliticanter, double-blind, randomized, placebo-controlled study of the efficacy and safety of botulinum toxin type A in the treatment of glabellar lines. *J Am Acad Dermatol* 2002;46:840–9

18. Hankins CL, Strimling R, Rogers GS. Botulinum A toxin for glabellar wrinkles: dose and response. *Dermatol Surg* 1998;24:1181–3

19. Lowe NJ, Maxwell A, Harper H. Botulinum A exotoxin for glabellar folds; a double-blind, placebo-controlled study with a electromyographic injection technique. *J Am Acad Dermatol* 1996;35:569–72

20. Pribitkin EA, Greco TM, Goode RL, Keane WM. Patient selection in the treatment of glabellar wrinkles with botulinum toxin type A injection. *Arch Otolaryngol Head Neck Surg* 1997;123:321–6

21. Roth JM, Metzinger SE. Quantifying the arch position of the female eyebrow. *Arch Facial Plast Surg* 2003;5:235–9

22. Benedetto AV, Lahti JG. Measurements of the anatomical position of the corrugator supercilii. *Derm Surg* 2005;31:923–7

23. Macdonald MR, Spiegel J, Raven RB *et al.* An anatomical approach to glabellar rhytides. *Arch Otolaryngol Head Neck Surg* 1998;124:1315–20

24. Daniel RK, Landon B. Endoscopic forehead lift. Anatomic basis. *Aesthet Surg* 1997;17:97–104

25. Cook, Jr. BE, Lucarelli MJ, Lemke BN. Depressor supercilii muscle: anatomy, histology, and cosmetic implications. *Opthalmic Plast Reconstr Surg* 2001;17:404–11

26. Botox Cosmetic [package insert]. Irvine, CA: Allergan, Inc., 2002

27. Alam M, Dover JS, Arndt KA. Pain associated with injection of botulinum A exotoxin reconstituted using isotonic sodium chloride with and with out preservative: a double-blind, randomized controlled trial. *Arch Dermatol* 2002;138:510–14

28. Klein AW, Mantell A. Electromyographic guidance in injecting botulinum toxin. *Dermatol Surg* 1998;24:1184–6

29. Blitzer A, Binder WJ, Aviv JE. The management of hyperfunctional facial lines with botulinum toxin: a collaborative study of 210 injection sites in 162 patients. *Arch Otolaryngol Head Neck Surg* 1997;123:389–92

30. Fagien S. Botulinum toxin type A for facial aesthetic enhancement: role in facial shaping. *Plast Reconstr Surg* 2003;112:6S–18S

31. Binder WJ, Blitzer A, Brin MF. Treatment of hyperfunctional lines of the face with botulinum toxin A. *Derm Surg* 1998;24:1198–205

32. Carruthers A, Carruthers J. Botulinum A exotoxin in clinical ophthalmology. *Can J Ophthalmol* 1996;30:389–400

33. Carruthers J, Fagien S, Matarasso SL. The Botox Consensus Group: Consensus Recommendations on the use of Botulinum Toxin Type A in facial aestletics. *Plast Reconstr Surg* 2004(6) supp. 1S–22S.

34. Huang W, Rogachefsky AS, Foster JA. Browlift with botulinum toxin. *Dermatol Surg* 2000;26:55–60

35. Frankel AS, Kamer FM. Chemical browlift. *Arch Otolaryngol Head Neck Surg* 1998;124:321–3

36. Ahn MS, Cotton M, Maas CS. Temporal browlift using botulinum toxin A. *Plast Reconstr Surg* 2000;105:1129–35

37. Huigol SC, Carruthers A, Carruthers J. Raising eyebrows with botulinum toxin. *Dermatol Surg* 1999;25:373–5

38. Chen AH, Frankel AS. Altering brow contour with botulinum toxin. *Facial Plast Surg Clin N Am* 2003;II:457–64

39. Matarasso SL. Complications of botulinum A exotoxin for hyperfuntional lines. *Derm Surg* 1998;24:1249–54

40. Frankel AS. BOTOX for rejuvenation of the periorbital region. *Facial Plast Surg* 1999;15:255–62

41. Fagien S. Botox for the treatment of dynamic and hyperkinetic facial lines and furrows; adjunctive use in facial aesthetic surgery. *Plast Reconstr Surg* 1999;103:701–13

42. Lowe NJ, Lask G, Yamanchi P *et al.* Bilateral, double-blind, randomized comparison of three doses of botulinum toxin type A and placebo in patient's with crow's feet. *J Am Acad Dermatol* 2002;47:834–40

43. Guerrissi JO. Intraoperative injection of botulinum toxin A into the orbicularis oculi muscle for the treatment of crow's feet. *Plast Reconstr Surg* 2003;112(5 Suppl):161S–163S

44. Matarasso SL. Comparison of botulinum toxin types A and B: bilateral and double-blind randomized evaluation in the treatment of canthal ryytides. *Dermatol Surg* 2003;29:7–13

45. Kane MA. Classification of crow's feet patterns among Caucasian women: the key to individualizing treatment. *Plast Reconstr Surg* 2003;112:33S–39S

46. Matarasso SL, Matarasso A. Treatment guidelines for botulinum toxin type A for the periocular region and a report on partial upper lip ptosis following injections to the lateral canthal rhytides. *Plast Reconstr Surg* 2001;108:208

47. Northington ME, Huang CC. Dry eyes and superficial punctuate keratitis: a complication of treatment of glabellar dynamic rhytides with botulinum exotoxin A. *Dermatol Surg* 2004;30:1515–17

48. Goldman M. Festoon formation after intraorbital botulinum A toxin: a case report. *Dermatol Surg* 2003;29:560–1

49. Yamauchi P, Lask. G, Lowe NJ, Botulinum toxin type A gives adjunctive benefit to periorbital laser resurfacing. *J Cosmet Laser Ther* 2004:6(3)145–48

50. Kadunc BV. Periorbital wrinkles. In: Hexsel D, Almeida AT de (eds) *Cosmetic Use of Botulinum Toxin.* Porto Alegre, Brazil: AGE Editora, 2002:149–54

51. Flynn TC, Carruthers J, Carruthers A. Botulinum A toxin treatment of the lower eyelids improves infraorbital rhytides and widens the eye. *Dermatol Surg* 2001;27:703–8

52. Flynn TC, Carruthers JA, Clark RE. Botulinum A toxin (BOTOX) in the lower eyelid: dose-finding study *Dermatol Surg* 2003;29:943–50

4 COSMETIC USES OF BOTULINUM TOXIN A IN THE MID FACE

Anthony V Benedetto

Mid face

Introduction

With the increased demand for facial rejuvenation done by non-invasive techniques, many experienced injectors of BOTOX® now are venturing below the upper face with their treatments[1]. As with any other part of the face, one must be completely knowledgeable of the levator and depressor action of the mimetic musculature. In the mid and lower face the reciprocating action of opposing mimetic muscles can prove to be a bit more complicated and challenging than in the upper face. Specifically, the muscles of the upper face are easily distinguishable from one another because of various topographic landmarks, making it easy to inject them with BOTOX®. However, in the mid and lower face, there is an interdependence of the superficial and deep muscles of facial expression, which also are adjacent to some of the muscles surrounding the mouth that function in the articulation of sounds or in mastication and deglutition. These muscles of facial expression are interlaced with and even help form the superficial muscular aponeurotic system (SMAS) and many of them perform complementary and, at times, unrelated functions. Nevertheless, the mimetic muscles of the mid and lower face have very specific functions, mostly centered around the mouth, sometimes acting as agonists, sometimes as antagonists, but always in a complex, synergistic manner. This allows a person to smile and laugh, grimace, or pucker the lips, or to make any other overt or subtle gesture with the mouth, or even to hold solids, liquid, and air within the mouth without loss of contents or to release at will the contents slowly or forcibly out of the mouth. These muscles allow for the fine motor movements necessary to produce subtle whispering sounds or thunderous clammer. They also facilitate the actions of chewing and swallowing and a myriad of other simple and complex movements that either explicitly or implicitly function in voluntary and involuntary motor movements that are so particular of an individual's mannerisms. In addition, many of these superficial and deep muscles overlie a thicker mass of soft tissue as well as each other, creating an anatomy that is quite different from the forehead and brow (Figure 4.1). Consequently, in the mid and lower face, it then is understandable why, if injected BOTOX® migrates beyond the targeted muscles, unintended results and complications can occur more readily. Therefore, when treating anyone with BOTOX® in the mid and lower face, a little bit of BOTOX® may be good, but a little bit more usually is not necessarily better.

There are additional factors that contribute to the differences in the anatomy of the upper face as compared to that of the mid and lower face which will reflect how one is to utilize injections of BOTOX® when rejuvenating the face[2]. In the upper face the skin can be thicker and more tightly adherent to the underlying muscles of facial expression and complications, if and

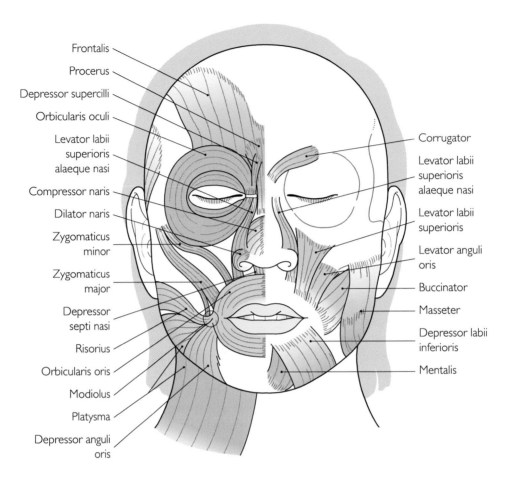

Frontalis
Procerus
Depressor supercilli
Orbicularis oculi
Levator labii superioris alaeque nasi
Compressor naris
Dilator naris
Zygomaticus minor
Zygomaticus major
Depressor septi nasi
Risorius
Orbicularis oris
Modiolus
Platysma
Depressor anguli oris

Corrugator
Levator labii superioris alaeque nasi
Levator labii superioris
Levator anguli oris
Buccinator
Masseter
Depressor labii inferioris
Mentalis

Figure 4.1   Mimetic muscles of facial expression. Right side depicts the superficial and left side depicts the deeper muscles

when they occur, often are related to BOTOX® diffusion. Usually much higher doses of BOTOX® are injected into the upper face musculature to produce more extensive muscle weakness, but BOTOX® treatments there rarely cause functional imbalance. On the other hand, the lower facial musculature should be treated with lower doses of BOTOX® to lightly weaken their activity. Deep longstanding wrinkles and furrows on many occasions cannot be totally effaced; otherwise, anatomic aberrations and functional imbalance can result. In order to maintain the functional as well as an anatomic balance in the mid and lower face when treating a patient with injections of BOTOX®, it is absolutely necessary, more so than in the upper face, that minimal volumes, accurately measured, of low doses of BOTOX® be precisely placed and injected into specifically targeted muscles. Particularly during treatment of the mid face, the upper lip levators are easily affected by the slightest diffusion of BOTOX®, which can readily cause a disruption in one or many of the complex motor functions of the lips (e.g. eating, drinking, and speaking). Also, because of the intermingling of the muscle fibers of the upper lip levators with the orbicularis oris, which overlie a thicker mass of subcutaneous soft tissue, BOTOX® injections to the mid face usually are best performed with electromyographic guidance.

In many areas of the mid and lower face, however, better overall cosmetic results can be achieved with soft tissue implants and fillers, or resurfacing techniques and many other types of invasive procedures (i.e. rhytidectomy and different soft tissue suspension techniques), while supplementary treatments with BOTOX® injections can be used to enhance and prolong the final esthetic outcomes[3].

Nasoglabellar lines
Introduction: problem assessment and patient selection

There are many individuals who form diagonal nasoglabellar lines over the lateral walls of the nasal bridge near the radix that radiate downward, toward the alae, and accentuate when they speak, smile, laugh, or frown. These wrinkles are produced by the contraction of the transverse nasalis (Figure 4.2). They are anatomically different both in location and source from the horizontal lines that span transversely across the nasal radix which are produced by the downward pull of the procerus. When this radial fanning of longitudinal wrinkles of the upper lateral aspect of the nasal bridge occurs as a compensatory maneuver after treatment of glabellar frown lines with BOTOX®, these lines are identified as the 'BOTOX® sign' (Figure 4.3a). On the other hand, when these nasoglabellar lines occur naturally, they are referred to as 'bunny lines' or a 'nasal scrunch'[3,4] (Figure 4.3b). They are annoyingly unsightly and unwanted by those

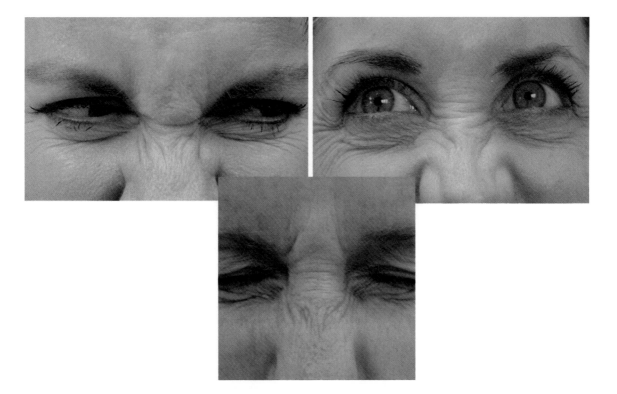

Figure 4.2 'Nasal scrunch' or 'bunny lines' produced by the transverse nasalis, are those vertical lines emanating from the lateral sides of the root the nose before a treatment with BOTOX®. The transverse or horizontal lines across the root of the nose are produced by the procerus. Different patients have different wrinkle patterns

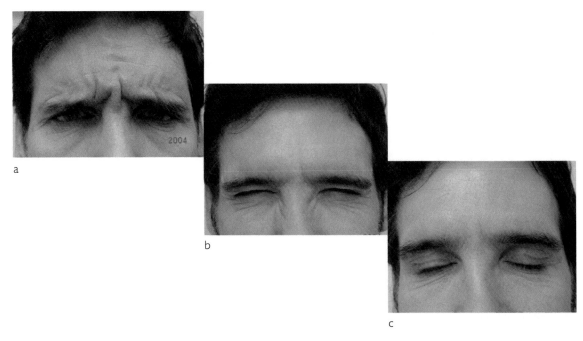

Figure 4.3a 'BOTOX® sign'. a) This 52 year old patient frowning and without nasoglabellar lines prior to a treatment with BOTOX®. b) Same patient frowning 3 weeks after BOTOX® treatment of his glabellar frown lines. Note the compensatory nasoglabellar lines, i.e. BOTOX® sign. c) Two weeks after a touch-up injection of BOTOX® in the transverse nasalis and 5 weeks after the original BOTOX® treatment. Note the compensatory nasoglabellar lines are gone

women who possess nasoglabellar wrinkles, and they should be treated with injections of BOTOX® along with the glabellar frown lines.

Functional anatomy

Nasoglabellar lines are the result of the contraction of the upper or transverse portion of the nasalis, also known as the compressor naris. The transverse nasalis originates from the maxilla, superior and lateral to the incisive fossa (Figure 4.4). Its fibers course medially and superiorly and expand into the aponeurosis over the bridge of the nose, inserting into the fibers of its paired muscle of the opposite side and into the aponeurosis of the procerus (Figure 4.5). The transverse nasalis or compressor naris depresses the cartilaginous part of the nose, drawing the ala toward the nasal septum. These nasoglabellar lines are produced by asking the patient to squint forcibly, as if intense light is shining in the eyes. If these lines become prominent, the patient will most likely produce them readily after their glabellar lines are treated with BOTOX® (Figure 4.3b). Therefore, such naturally occurring nasoglabellar lines should be treated automatically with injections of BOTOX® at the same treatment session when glabellar frown lines are treated. If they are not treated, whether or not the patient is aware of the existence of their nasoglabellar lines before a treatment of BOTOX®, the patient more than likely will blame the physician and BOTOX® for their presence after treatment. Therefore, it behooves the physician to disclose their presence to the patient prior to any treatment with BOTOX®, underscoring the necessity to include these nasoglabellar frown lines as part and parcel of the treatment of glabellar frown lines.

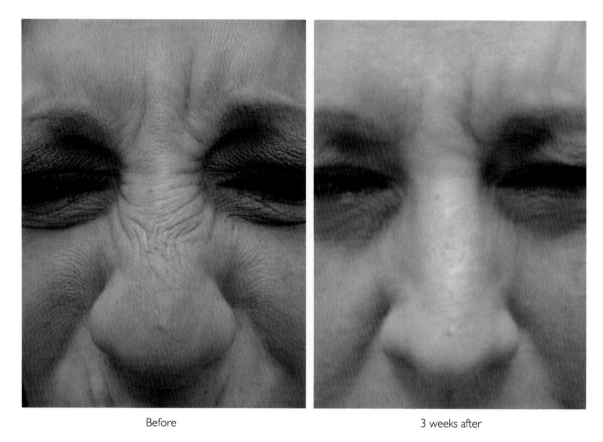

Before   3 weeks after

Figure 4.3b   This 49-year-old patient is shown frowning before and 3 weeks after a treatment with BOTOX®. Note the diminished nasoglabellar 'bunny lines'

If these lines become evident after the patient's glabellar frown lines are treated with BOTOX®, then they should be identified and treated during the obligatory follow-up visit 2–3 weeks after a BOTOX® treatment session (Figure 4.3a). (See Appendix 4).

Dilution

In order to prevent the unintended widespread diffusion of BOTOX®, it is necessary that a minimum amount of BOTOX® be injected when treating the nasoglabellar lines. Therefore, 1ml of normal saline should be used to reconstitute the 100 U vial of BOTOX® when injecting nasoglabellar lines (see Appendix 1).

Dosing: how to correct the problem (what to do and what not to do)

With the patient in the upright sitting or semirecumbent position, nasoglabellar lines can be relaxed by injecting 2–5 U of BOTOX® subcutaneously or intramuscularly into the lateral walls of the nasal bridge, just inferior to the nasal radix and anterior and superior to the nasofacial angle (Figure 4.6). This technique should position the needle well above the angular vessels[5–8]. The soft

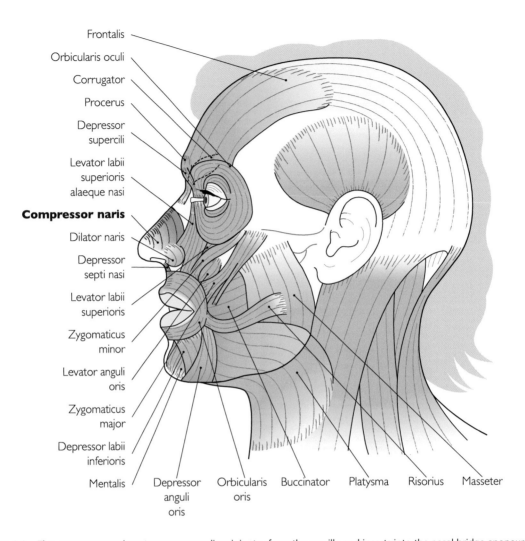

Frontalis
Orbicularis oculi
Corrugator
Procerus
Depressor supercili
Levator labii superioris alaeque nasi
Compressor naris
Dilator naris
Depressor septi nasi
Levator labii superioris
Zygomaticus minor
Levator anguli oris
Zygomaticus major
Depressor labii inferioris
Mentalis
Depressor anguli oris
Orbicularis oris
Buccinator
Platysma
Risorius
Masseter

Figure 4.4   The compressor naris or transverse nasalis originates from the maxilla and inserts into the nasal bridge aponeurosis

tissue is extremely thin and vascular in this area and advancing the needle tip a few millimeters here goes a long way. It is most important to avoid injecting too low along the nasal sidewalls and into the nasofacial sulcus (Figure 4.7a). Otherwise, either the levator labii superioris alaeque nasi or the levator labii superioris, or both, may be weakened by the injected BOTOX®, since they both originate along the medial aspect of the malar prominence. If either of these levators is affected then upper lip ptosis, asymmetry, and resultant functional changes of the mouth can occur.

It appears men are not treated for this problem as frequently as women. Dose of BOTOX® depends on the overall depth and location of the lines and strength of the transverse nasalis. Higher doses by 1 or 2 U more than 5 U of BOTOX® injected on each side may be necessary to diminish these lines, especially in those men and women who spend the better part of the day outdoors and whose nasalis is hypertrophic and hyperkinetic from constant squinting. The effects of BOTOX® can last at least 3 months and usually longer. In patients who previously have had a rhinoplasty, the results may be somewhat less than expected[6–10] (see Appendix 2).

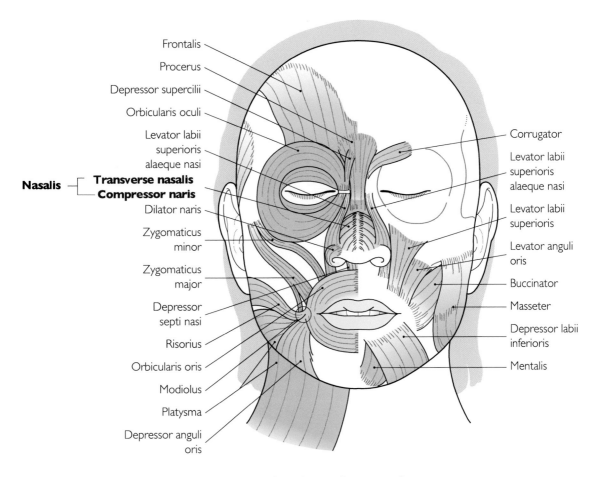

Frontalis
Procerus
Depressor supercilii
Orbicularis oculi
Levator labii superioris alaeque nasi

Nasalis — **Transverse nasalis**
Compressor naris

Dilator naris
Zygomaticus minor
Zygomaticus major
Depressor septi nasi
Risorius
Orbicularis oris
Modiolus
Platysma
Depressor anguli oris

Corrugator
Levator labii superioris alaeque nasi
Levator labii superioris
Levator anguli oris
Buccinator
Masseter
Depressor labii inferioris
Mentalis

Figure 4.5   Compressor naris or transverse nasalis – its relationship to adjacent musculature

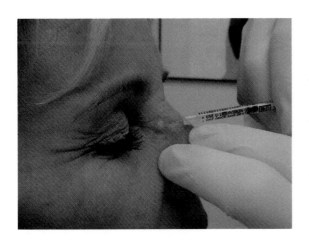
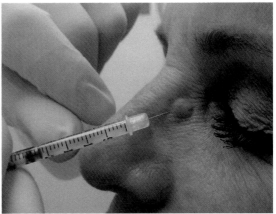

Figure 4.6   Injecting the transverse nasalis anterior and superior to the nasofacial angle. Note the wheal of injected BOTOX®

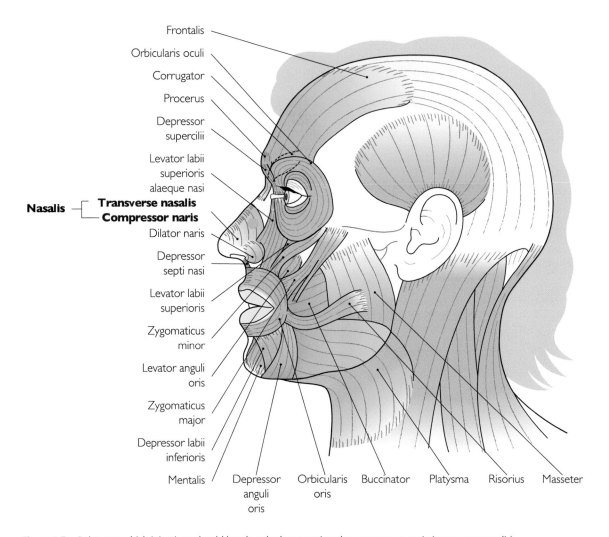

Figure 4.7a Point • at which injections should be placed when treating the compressor naris (transverse nasalis)

Outcomes (results)

Eliminating nasoglabellar lines along with glabellar frown lines gives an individual a relaxed, youthful appearance. When the nasoglabellar lines are not treated and the glabellar frown lines are, nasoglabellar lines in the presence of a smooth glabella produce an exceptionally unsightly effect (Figure 4.3a,b) (see Appendix 3). Recently, Tamuro et al[11] found that they were able to successfully treat approximately 40% of their patients with nasoglabellar lines by injecting them with 3 U of BOTOX® on either side of the nasal side wall in the belly of the transverse nasalis. The other 60% of the patients in their study had persistent bunny lines that exhibited different linear patterns along the proximal and distal nasal bridge. They found that in order to further diminish these persistent bunny lines an additional 2 U of BOTOX® needed to be injected at different sites along either side of the nasal bridge according to the three different patterns they identified as the naso-alar rhytides, naso-orbicular rhytides, and naso-ciliary rhytides. These additional BOTOX® treatments were given at four weeks during the first follow up visit. There

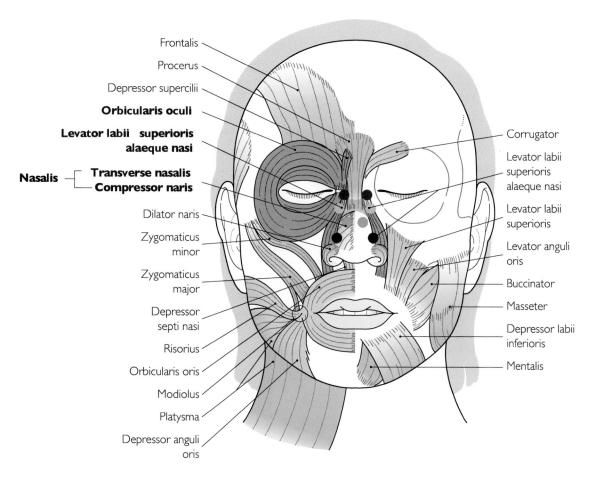

Frontalis
Procerus
Depressor supercilii
Orbicularis oculi
Levator labii superioris alaeque nasi
Nasalis — **Transverse nasalis** **Compressor naris**
Dilator naris
Zygomaticus minor
Zygomaticus major
Depressor septi nasi
Risorius
Orbicularis oris
Modiolus
Platysma
Depressor anguli oris

Corrugator
Levator labii superioris alaeque nasi
Levator labii superioris
Levator anguli oris
Buccinator
Masseter
Depressor labii inferioris
Mentalis

Figure 4.7b Additional injection sites to diminish persistent nasoglabellar lines. Red dot for nasocilliary rhytides; green dot for nasoorbicular rhytides; purple dot for naso-alar rhytides

were approximately 30% of the patients who had persistent wrinkling of the root of the nose owing to contraction of the nasal portion of the orbicularis oculi, so these patients were identified as having naso-orbicular rhytides (Figures 4.7b,c). Another 30% of the patients had persistent wrinkling at the root of the nose which extended superiorly toward the medial margin of the eyebrow and glabella caused also by contraction of the orbicularis oculi, but adjacent to the ciliary arch so they were identified as having naso-ciliary rhytides (Figures 4.7b,c). The third pattern identified as naso-alar persistent wrinkles occured in both subgroups and were felt to be the result of the contraction of the alar portion of the levator labii superioris alaeque nasi. Each area of persistent wrinkling, was produced by unaffected fibers of the underlying muscles which required the additional 2 U of BOTOX® on either side of the nasal bridge to completely eliminate any residual nasoglabellar 'bunny lines'[11].

Complications (adverse sequelae) (see Appendix 5)

Injecting BOTOX® too low along the nasal sidewalls and allowing it to diffuse into the upper lip levators (i.e. levator labii superioris alaeque nasi and levator labii superioris) can produce asymmetry and even ptosis of the upper lip, including sphincter incompetence and functional

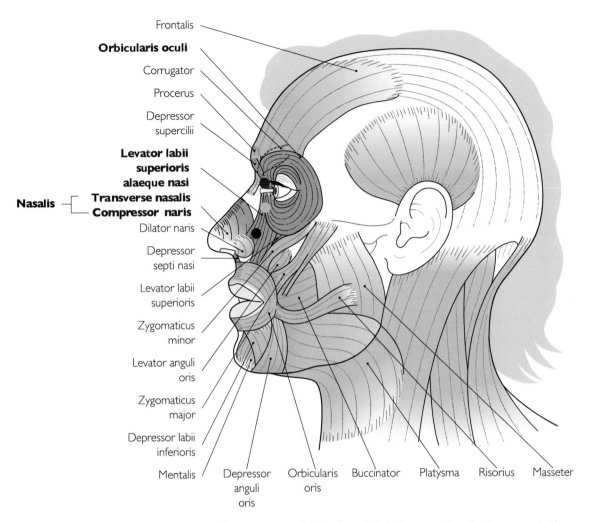

Figure 4.7c Additional injection sites to diminish persistent nasoglabellar lines. Red dot for nasocilliary rhytides; green dot for naso orbicular rhytides; purple dot for naso-alar rhytides

difficulties with speaking and eating. Also, if the medial palpebral portion of the orbicularis oculi is weakened as the result of the unintended diffusion of BOTOX®, a diminution in the action of the lacrimal pump can occur, causing epiphora (excessive tearing)[10]. Diplopia also can result if the medial rectus is weakened by the BOTOX®. Vigorous massage to the area after the injection of BOTOX® can produce the same adverse results, even if dosing and the injection technique are flawless. There is no antidote for any of these unwanted post-treatment adverse sequelae, and the patient is obligated to endure them until the effects of the BOTOX® remit. In the meantime, consultation with an ophthalmologist to help the patient cope with these ocular problems is advisable.

It is important also to keep in mind that the angular artery and vein sit in the nasofacial angle and injections placed deeply can result in an intravascular injection of the BOTOX®. Therefore, subcutaneous placement of the needle tip is all that is necessary when injecting this area with BOTOX®.

Treatment implications when injecting nasoglabellar lines

1. Nasoglabellar lines can occur naturally in some individuals or they can be produced by treating glabellar frown lines with injections of BOTOX®.
2. Squinting will elicit the presence or absence of nasoglabellar lines before treating the glabellar frown lines with BOTOX®.
3. Treat nasoglabellar frown lines along with horizontal glabellar frown lines (i.e. those produced by the contraction of the procerus).
4. Injections too low and into the nasofacial sulcus may result in upper lip ptosis, asymmetry, or even upper lip incompetence and functional difficulties of the sphincteric action of the mouth.
5. Inject additional units of BOTOX® along the proximal and distal nasal bridge in different patterns to attenuate all the nasoglabellar lines in certain patients.

Nasal flare

Introduction: problem assessment and patient selection

There are some individuals who, either naturally or when they are under physical or emotional stress, flare their nostrils and widen their nasal aperture repeatedly as they inspire. Many individuals, who possess a broad nasal bridge with wide nasal alae, also may have a well-developed muscle of the distal nose (i.e. nasalis), which will allow them to dilate their nostrils voluntarily and involuntarily. This noticeable movement of the nostrils can impart a negative sentiment to observers which may include anger, fear, exhaustion, concern, disapproval, or personal distress.

Functional anatomy

Nasal flaring is the result of the involuntary contraction of the lower portion of the nasalis or the alar nasalis also called the dilator naris, causing the alae nasi to dilate repeatedly (Figure 4.8). The alar nasalis originates from the maxilla above the lateral incisor and medial to the transverse nasalis under the nasolabial fold, and inserts into the lower portion of the nasal cartilage and skin near the margin of the nasal aperature. Its medial fibers can blend with the fibers of the depressor septi nasi. The alar nasalis or dilator naris draws the ala of the nose downward and laterally, dilating the nostrils, thereby preventing the alae nasi from collapsing during inspiration. (See Appendix 4).

Dilution

Moderate diffusion of BOTOX® is encouraged when treating the lower nasalis. Therefore, reconstituting a 100 U vial of BOTOX® with 1–2.5 ml of normal saline to inject into this area is acceptable (see Appendix 1).

Dosing: how to correct the problem (what to do and what not to do)

Injections of 5–10 U of BOTOX® subcutaneously into the center of each ala toward the alar rim along the lateral fibers of the alar nasalis will weaken involuntary muscle contractions of the nostrils[12]. This can be useful in African-American patients or other ethnic groups who have a

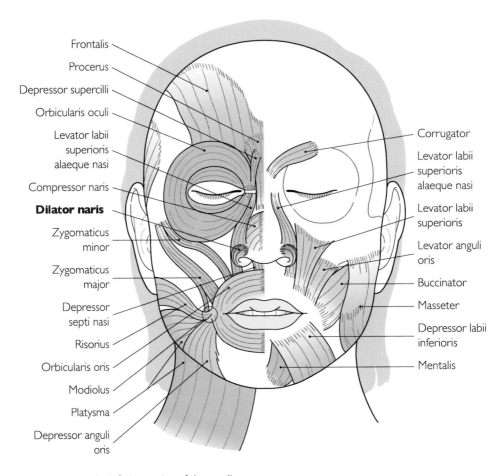

Figure 4.8   Dilator naris is the inferior portion of the nasalis

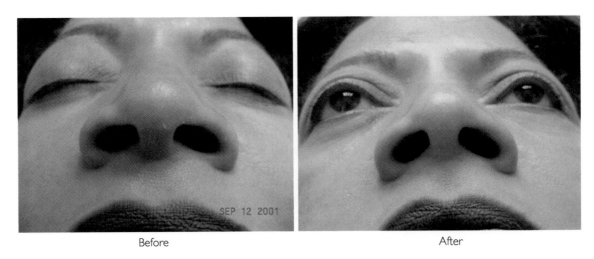

Before   After

Figure 4.9   Patient at rest before and 4 weeks after a treatment with BOTOX®. A slight reduction of a nasal flare was achieved with 5 U of BOTOX® injected into the dilator naris (alar nasalis) bilaterally

characteristically similar, broad nasal bridge and wide alae that flare easily because of a hyperkinetic alar nasalis (Figure 4.9). For some individuals, 10–15 U of BOTOX® may be necessary to relax each ala nasi. Only those patients who can voluntarily and actively flare their nostrils are candidates for BOTOX® injections. For those individuals, especially patients of African and Asian descent, who have a characteristically broad nasal bridge and wide alar base, but who cannot actively flare their nostrils at will, injections of BOTOX® will have no effect in narrowing the nasal aperture and should not be performed (see Appendix 1).

Outcomes (results)

For those individuals who voluntarily can flare or dilate their alae nasi, injections of BOTOX® will decrease the frontal diameter of the nostril and give their nose a narrower, more Caucasian appearance, without interfering with inspiration (see Appendix 1).

Complications (adverse sequelae) (see Appendix 5)

If patients are not selected properly, injections of BOTOX® will produce no effect, and time, effort, and expense will have been wasted. Otherwise, these patients experience no other adverse sequelae, except the usual ones that occur with intracutaneous injections, including pain, edema, and possible ecchymoses.

Treatment implications when injecting the nose for nasal flare

1. Treat only those patients who can actively flare their nostrils.
2. Injections of 5–10 U of BOTOX® in the center or along the alar rim of each ala nasi into the dilator naris will relax flaring nostrils.
3. No adverse side effects have been identified with this injection technique.

Nasal tip drop

Introduction: problem assessment and patient selection

With age, the nasal tip in some individuals naturally rotates downward, partly because of the pull of gravity and partly because of the pull of a hyperkinetic muscle of the nasal septum (i.e. depressor septi nasi). When this occurs, a person may possess the appearance of senility and decrepitude, projecting an evil and sinister demeanor (Figure 4.10).

Recently, BOTOX® therapy has provided a non-invasive means to elevate the nasal tip and produce tip projection, an effect that usually only can be accomplished by surgical rhinoplasty.

Functional anatomy

The depressor septi nasi is often considered a component part of the dilator naris, which originates from the center of the incisor fossa of the maxilla deep to the orbicularis oris. Its fibers course upward and insert into both the cartilaginous nasal septum (its mobile part) and the mucous membrane undersurface of the ala nasi, and the superficial muscle fibers of the orbicularis oris and mucous membrane of the upper lip (Figure 4.11).

Figure 4.10 Downward
projected nasal tip

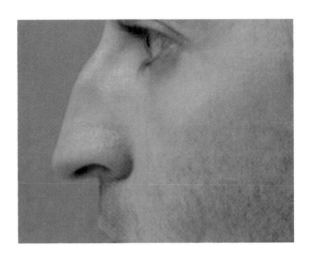

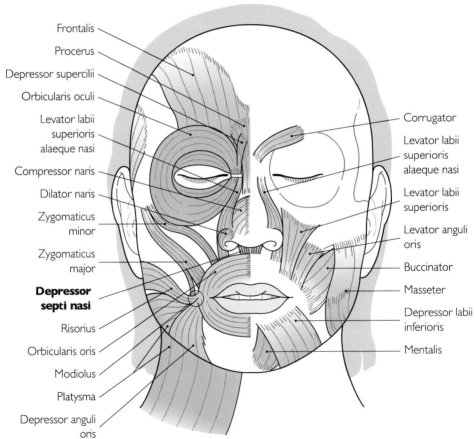

Frontalis

Procerus

Depressor supercilii

Orbicularis oculi

Levator labii
superioris
alaeque nasi

Compressor naris

Dilator naris

Zygomaticus
minor

Zygomaticus
major

**Depressor
septi nasi**

Risorius

Orbicularis oris

Modiolus

Platysma

Depressor anguli
oris

Corrugator

Levator labii
superioris
alaeque nasi

Levator labii
superioris

Levator anguli
oris

Buccinator

Masseter

Depressor labii
inferioris

Mentalis

Figure 4.11 Depressor septi nasi may intermingle with the dilator naris

The depressor septi nasi pulls the nasal septum downward, draws the ala inferiorly, and narrows the nostril. In some individuals, on the other hand, fibers of the dilator naris have been found to interdigitate with those of the depressor septi nasi. Consequently, when the depressor septi nasi contracts in unison with the dilator naris, a paradoxical widening of the nasal aperture will then occur. Because of the variability in the anatomy and the multifactorial etiology of nasal tip depression, elevation and projection of the nasal tip usually is not as simple to produce with injections of BOTOX® as might be thought. (See Appendix 4).

Dilution

In the paranasal area, minimum amounts of BOTOX® should be used so as not to accidentally affect the levators of the upper lip by inadvertent diffusion of BOTOX®. Therefore, a 100 U vial of BOTOX® should be reconstituted with 1 ml of normal saline (see Appendix 1).

Dosing: how to correct the problem (what to do and what not to do)

For those patients who can intentionally depress the tip of their nose downward by lowering their upper lip, injections of BOTOX® can be helpful in raising and projecting their nasal tip. To effectively treat a dropped nasal tip, have the patient depress their upper lip downward, widening the junction between the base of the nasal columella and the upper lip. This maneuver elongates the depressor septi nasi, separating it functionally and anatomically away from the orbicularis oris. This allows one to place the needle precisely into the depressor septi nasi, and not into fibers of the orbicularis oris, before injecting the BOTOX®.

Depending on the strength of the depressor septi nasi, 2–4 U of BOTOX® can be injected just superior to this columella–labial juncture. An additional 2–4 U of BOTOX® also can be injected into the middle of the columella, depending on the strength and whether or not the depressor septi nasi is visibly functional. Stronger muscles can be injected with higher doses of BOTOX®[13]. In some patients whose dilator naris also interdigitates with the depressor septi nasi, an additional injection of 4–5 U of BOTOX® into each side of the dorsum of the ala nasi, i.e. into the dilator naris (as described previously on page 132), will be necessary to effectively project the nasal tip. The combination of injecting both the depressor septi nasi and the dilator naris with BOTOX® will relax the lower end and base of the nose, producing additional lifting of the nasal tip[14]. If, when depressing the upper lip, one can see an obvious downward rotation of the nasal tip, then injections of BOTOX® will be effective. If there is no movement of the nasal tip when the upper lip is depressed, BOTOX® injections should not be performed.

Atamoros has devised a therapeutic dosing scheme whereby he can predict the height change in the nasal tip elevation in the patients he treats with BOTOX®[14]. Injecting 2 U of BOTOX® into each of the right and left dilator naris and 2 U of BOTOX® into the depressor septi nasi (total of 6 U of BOTOX®) produces a slight elevation of the nasal tip. Approximately 4 U of BOTOX® injected into each of the right and left alae nasi and the depressor septi (total of 12 U of BOTOX®) produces a medium elevation of the nasal tip. For a high elevation and projection of the nasal tip, 6 U of BOTOX® into each of the right and left dilator naris and depressor septi (total of 18 U of BOTOX®) may be needed[14] (Figure 4.12) (see Appendix 3).

Outcomes (results)

Injecting BOTOX® into the depressor septi nasi will relax the muscle, lifting and projecting the nasal tip (Figure 4.13). Injecting the depressor septi nasi with BOTOX® also can provide an apparent increase in the distance between the columella and vermillion border, occasionally creating a fuller, more voluminous upper lip for some patients[13]. Consequently, the depressor septi nasi is one of the muscles which might need to be weakened when treating a patient for exaggerated upper gum smile (see p. 148) (see Appendix 3).

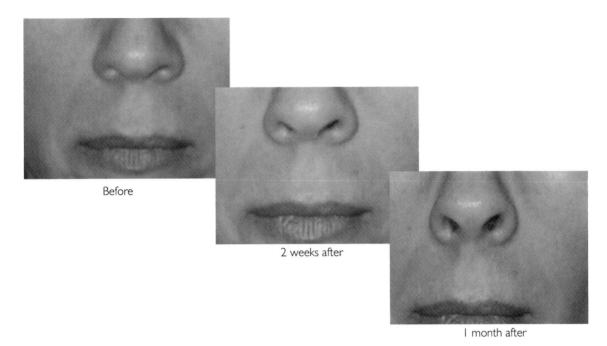

Before

2 weeks after

1 month after

Figure 4.12 Exaggerated elevation of the nasal tip, flattening of the tip projection, and excessive widening of the nostralis can be seen in this patient, who was injected with a total of 18 U of BOTOX® (6 U into each dilator naris and 6 U into the depressor septi nasi). (Courtesy of Dr Francisco Atamoros Perez)

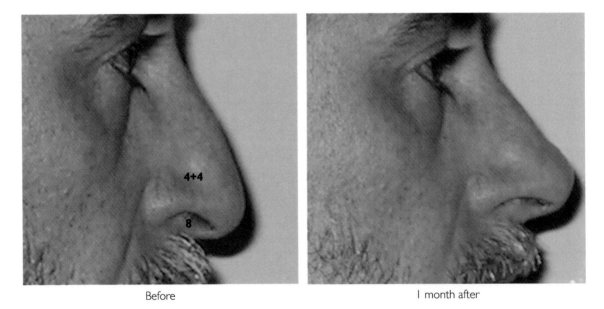

Before

1 month after

Figure 4.13 Nasal tip before and 1 month after a treatment with BOTOX®. To achieve these results, a total of 8 U of BOTOX® was injected into the lower nasalis (4 U on each side) and 8 U into the depressor septi nasi, for an overall total of 16 U. (Courtesy of Dr Francisco Atamoros Perez)

Treatment implications when injecting the nose for a drop of the nasal tip

1. The tip of the nose can drop because of muscle contraction, age, and gravity.
2. BOTOX® injections of the depressor septi nasi will elevate and project the nasal tip.
3. In some patients, the dilator naris also may need to be injected with BOTOX® for nasal tip elevation and projection.
4. Overtreatment with BOTOX® can cause excessive nostril widening and an exaggerated elevation and a flattening of the nasal tip projection.
5. Diffusion of BOTOX® lateral to the columella can affect the upper lip levators, elongating the upper lip and blunting the contour of the philtrum. Upper lip asymmetry and oral sphincter weakness can result from injecting too high a dose of BOTOX® at the base of the columella.

Complications (adverse sequelae) (see Appendix 5)

Higher doses of injected BOTOX® produce a relaxation of the alar nasalis and depressor septi nasi which can result in an unattractive, prolonged widening of the nostrils along with the projection and elevation of the nasal tip (Figure 4.12). This forced widening of the nostrils was accompanied in some patients by persistent pain and soreness over the nasal tip that lasted for over 2 weeks[14]. The duration of the effect of the injected BOTOX® in this area sometimes can last for only 2 months, and even less in some patients.

Weakening only the depressor septi nasi may just elevate the nasal tip. However, if the BOTOX® diffuses laterally from the midpoint of the base of the nasal columella and into the central upper lip levators (i.e. levator labii superioris, levator labii superioris alaeque nasi), then the upper lip can become elongated and thinned, obliterating the contour and depth of the philtrum. Unless there is an obvious downward displacement of the anterior aspect of the nose and nasal tip when a patient forcibly lowers their upper lip, injections of the depressor septi nasi should not be attempted.

Melolabial grooves and folds

Introduction: problem assessment and patient selection

Chronological aging and a downward shift of soft tissue can deepen a nasolabial sulcus, which, in turn, augments its fold. Accentuated by side lighting and shadows, the nasolabial fold is enhanced by the descent of the soft tissue mass of the cheek by the incessant effects of gravity. This descent of cheek mass is in the infraorbital area at different depths and shapes and varies with each individual. As the descent of the soft tissue mass intensifies, hooding or folds over the lateral labial commissures appears. The appearance of the so-called nasolabial folds probably is more frequently seen in genetically predisposed individuals, but more than likely they also can be acquired by those whose mid facial movements are constant and excessively intense. Deep, diagonal folds from the sides of the nose that progress downward toward the angle of the mouth, and at times even lower, portray an attitude of disgust and dismay and are a characteristic sign of senescence and dotage. These deep furrows and folds remain as one of the still barely correctable harbingers of decrepitude in the treatment of the aging face. In the past, different surgical procedures have been attempted to efface the outline of the groove, thereby flattening the fold. These procedures were fraught with scars and failure. Recently, injections of permanent and absorbable soft tissue fillers have been the most useful in achieving a modicum of success, and probably are still the best technique for softening and filling this defect, considering the reason for its presence. Nevertheless, injections of BOTOX® also have been employed in an attempt to reduce the appearance of the nasolabial folds. Unfortunately, intramuscular injections of BOTOX® appear not to be the long sought after panacea for this problem and they too have proven to be fraught with complications and failure in this area of the mid face.

Functional anatomy

There is significant variation in the anatomy that creates the nasolabial fold, which extends from the lateral nasal ala to a point lateral to or lower than the oral commissure. A prominent nasolabial fold may have a mutifactorial etiology with contributing influences of varying degrees from skin, bone, muscles, and fat. The cutaneous insertions of the different mimetic facial muscles along this fold may promote the early appearance of the nasolabial fold and sulcus, starting in those so predisposed persons in their mid to late thirties. In older patients, a combination of any of the following also may contribute to their prominent appearance:

- Loss of skin thickness over the sulcus;
- Redundant skin lateral to the sulcus;

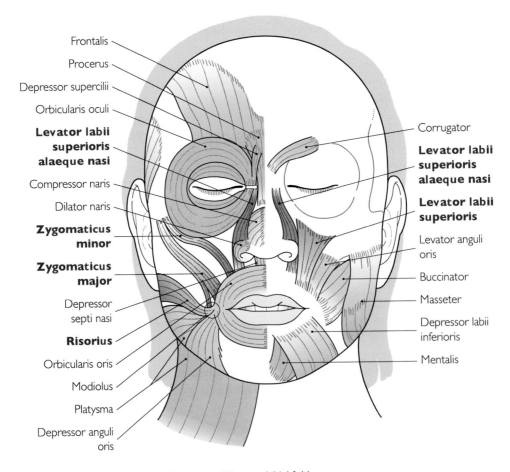

Figure 4.14 Muscles that contribute to the formation of the nasolabial fold

- Excessive fat deposits or ptosis of the malar fat laterally as a result of a weakening of the SMAS in the mid upper cheek.

Aging and frequent mimetic action of the causative facial muscles can intensify the vertical sulcus that runs from the upper border of the nasofacial angle downward and laterally toward the commissures of the mouth. Dependent on idiosyncratic and anatomic variations of an individual, it is the set of facial muscles responsible for elevating the upper lip and producing a smile (zygomatic complex, the central upper lip elevators, and the risorius) that contributes significantly to the initial formation and perpetuation of the nasolabial folds (Figure 4.14).

According to some authors, in many patients it is the levator labii superioris alaeque nasi that is the muscle most responsible for producing the upper, medial portion of the nasolabial fold[15]. It is the zygomatic muscle complex and the levator labii superioris that are primarily responsible for elevating the lip and producing a smile[16]. In some individuals, however, the levator labii superioris alaeque nasi is less important in the formation of a smile, especially if elevating the medial aspect of the upper lip is minimal when they do smile. In many other individuals, the zygomaticus complex, along with a contribution from the levator labii superioris, can deepen the middle portion of the nasolabial fold and even exaggerate lateral canthal wrinkles, extending crow's feet downward over the surface of the mid and lateral cheeks (Figure 4.15). In most individuals the zygomaticus major helps to elevate the corner of the mouth and move it laterally with smiling, but, in so doing, it can mobilize lateral cheek skin downward and medially, extending the lower crow's feet down the face, especially in individuals who have inelastic, loose, redundant skin.

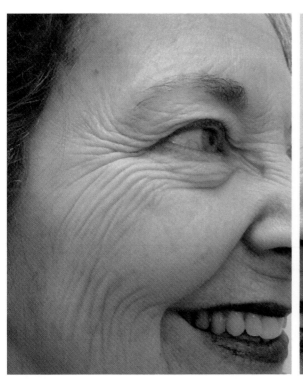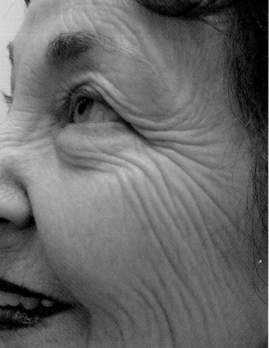

Figure 4.15 Lower crow's feet and lateral cheek rhytides

The zygomaticus major originates on the zygomatic bone, just anterior to the zygomaticotemporal suture line, and then continues downward toward the angle of the mouth and joins other muscle fibers of the modiolus before its fibers reach the oral commissure, where they interdigitate with the fibers of the levator anguli oris and superficial and deep fibers of the orbicularis oris. The zygomaticus minor, on the other hand, originates more medially on the zygoma than the zygomaticus major just behind the zygomaticomaxillary suture line. Its fibers move downward to insert more medially and directly into the upper lip, interdigitating with fibers of the levator labii superioris. The zygomaticus minor helps elevate the center of the upper lip, exposing the maxillary teeth. Both muscles of the zygomatic complex can deepen the nasolabial fold when they contract. In most individuals, when the zygomaticus minor contracts together with the central upper lip levators (i.e. levator labii superioris alaeque nasi and levator labii superioris) they will cause the upper lip to curl when expressing smugness, contempt, or disdain (see Appendix 4).

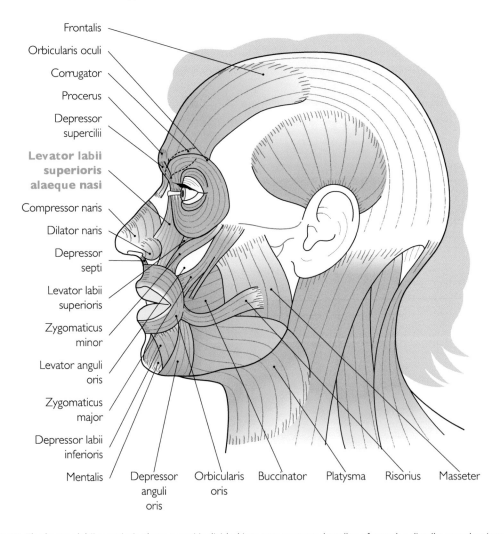

Figure 4.16 The levator labii superioris alaeque nasi is divided into two separate bundles of muscles distally; one that inserts over the ala and skin of the nose, the other that inserts in the upper lip, skin, and mucosa

The levator labii superioris alaeque nasi originates from the superior part of the frontal process of the maxilla close to the side of the nose (Figure 4.16). It travels obliquely downward and laterally, dividing itself into two separate muscle bundles. The one smaller bundle inserts medially into the greater alar cartilage and skin of the nose. The other larger bundle continues downward toward the lateral aspect of the upper lip and crosses over the front of the levator labii superioris, merging with fibers of the levator labii superioris and orbicularis oris. It inserts along the floor of the dermis into the overlying skin of the ipsilateral aspect of the upper lip near the upper part of the nasolabial furrow and fold. The lateral labial muscle bundle raises and everts the upper lip and increases the curvature of the upper part of the nasolabial sulcus. The medial nasal muscle bundle dilates the nostrils and displaces the circumalar facial sulcus laterally, elevating the nasolabial fold (see Appendix 4).

The levator labii superioris originates from the maxilla at the lower margin of the orbit, just above the infraorbital foramen, deep to the orbicularis oculi (Figure 4.17). Coursing downward between the lateral bundle of the levator labii superioris alaeque, the zygomaticus minor, and the levator anguli oris, some of its fibers insert directly into the skin overlying these muscles in the central and lateral aspect of the upper lip and other fibers interdigitate with those of the orbicularis oris. Its function is to raise and evert the central aspect of the upper lip. In

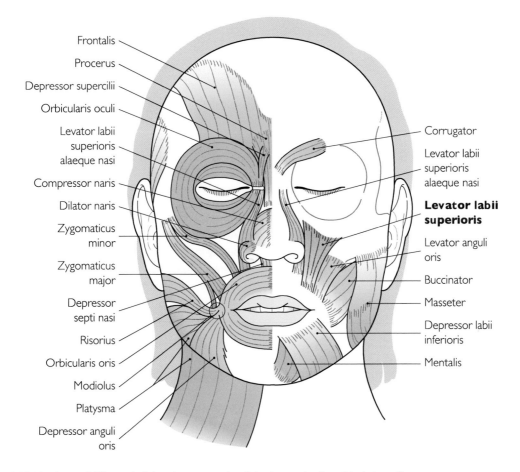

Figure 4.17 The levator labii superioris is a deeper muscle originating under the orbicularis oculi

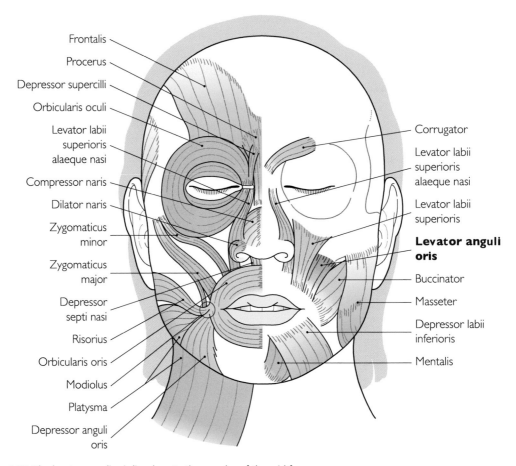

Figure 4.18 The levator anguli oris lies deep to the muscles of the mid face

conjunction with other muscles, it moves and deepens the nasolabial sulcus, especially during expressions of seriousness and sadness (see Appendix 4).

The levator anguli oris originates more deeply in the canine fossa of the maxilla, just below the infraorbital foramen (Figure 4.18). It lies beneath and deep to the upper lip levators and the zygomaticus complex. Its muscle fibers travel downward into the modiolus and then decussate with those of the zygomaticus major while wrapping around the oral commissure to inter-digitate with the fibers of the orbicularis oris and the depressor anguli oris. The levator anguli oris then inserts into the overlying skin at and just below the angle of the mouth into the lower portion of the nasolabial sulcus. It raises the lateral aspect of the upper lip, and the lateral corners of the mouth when smiling or laughing. It also deepens and shifts the contour of the nasolabial sulcus (see Appendix 4).

The previous group of four muscles was formerly identified as the quadratus labii superioris, which, when contracted, was felt to cause the nasolabial sulcus to deepen. The quadratus labii superioris was described as comprising four muscle heads: the angular head or the levator labii superioris alaeque nasi, the infraorbital head or the levator labii superioris, the zygomatic head or the zygomaticus minor, and the canine head or the levator anguli oris. (See Appendix 4).

Dilution

Injecting minimal volumes of BOTOX® in this area is of paramount importance so as not to have unintended diffusion of the BOTOX® affect the surrounding muscles of the mid face. Therefore, a 100 U vial of BOTOX® should be reconstituted with only 1 ml of normal saline (see Appendix 1).

Dosing: how to correct the problem (what to do and what not to do)

Injecting 1 and not more than 2 U of BOTOX® into the mid nasofacial angle just lateral to the upper border of the ala nasi will weaken the upper nasal fibers of the levator labii superioris alaeque nasi and flatten the upper and medial aspect of the nasolabial fold (Figures 4.19 and 4.20a). Depending on the depth of the nasolabial sulcus and the height of the nasolabial fold, another technique is to inject 1 and not more than 2 U of BOTOX® lateral and slightly inferior to this point to weaken the lower fibers of the levator labii superioris and zygomaticus minor (Figure 4.20a,b). These injection techniques should be performed only by the very experienced physician whose patient produces innumerable wrinkles of the mid cheek with smiling or squinting or both, and whose nasolabial folds are exaggerated with a simple upward movement of the upper lip, as in sniffing and smiling. Proper patient selection is of paramount importance, because untoward sequelae can occur very easily and be devasting to the patient. The use of electromyographic guidance when treating this area is of inestimable value.

An injection of 1–2 U and not more than 3 U of BOTOX® near the origins of the zygomatic complex along the zygomatic arch at the inferior border of the orbicularis oculi of the lower eyelid (Figure 4.21) can achieve an additive effect of diminishing lower lateral canthal rhytides along with effacing nasolabial folds. Depending on the idiosyncratic anatomy of a particular individual, the shape of the face, and the strength of the muscles, it might be necessary to administer one or two injections of BOTOX®, each over the mid to lateral malar prominence, to obtain the consistent results desired (Figure 4.21) (see Appendix 2).

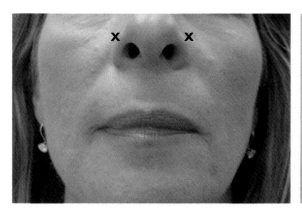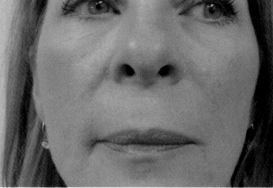

Figure 4.19 'X' marks the point where 1 U of BOTOX® was injected into this 53-year-old to diminish the depth of the nasolabial sulcus. Note the elongation of the upper lip, flattening of the philtrum, and thinning of the vermillion in this patient at rest

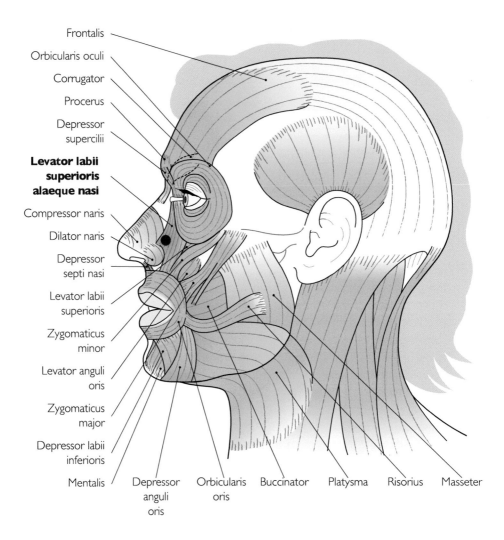

Frontalis
Orbicularis oculi
Corrugator
Procerus
Depressor
supercilii
**Levator labii
superioris
alaeque nasi**
Compressor naris
Dilator naris
Depressor
septi nasi
Levator labii
superioris
Zygomaticus
minor
Levator anguli
oris
Zygomaticus
major
Depressor labii
inferioris
Mentalis
Depressor
anguli
oris
Orbicularis
oris
Buccinator
Platysma
Risorius
Masseter

Figure 4.20a ● marks the point where 1–2 U of BOTOX® can be injected to weaken the nasal fibers of the levator labii superioris alaeque nasi to diminish the nasolabial fold

Outcomes (results)

There have been a few attempts to establish a fail-safe technique in which some of the upper lip levators could be treated with BOTOX® to reduce a deep nasolabial sulcus and fold without subsequent adverse effects.

If one considers the levator labii superioris alaeque nasi the principal muscle that creates the nasolabial fold, and the other central and lateral lip levators (the levator labii superioris, zygomaticus complex, and levator anguli oris) and risorius responsible for deepening the nasolabial sulcus when they contract, then precisely placed low-volume injections of BOTOX® should be able to reduce the appearance of the nasolabial fold and the depth of its sulcus. Because this is not the only or primary function of these muscles, injections of BOTOX® can unwittingly produce secondary changes that interfere with the primary function of these muscles, i.e. elevating the upper lip and laterally abducting the corners of the mouth, which are

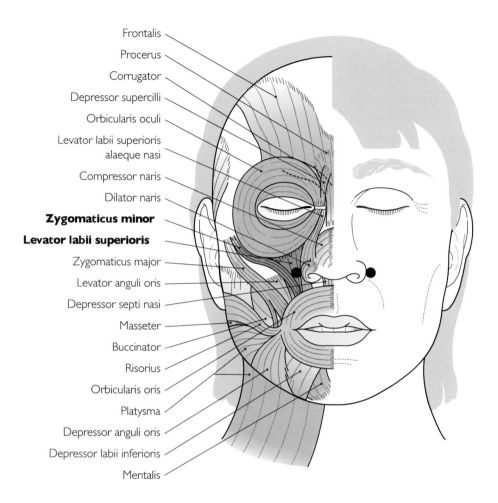

Frontalis
Procerus
Corrugator
Depressor supercilli
Orbicularis oculi
Levator labii superioris
alaeque nasi
Compressor naris
Dilator naris
Zygomaticus minor
Levator labii superioris
Zygomaticus major
Levator anguli oris
Depressor septi nasi
Masseter
Buccinator
Risorius
Orbicularis oris
Platysma
Depressor anguli oris
Depressor labii inferioris
Mentalis

Figure 4.20b ● marks the point where 1–2 U of BOTOX® can be injected to weaken the levator labii superioris and zygomatic minor to diminish the nasolabial fold

necessary movements when one speaks, smiles, laughs, yawns, or forcibly breathes by mouth (see Appendix 3).

Complications (adverse sequalae) (see Appendix 5)

Just 1 to 3 U of BOTOX® into each lip levator complex in the lower nasofacial sulcus will collapse the upper extent of the nasolabial fold and also elongate the upper lip, with fairly long lasting results[1]. However, injecting this area can result in a flat mid face with elongation of the upper lip, effacement of the philtrum, and narrowing and diminishing the fullness of the upper vermillion, an appearance that is not well accepted by most individuals, especially those who already have a naturally longer upper lip (Figure 4.19). Overzealous treatment of this area can result in an asymmetric smile and a ptotic upper lip, causing drooling and fluid incontinence when drinking from a glass or cup. In most patients, these nasolabial lines are best treated with implants and fillers, and not with BOTOX®.

Overinjecting BOTOX® any lower than the upper alar facial border, i.e. closer to the alar labial sulcus or along the nasal sill, can produce a weakening of the central upper lip levators

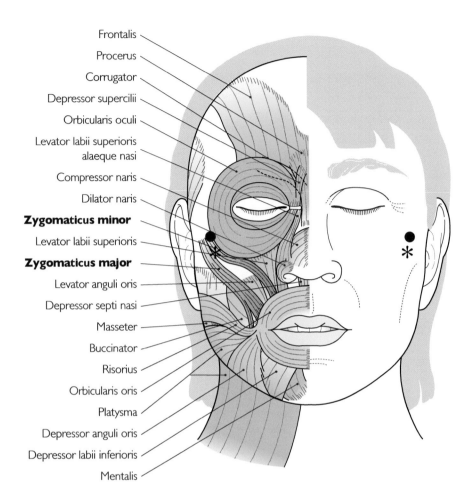

Frontalis
Procerus
Corrugator
Depressor supercilii
Orbicularis oculi
Levator labii superioris alaeque nasi
Compressor naris
Dilator naris
Zygomaticus minor
Levator labii superioris
Zygomaticus major
Levator anguli oris
Depressor septi nasi
Masseter
Buccinator
Risorius
Orbicularis oris
Platysma
Depressor anguli oris
Depressor labii inferioris
Mentalis

Figure 4.21 Injection of 1–3 U of BOTOX® at the lateral zygomatic arch near the origin of the zygomaticus complex can diminish lower crow's feet and help efface the upper and mid nasolabial sulcus and fold. Depending on the individual's anatomy, shape of face, and strength of the muscles, a second injection point (*) might be necessary to produce the same results

that can produce an inability to elevate the upper lip, elongating its overall dimensions. This is a common technique used to drop the upper lip and correct a gummy smile, but is not appropriate in most patients seeking a reduction in the fullness of their nasolabial folds (see p. 148).

Usually, injecting only 1–2 U of BOTOX® away from the mouth, and near the origins of the zygomaticus major et minor and levator labii superioris, can help reduce both the nasolabial fold and the lower lateral canthal wrinkles and lower lateral cheek rhytides, usually with minimal effect to the strength of the upper lip sphincter competence and smile symmetry[3,17]. It is extremely important, however, that minimal volume BOTOX® is injected precisely into the fibers of the targeted muscles. The objective is to inject minimal amounts of BOTOX® to lightly weaken and not paralyze these muscles. Even with a light weakening of the levator labii superioris and the zygomatic complex, a certain amount of lip ptosis will occur, and is actually expected. This should be discussed with the patient before treatment, and should not be considered a true adverse outcome or complication[2,18] (Figure 4.19).

In older patients who have a large amount of excessive fat deposition or ptotic malar fat along with redundant skin lateral to the nasolabial sulcus, weakening the central upper lip levators will have no effect on the extent and depth of the nasolabial folds. The nasolabial folds might even be enhanced if the lateral upper lip levators are weakened, causing a reduction in the lateral muscle support, which in turn will allow the ptotic fat and redundant skin to sag even more so. On the other hand, in younger patients with good cutaneous elasticity and soft tissue support (i.e. those in their early thirties to late fifties) much of the appearance of the nasolabial fold is caused by mimetic muscle contraction, the bulk of which can be attributed to the levator labii superioris alaeque nasi. When this muscle is weakened in younger persons, the nasolabial fold is diminished, usually uneventfully. Attempting to weaken some of the other upper lip levators may cause unexpected sequelae, e.g. upper lip ptosis, asymmetry, and even oral sphincter incompetence. For example, weakening the zygomatic muscles also can soften the nasolabial folds, but the smile may be changed, reducing the extent of its upward and lateral expansion. However, for those patients with an exaggerated gingival smile, weakening of the central upper lip levators may actually function in a positive fashion, reducing the full upward movement of the upper lip, thereby not allowing overexposure of the crown and gums of the anterior upper teeth to occur when smiling or laughing (see p. 148).

Injecting BOTOX® in the mid face in an attempt to diminish the nasolabial folds and to eliminate the random wrinkling of the center of the cheeks produced by squinting or smiling should only be attempted by the most experienced physician injector. Selecting the right patient can be more important, at times, than any other aspect of a BOTOX® injection. Understanding how certain facial and cheek wrinkles and folds are produced, and how to palpate and identify the offending muscles for injection, is the key to success or failure. Attempting to reduce mid cheek wrinkling and nasolabial folds with injections of BOTOX® can result in not only a flattening of the nasolabial fold, but also an overall flattening of the cheek and an elongation of

Treatment implications when injecting nasolabial folds

1. Nasolabial folds are best reduced by injections of soft tissue fillers and implants rather than with injections of BOTOX®.
2. The levator labii superioris alaeque nasi is the muscle primarily responsible for the creation of the nasolabial sulcus and fold.
3. Injections of 1–2 U of BOTOX® should be given in the lower nasofacial or upper alar facial sulcus in an attempt to flatten the nasolabial fold.
4. Injections of BOTOX® too low along the alar facial angle will produce an elongation or ptosis of the upper lip, an asymmetric smile, and functional incompetence of the oral sphincter.
5. Injections of BOTOX® too lateral to the nasofacial angle will produce an overall flattening of the mid cheek and a drop in the soft tissue support of the malar fat pad.
6. In the properly selected patient, a combination of injections of BOTOX® and soft tissue fillers and implants will produce longer lasting results than if the nasolabial folds were treated solely with either alone.
7. Successful treatment of the nasolabial fold is absolutely dependent upon proper patient assessment of what actually is causing and increasing the fold and sulcus.

the upper lip, an eklabion or lip ptosis as well as lip asymmetry and lack of oral sphincter control. For these reasons, it is probably most advisable not to treat this area of the mid face with BOTOX® unless the patient is willing to endure unconditionally the expected untoward sequelae. Injecting the melolabial sulcus with a soft tissue filler and resurfacing the cheeks by chemical peeling, dermabrasion, or laser abrasion is probably a more dependable way to address these problems and produce the best consistent results most of the time.

Exaggerated upper gum smile

Introduction: problem assessment and patient selection

Some individuals have a tendency to reveal an excessive amount of their upper gum mucosa when they smile or laugh. This commonly is seen as a familial trait, which is especially disconcerting in women who display this type of smile. Most of the time, since this is a source of considerable embarrassment, one can observe these individuals concealing with their fingertips the appearance of their teeth when they smile or laugh. Also, while speaking in an animated fashion which causes them to smile or laugh during the conversation, they can be seen covering their mouths in whatever way possible. No matter how hard they try, it is impossible for these individuals to smile or laugh without revealing their upper gum mucosa. Consequently, they attempt only to smile partially when being photographed or during social interactions, which creates a certain amount of anxiety for those affected and who are more self-conscious. These individuals commonly tend to have sharply defined nasolabial folds with deep furrows (Figure 4.22).

Some patients, in conjunction with the inadvertent shortening of their upper lip causing an exaggerated gingival smile, also are plagued with exhibiting an involuntary lowering of the tip of their nose. There are still others who also form a transverse furrow across the philtrum of their upper lip when they speak, laugh, or smile. Occasionally, the same person will exhibit a combination of these changes. A horizontal furrow across the upper lip usually is seen in older individuals or in those whose photodamaged skin has reduced elasticity and soft tissue bulk, causing the lax upper lip skin to wrinkle easily with every lip movement (Figure 4.23). Many of these individuals have a long history of smoking tobacco.

Functional anatomy

The ideal tooth exposure when smiling has been calculated to be three-quarters of the dental crown height of the upper incisors and no more exposure than 1–2 mm of upper gum mucosa.

Figure 4.22 Individuals with a gummy smile commonly will have deep nasolabial folds and furrows as seen in this 23 year old

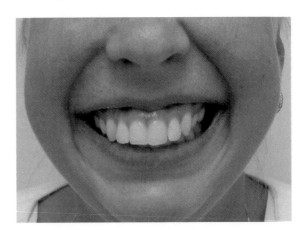

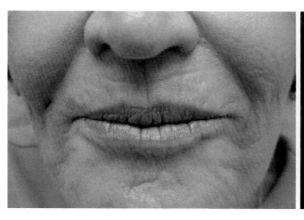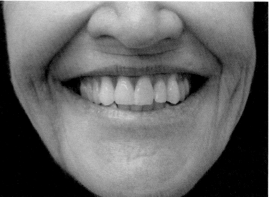

Figure 4.23 A transverse rhytide is seen across the philtrum of the upper lip at rest, which is intensified with smiling in this 68-year-old non-cigarette smoker with extensive photodamage. Note the minimal gummy smile and the slight nasal tip depression with smiling

Generally, men show less gum and interlabial excursion than women[19,20]. There are many reasons for this 'gingival smile,' which is the result of an increase in the interlabial space combined with an excessive contraction of the upper lip levators, producing an excessive amount of exposure of the gums upon smiling or laughing[19,20]. Additional causes of this exaggerated upper gum smile, include an elongation of facial height created by an excessive vertical length of the maxilla, a genetically short upper lip, and a short crown length with or without malpositioning of the incisors.

Functionally, according to Rubin, there are three patterns of smiles by which an individual is identified[21,22]. The first and most commonly encountered type of smile (67 per cent of the patients studied) is when the zygomaticus major dominates the movement of the lips. This is called the 'Mona Lisa' smile and is initiated with a sharp elevation and outward pull of the corners of the mouth and then a soft elevation of the center of the upper lip, revealing approximately 80 per cent of the incisors (Figure 4.24). This type of smile is produced predominantly by the pull of the zygomaticus major.

The canine smile is the second most commonly identified smile pattern (35 per cent of the patients studied) and is characterized by a high elevation of the center of the upper lip, exposing

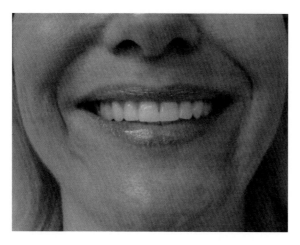

Figure 4.24 The most common type of smile is produced primarily by the pull of the zygomaticus major

Figure 4.25 The canine smile exposes the canine teeth before the rest of the upper lip is elevated

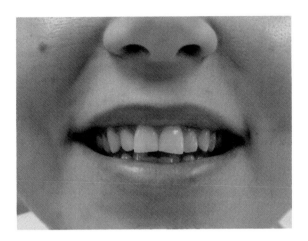

the canine teeth first before the rest of the upper lip is elevated (Figure 4.25). The canine smile can produce anywhere from a partial central dental reveal to an exaggerated full denture show with a certain amount of gingival exposure (Figure 4.22). This pattern of smile is produced predominantly by a contraction of the levator labii superioris elevating the upper lip. When the contraction of the levator labii superioris is intense and severe, a gummy smile results.

The third and least commonly seen smile pattern is the full denture smile, which was seen in about 2 per cent of the patients studied. The full denture smile is characterized by the simultaneous separation of both the upper and lower lips in which both the upper and lower dentures have partial or full exposure. This type of smile is the result of the contraction of all the upper lip levators and lower lip depressors around the mouth at the same time (Figure 4.26).

Commonly found with a simple canine or an exaggerated canine smile, i.e a 'gummy smile', are individuals with deep nasolabial furrows and highly mounded nasolabial folds (Figure 4.22). These two conditions usually are found together, because contraction of the levator labii superioris alaeque nasi creates a steep medial nasolabial fold while lifting the central upper lip a few extra millimeters, which also can expose gingiva. With such hyperkinetic upper lip levators, asymmetric smiles usually are not uncommon (Figures 4.27 and 4.28). (See Appendix 4)

Figure 4.26 The full denture smile is characterized by the simultaneous partial or full exposure of both upper and lower dentures

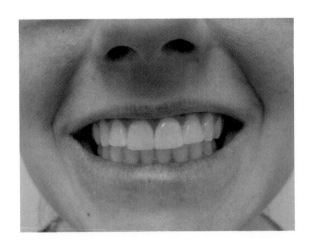

Dilution

Injecting minimal amounts of low-volume BOTOX® in the central face is of paramount importance. The least amount of unintended diffusion of BOTOX® in this area of stratified tiers of different muscle bundles can be disastrous to the overall therapeutic success and cosmetic appearance of the patient and the tenure of reputation of a physician injector. Therefore, most qualified physicians treating this area of the face will reconstitute a 100 U vial of BOTOX® with only 1ml of normal saline (see Appendix 1).

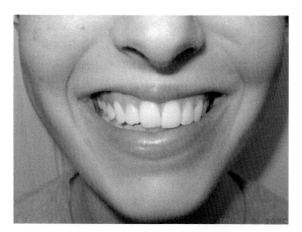

Figure 4.27 Hyperkinetic upper lip levators create a slight gummy smile, that is asymmetrically higher on the upper right side in this 20-year-old. Note the deep nasolabial folds

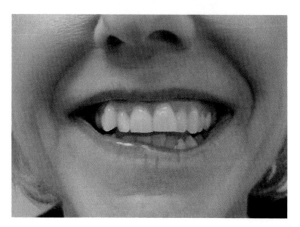

Figure 4.28 Hyperkinetic upper lip levators create a slight gummy smile in this 47-year-old who also has an asymmetric smile caused by her left depressor labii inferioris. Note the deep nasolabial folds

Dosing: how to correct the problem (what to do and what not to do)

To non-surgically elongate the upper lip, especially during a smile, the central upper lip levators need to be gently relaxed (not paralyzed) with injections of BOTOX®. With the patient in a sitting or semireclined position, injections of 1–2 U of BOTOX® applied perpendicularly to the surface of the skin and deeply into the nasofacial groove can be administered (Figures 4.19 and 4.20). This can be accomplished by palpating the nasomaxillary groove with the fingertip of the index finger of the non-dominant hand, until the finger tip pad straddles the lower lateral aspect of

Figure 4.29 Place the needle perpendicular to the skin surface and inject 1–2 U of BOTOX® deeply into the belly of the muscle at the nasomaxillary groove while the patient smiles excessively

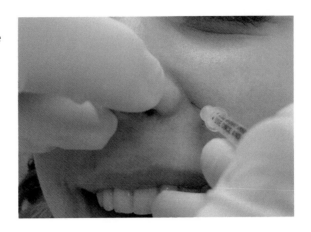

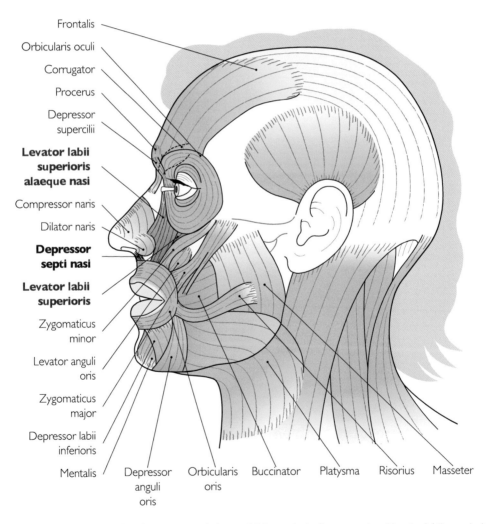

Figure 4.30 The central lip levators (i.e. direct retractors): levator labii superioris alaeque nasi and levator labii superioris and the indirect retractor, depressor septi nasi

the alar facial sulcus and the superior edge of the maxillary alveolar process. Excessive pressure with palpation in this area can cause some discomfort to the patient, so this maneuver should be done as expeditiously as possible. As the patient smiles with the finger in this position, contraction of the levator labii superioris alaeque nasi can be felt. At the point of maximum thickness of the muscle, 1–2 U of BOTOX® can be injected deeply intramuscularly and just above the periosteum (Figure 4.29). Remember to reserve this injection technique only for those patients who have an exaggerated gingival smile, and in whom the levator labii superioris alaeque nasi can be palpated. Also, remember that injecting BOTOX® at this site may reduce the height and extent of the nasolabial fold by weakening the levator labii superioris and the levator labii superioris alaeque nasi (Figure 4.30). The more laterally located muscles, i.e. zygomaticus major and minor, levator anguli oris, and risorius, are to be avoided; otherwise, either an adynamic or asymmetric smile can result. If migration of BOTOX® extends into the superficial fibers of the orbicularis oris an inability to fully pucker the lips also will occur. Another technique is to inject 1–2 U of BOTOX® intraorally into the bellies of the two central upper lip levators[19] (Figure 4.31) by passing the needle through the gingivo-labial sulcus above the alveolar ridge at the same point in the nasofacial groove as described above. A minimum dose of low-volume BOTOX® should just barely relax the central upper lip levators so that the upper lip cannot fully retract upward (Figure 4.32) (see Appendix 2). If the excessive gummy show is at its highest in the center of the upper lip, then 1 U of BOTOX® may need to be injected into the distal half of the depressor septi nasi (Figure 4.30).

Outcomes (results)

Because of the anatomy of the different co-dependent muscles and their attachments in the area of the upper lip skin and orbicularis oris, the risk–benefit ratio of treating a patient with a gingival smile is high and the potential co-morbidity is significant. Treating those patients with an exaggerated gingival smile can produce a variety of anatomic and functional changes. By limiting the exaggerated upward movement of the upper lip with injections of BOTOX® an obvious reduction in the amount of upper gingival and dental show will result, along with an elongation of the upper lip, a flattening of the philtrum, a thinning of the vermillion, and an effacement of the medial aspect of the nasolabial fold and sulcus (Figure 4.19). In addition, it is

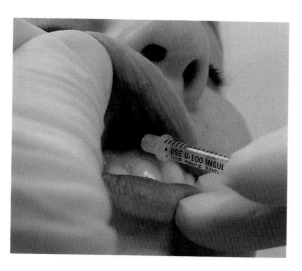

Figure 4.31 The intraoral injection of the central lip levators may be less painful to the patient, but a less precise way of injecting by the physician

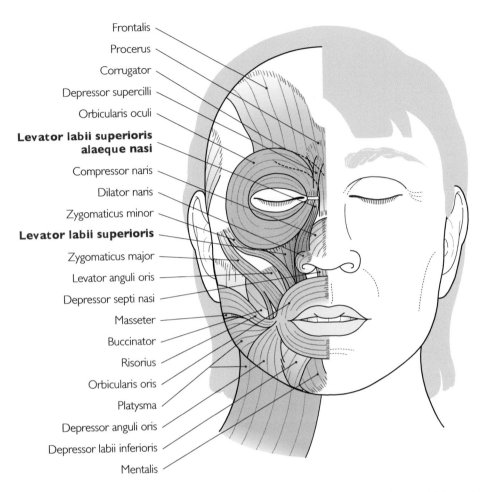

Frontalis
Procerus
Corrugator
Depressor supercilli
Orbicularis oculi
Levator labii superioris alaeque nasi
Compressor naris
Dilator naris
Zygomaticus minor
Levator labii superioris
Zygomaticus major
Levator anguli oris
Depressor septi nasi
Masseter
Buccinator
Risorius
Orbicularis oris
Platysma
Depressor anguli oris
Depressor labii inferioris
Mentalis

Figure 4.32 The central lip levators (i.e. direct retractors): levator labii superioris alaeque nasi and levator labii superioris

possible to diminish the appearance of an idiosyncratic horizontal rhytid when and if it is present across the transverse aspect of the upper lip. An additional 1–2 U of BOTOX® at the base of the columella into the depressor septi nasi by the technique described above (p. 134) may be necessary to further eliminate the central aspect of this horizontal upper lip rhytid (Figure 4.23). Remember to avoid injecting and affecting the deep fibers of the orbicularis oris, otherwise lip incompetence and asymmetry will occur. No more than 2 U of BOTOX® at each injection site should be attempted, especially during the initial treatment session.

In patients with extremely thin and atrophic lips, the transverse lip rhytides may not be amenable to treatments of BOTOX®, because atrophic skin will readily crease and develop wrinkling superficially with the least bit of lip movement. The majority of patients who develop the transverse rhytides across their upper lip seem to be those over the age of 60 years who are of light complexion (usually of skin type I–III), have spent a lot of time outdoors, and may or may not have a history of smoking tobacco (Figure 4.23) (see Appendix 3).

Complications (adverse sequelae) (see Appendix 5)

Assistance with an electromyograph (EMG) might ensure a more accurate needle placement and avoid untoward results when attempting to treat an exaggerated upper gum smile with injections of BOTOX®. Inaccurate needle placement or overzealous dosing in this area is subject to upper lip ptosis, which, in turn, might be coupled with buccal sphincter incompetence, difficulty with producing particular sounds and articulating certain words, and an inability to move the upper lip in a full smile or pucker, because the upper lip levators (i.e. levator labii superioris alaeque, levator labii superioris, the zygomaticus complex, risorius, levator anguli oris, and orbicularis oris) (Figure 4.33) can easily be affected by the least amount of diffusion of the BOTOX®. Buccal sphincter incompetence can result in an embarrassing incontinence of liquid or solids.

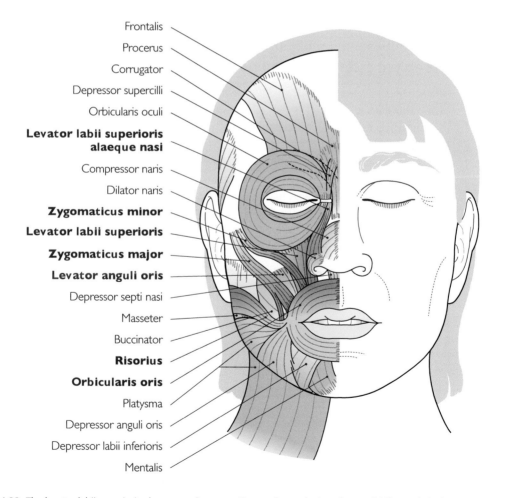

Figure 4.33 The levator labii superioris alaeque nasi, zygomaticus major and minor, levator labii superioris, levator anguli oris, risorius and obicularis oris participate in buccal sphincter competence

Treatment implications when injecting a gummy smile

1. Injecting the levator labii superioris alaeque nasi can reduce exaggerated gingival show by elongating the upper lip. It also will efface the nasolabial sulcus and fold and flatten the philtrum and vermillion.
2. Only inject the levator labii superioris alaeque nasi when it can be palpated, otherwise, non-targeted muscles will be affected, and lip competence and symmetry will be compromised.
3. Prior to any treatment with BOTOX®, inform the patient of the risk to benefit ratio, potential co-morbidities, and inherent topographical and cosmetic changes expected when perioral mimetic muscles are weakened.
4. Patients with either a zygomatic ('Mona Lisa') smile, a full denture or a canine smile without exaggerated gingival exposure should not be treated with BOTOX® injections to reduce the nasolabial folds (see previous section).

Asymmetric smile

Introduction: problem assessment and patient selection

Many men and women are born with an asymmetric smile (idiopathic asymmetry) (Figure 4.27, 4.28, and 4.34 to 4.36). This also can be manifested as a familial trait, which is especially disconcerting for women who display this type of smile (Figure 4.37). For many of these individuals this is a source of considerable embarrassment, especially when they are in a socially interactive situation. Just like those with a gummy smile, but not as frequently, they are reticent to openly show their smile in public, and seek ways to hide their mouths when laughing or smiling with others. Those who have a prominent position in the workplace are especially self-conscious of an obviously 'crooked smile', and prefer not to smile when being photographed.

Functional anatomy

No matter what type of smile one has (zygomatic, canine, or full denture) if it is asymmetrical or 'crooked' it is always a source of anxiety and self-consciousness for the bearer, whether male or

Figure 4.34 In this 55-year-old female an asymmetric smile is caused by hyperkinetic lateral levators of the left side of the upper lip

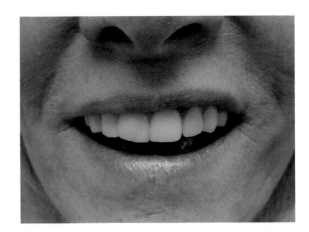

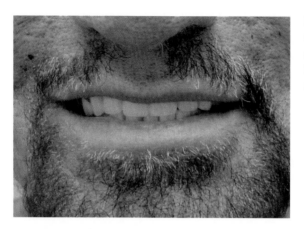

Figure 4.35 In this 62-year-old male an asymmetric smile is caused by hyperkinetic central levators of the right side of the upper lip

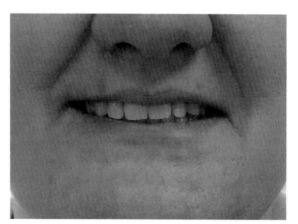

Figure 4.36 In this 46-year-old female an asymmetric smile is caused by weakened elevators of the left lateral upper lip and angle of the mouth (zygomaticus, levator anguli oris, risorius). Note the down turned commissure on the left

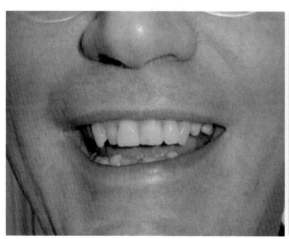
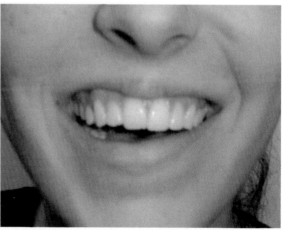

Figure 4.37 Father (55 years old) and daughter (20 years old) manifesting the same type of idiosyncratic, asymmetric smile caused by a hyperkinetic right depressor labii inferioris. The daughter also has a mild gummy smile with deep nasolabial grooves and folds

female. Aside from a segmental weakening of the upper lip levators or the orbicularis oris, an asymmetric smile can be created by the unilateral malfunctioning of a lower lip depressor that is usually weaker or stronger than its contralateral paired muscle. This commonly occurs with either the depressor anguli oris or the depressor labii inferioris, or both, and also with isolated, portions of muscle fibers of the upper or lower orbicularis oris.

The depressor labii inferioris is a quadrilateral muscle that originates from the oblique line of the mandible between the symphysis menti and the mental foramen (Figure 4.38). Its fibers travel upward and medially to insert into the skin and mucosa of the lower lip, decussating with fibers of its paired muscle from the opposite side along with some muscle fibers of the orbicularis oris. Inferiorly and laterally it is continuous with the platysma (pars labialis) (Figure 4.39).

The function of the depressor labii inferioris is to pull the lower lip downward and slightly laterally when a person is chewing, smiling, laughing, or speaking, and it can help evert the lower lip when necessary. It should act in unison with its paired counterpart on the opposite side of the chin, and therefore in a symmetric fashion, which is not always the case in some individuals. The depressor labii inferioris is one of the muscles used when expressing sorrow, irony, melancholy, and doubt. (See Appendix 4).

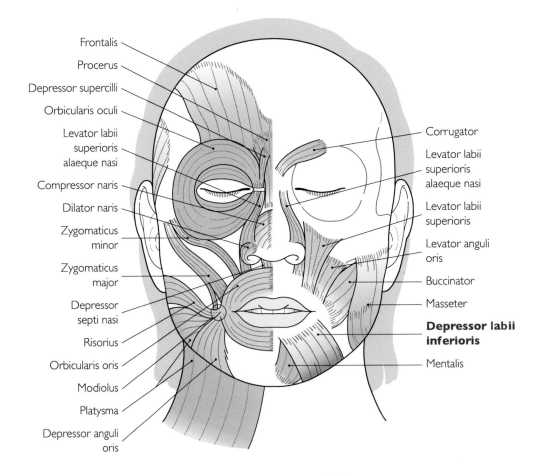

Figure 4.38 Depressor labii inferioris is a square, deeply situated muscle on the chin

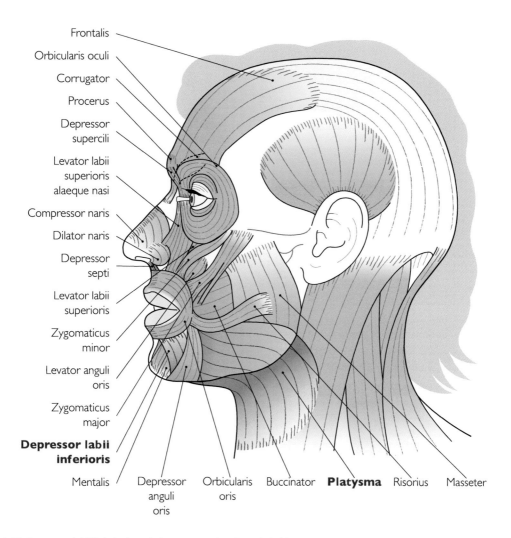

Frontalis
Orbicularis oculi
Corrugator
Procerus
Depressor
supercili
Levator labii
superioris
alaeque nasi
Compressor naris
Dilator naris
Depressor
septi
Levator labii
superioris
Zygomaticus
minor
Levator anguli
oris
Zygomaticus
major
**Depressor labii
inferioris**
Mentalis   Depressor   Orbicularis   Buccinator   **Platysma**   Risorius   Masseter
              anguli   oris
              oris

Figure 4.39 Depressor labii inferioris and platysma can interlace their fibers in some individuals

Dilution

Because of the widespread interlacing of muscle fibers in the perioral area, the success of treating a particular muscle in the lower face is predicated upon not having the BOTOX® diffuse beyond the area of injection. Consequently, minimal amounts of low-volume, highly concentrated BOTOX® should be used when targeting a perioral muscle for treatment. Therefore, experienced physicians will reconstitute a 100 U vial of BOTOX® with only 1 ml of normal saline (see Appendix 1).

Dosing: how to correct the problem (what to do and what not to do)

Depending on the particular situation, the type of asymmetry to be corrected and the location and strength of the muscle to be weakened it is usually advisable for the injector to determine the appropriate dose of BOTOX® necessary for injection at the time of treatment. Ordinarily, the

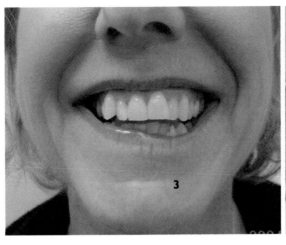
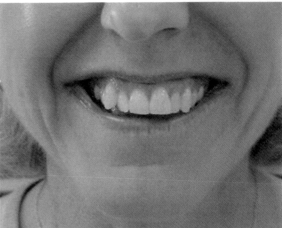

Figure 4.40 This 47-year-old with an idiosyncratic asymmetric smile is shown before and 3 weeks after 3 U of BOTOX® were injected into her left depressor labii inferioris

stronger side of the face is weakened with injections of BOTOX® to correct an asymmetry (Figure 4.40). Each patient's problem should be evaluated individually and a solution determined according to the patient's idiosyncratic anatomy.

Prior to injection the patient should be in the sitting position and contracting the muscle to be treated. The needle should pass perpendicular to the skin's surface and enter directly into the belly (thickest part) of the muscle (see Appendix 2).

Outcomes (results)

When the problem has been correctly assessed, and the proper conservative dose of BOTOX® determined, weakening the hyperkinetic muscle on the side of the face producing the asymmetry with injections of BOTOX® will correct the asymmetry (Figures 4.40 and 4.41). The

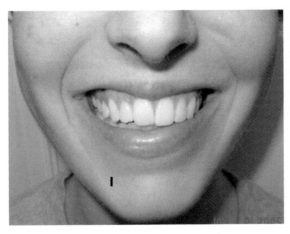
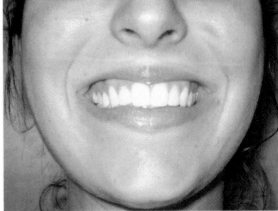

Figure 4.41 This 20-year-old with an idiosyncratic asymmetric smile is shown before and 1 month after 1 U of BOTOX® was injected into her right depressor labii inferioris

effect of the treatment should last at least 3 months, if not longer. It is best to attempt to correct an asymmetry with a lower dose, which can be increased by a touch-up treatment 2–3 weeks later when the patient returns for his or her obligatory post-treatment evaluation. It is better to correct a problem conservatively, albeit insufficiently, so that the appropriateness of the corrective action can be confirmed. Subsequently, additional units of BOTOX® can then be injected with confidence to adequately treat the problem to the satisfaction of the patient and physician (see Appendix 3).

Complications (adverse sequelae) (see Appendix 5)

A fallacious assessment and conclusion to a problem can produce incomplete and even improper results which can become an intolerable annoyance to the patient. Therefore, a thorough knowledge of the anatomy and function of the muscles of the face and area of the body to be treated is absolutely necessary when one is attempting to treat a patient with BOTOX®, whether or not the problem is a recognized commonly occurring complaint with well-established and approved techniques of treatment (i.e. glabellar frown lines) or an idiosyncratic or iatrogenic asymmetry. Overzealous treatment of any problem can only lead to adverse sequelae which are all dependent on the location and the particular muscle or muscles in which the problem resides. In the case of an asymmetric smile, the same complications of an adynamic smile and incompetent buccal sphincter causing difficulty with eating, drinking, swallowing, and speech articulation can occur.

Treatment implications when injecting an asymmetric smile

1. Know the anatomy and function of the muscle(s) to be treated.
2. Inject low-volume, minimal doses of BOTOX® directly into the muscle(s) in question.
3. First treatments should be conservative with low doses of BOTOX® to confirm the appropriateness of the treatment.
4. All first-time and repeatedly treated patients must be re-evaluated 2–3 weeks after a BOTOX® treatment session to assess their results and to monitor their satisfaction with the outcome.
5. Assess and treat each and every patient individually. No two patients or their problems are alike and therefore cannot be treated the same.

References

1. Carruthers J, Carruthers A. Botulinum toxin (BOTOX®) use in the mid and lower face and neck. *Semin Cutan Med Surg* 2001;20:85–92
2. Matarasso A. Discussion: new indications for botulinum toxin type A in cosmetics: mouth and neck. *Plast Reconstr Surg* 2003;110:86S–87S
3. Fagien S. BOTOX® for the treatment of dynamic and hyperkinetic facial lines and furrows: adjunctive use in facial aesthetic surgery. *Plast Reconstr Surg* 1999;103:701–7
4. Manaloto RM, Alster TS. Periorbital rejuvenation: a review of dermatologic treatments. *Dermatol Surg* 1999;25:1–9
5. Carruthers A, Kiene K, Carruthers J. Botulinum A exotoxin use in clinical dermatology. *J Am Acad Dermatol* 1996;34:788–97

6. Carruthers J, Carruthers A. Botulinum toxin (BOTOX®) chemodenervation for facial rejuvenation. *Facial Plast Surg* 2001;9:197–204

7. Carruthers J, Carruthers A. Practical cosmetic BOTOX® techniques. *J Cutaneous Med Surg* 1999;3 (Suppl 4):55–9

8. Blitzer A, Binder WJ. Current practices in the use of botulinum toxin in the management of facial lines and wrinkles. *Facial Plast Surg* 2001;9:395–404

9. Matarasso SL. Complications of botulinum A exotoxin for hyperfunctional lines. *Derm Surg* 1998;24:1249–54

10. Goldwyn R, Rohrich R. Consensus recommendations on the use of botulinum toxin type A in facial aesthetics. Supplement to *Plast Reconstr Surg* 2004;114:1S–22S

11. Tamura BM, Odo MY, Changi B et al. Treatment of nasal wrinkles with botulinum toxin. *Derm Surg* 2005;3:271–5

12. LeLouran C. Botulinum toxin A and facial lines: the variable concentration. *Aesthet Plast Surg* 2001;25:73–84

13. Almeida AT de Nose. In: Excel D, Almeida AT de (eds). *Cosmetic use of Botulinum Toxin*. Porto Allergre, Brazil: AGE Editora, 2002:158–63

14. Atamoros, PF. Botulinum toxin in the lower one-third of the face. *Clin Derm* 2003;21:505–12

15. Pessa JE, Brown F. Independent effect of various facial mimetic muscles on the nasolabial fold. *Aesth Plast Surg* 1992;16:167–71

16. Hoefflin SM. Anatomy of the platysma and lip depressor muscles. A simplified mnemonic approach. *Dermatol Surg* 1998;24:1225–31

17. Rohrich RJ, James JE, Fagien S *et al*. The cosmetic use of botulinum toxin. *Plast Reconstr Surg* 2003;112(Suppl):177S

18. Matarasso SL, Matarasso A. Treatment guidelines for botulinum toxin type A for the periocular region and a report on partial upper lip ptosis following injections to the lateral canthal rhytides. *Plast Reconstr Surg* 2001;108:208–14

19. Kokich V, Nappen D, Shapiro P. Gingival contour and clinical crown length: their effects on the esthetic appearance of maxillary anterior teeth. *Am J Orthod* 1984;86:89–94

20. Arnett GW, Bergman RJ. Facial key to orthodontic diagnosis and treatment planning. *Am J Orthod and Dentofac Orthop* 1993; Part I 103:299–312, Part II 395–411

21. Rubin LR. The anatomy of a smile: its importance in the treatment of facial paralysis. *Plast Reconstr Surg* 1974;53:384–7

22. Rubin LR. The anatomy of the nasolabial fold: the keystone of the smiling mechanism. *Plast Reconstr Surg* 1999;103:687–91

5 COSMETIC USES OF BOTULINUM TOXIN A IN THE LOWER FACE, NECK AND UPPER CHEST

Anthony V Benedetto

Introduction

Anatomic delineation of the lower face for our purpose encompasses the perioral region and chin, which is the area that includes the remainder of the superficial muscles of facial expression. The orbicularis oris provides motor function to the upper and lower lips, and the corners of the mouth. The remaining facial muscles consist mostly of the upper lip levators and the depressors of the lower lip, which are not necessarily antagonistic to each other, but act more synergistically with one another, opening and closing the mouth and performing essential buccal functions in unison with the orbicularis oris, such as maintaining sphincter control and lip competence with or without a mouth filled with solid material, liquid, or air. Other vital functions of the orbicularis oris together with its levators and depressors include the ability to make sounds and articulate them into speech, chew, and swallow solids and liquids. This is in direct contrast with the upper face where levators and depressors take on an antagonistic role and are in direct opposition to each another. In addition, by contracting the orbicularis oris along with its levators and depressors in a particularly idiosyncratic manner, a person consciously or unconsciously can express various and sundry emotions.

In the lower face some, if not all of the upper lip levators and the lower lip depressors interdigitate with the fibers of the orbicularis oris, which also can function as an antagonistic muscle to them and perform the opposite movement of either the levators and the depressors after they have moved in unison to separate or approximate the lips when opening or closing the mouth, as one does when blowing air or liquid out of the mouth. After the completion of a particular function by the labial levators and depressors, the orbicularis oris can move in the opposite direction to open or shut the mouth by pursing or puckering the lips.

This subtle but functional difference in the way the various perioral muscles operate plays a significant role in how to devise a treatment plan with BOTOX®. One cannot just identify a levator or a depressor in the lower face and weaken it like in the upper face with injections of BOTOX® without potential consequences of lip asymmetry, sphincter incompetence affecting mastication or deglutition, and a disturbance in sound production and word pronunciation. Because of these functional differences and the complex muscle interactions in the lower face, only the experienced physician should attempt to reduce various rhytides of the lower face or correct anatomic variations and asymmetries of this area with injections of BOTOX®. Otherwise, what was intended to be remedied might very easily be exacerbated.

Perioral lip lines or rhytides

Introduction: problem assessment and patient selection

As the eyes are the center of focus for the upper face, enabling an individual to express deep felt emotions and personal sentiment, the mouth also is the center of focus for the mid and lower face. A full lip with a smooth and distinct border of the vermillion delineating it from the rest of the lip is the hallmark of youth with all its pristine beauty. With time and sun exposure, the lips become thin, flaccid, elongated and wrinkled, lacking substance and contour. What once reflected a person's vitality and sensuality now reveals the passing years of trials and tribulation leaving one appearing weary and worn, evidenced by wrinkles on the face, and betrayed by perioral rhytides.

Both static and dynamic wrinkling can be found around the mouth appearing as vertical lip lines perpendicular to the vermillion border. It has been shown that static perioral wrinkles are caused not only by intrinsic aging and photodamage, but also are precipitated by tobacco smoking. Frequent and chronic cigarette smoking also can augment perioral dynamic wrinkles, probably because of the persistent lip puckering and pursing needed to hold a cigarette in the mouth while inhaling and exhaling tobacco smoke (Figure 5.1). Dynamic perioral wrinkles are found in those who are genetically predisposed and frequently pout and repetitively purse their lips, whether voluntarily or involuntarily. This is seen more commonly in women in the way they habitually move (i.e. pucker or purse) their lips during routine daily activities of eating, drinking, and speaking (Figure 5.2). Other activities, such as cigarette smoking, sipping liquids from a straw, and playing certain musical wind instruments, provide a supplemental role in the

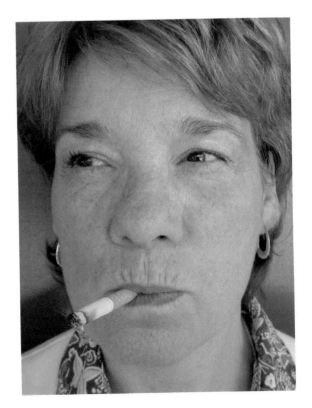

Figure 5.1 Note the perioral wrinkles that are produced when this 56 year old inhales on a cigarette

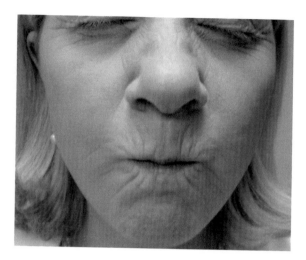

Figure 5.2   Note the perioral wrinkles in this 57-year-old woman expressing her displeasure and exasperation by pursing her lips

formation of dynamic perioral rhytides. Repeated purse-string-like movements of the orbicularis oris exaggerate and intensify the dynamic perioral lines on a daily basis. Men usually are not in the habit of pursing or puckering their lips as is commonly done by women. Consequently, men are less afflicted than women with perioral wrinkling, nor are they bothered by peribuccal rhytides when and if they occur. Women are particularly frustrated by these lines, especially when lipstick channels up and down these rhytides blurring the outline of the vermillion.

There are many other causes for these perioral vertical lines besides repetitive puckering of the orbicularis oris, which include chronological aging and environmental exposure, all of which can be manifested mostly as static wrinkling. Static wrinkling can be the result of identifiable causes, like age and sun exposure, and unknown causes like genetics, gender differences, intrinsic soft tissue characteristics, and anatomic idiosyncrasies like the shape of the mouth and how it functions on a daily basis. Much of the static wrinkling of the perioral area can be reduced by invasive surgical procedures such as facial skin resurfacing, either by laser, mechanical dermabrasion or chemical peeling, and other different types of surgical procedures like rhytidectomy, and various surgical plasties, implants, and excisions. It also can be reduced by non-invasive procedures such as injections of various soft tissue fillers.

It is important to distinguish the dynamic wrinkles of the lips from those that are static, which are intrinsically produced because of photodamage and chronologic aging. Static wrinkling usually is not affected by treatment with BOTOX®. Static wrinkles can be easily distinguished from dynamic wrinkles by asking a person to purse their lips. If there are rhytides present in the lips prior to pursing the lips and there is minimal change or intensification of these wrinkles with movement, especially in someone over the age of 60–65 years or in a younger person who possesses extensive solar elastosis of their exposed skin, then their perioral rhytides are primarily static and probably unamenable to treatment with BOTOX® (Figure 5.3). If the wrinkles intensify and deepen with lip movement and puckering no matter how young or old a person is, then these are dynamic wrinkles and can be diminished with injections of BOTOX® (Figure 5.4a,b).

Functional anatomy

The shape of the mouth and the position of the lips are controlled by a complex three-dimensional arrangement of interlacing and decussating bundles of different facial muscles.

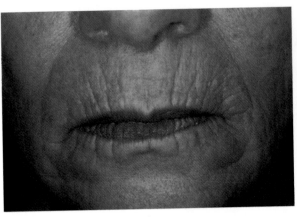 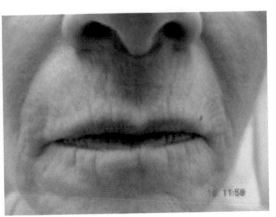

Before   1 month after

Figure 5.3   This 72-year-old has deep peribuccal rhytides and moderate solar elastosis of the face and lips at rest. Her peribuccal rhytides barely intensified with puckering. Note the presence of most of the peribuccal rhytides that persist 1 month after a treatment of BOTOX®, because the bulk of her wrinkles were age related and of the static type. Note also the eversion and fullness of the upper lip, that were intensified by puckering, seen 1 month after a treatment with BOTOX®

These include various levators (retractors and evertors) of the upper lip (i.e. levator labii superioris alaeque nasi, levator labii superioris, zygomaticus major et minor, levator anguli oris, and risorius), various depressors, retractors, and evertors of the lower lip (depressor labii inferioris, depressor anguli oris, and mentalis), a multilamellar, compound sphincter (the orbicularis oris), and the buccinator[1].

The orbicularis oris is not a simple sphincter like the orbicularis oculi. It is comprised of multiple lamellae of muscular fibers traversing in different directions around the orifice of the mouth. It is composed partly of muscle fibers from other facial muscles that insert into the lips and partly from fibers intrinsic to the lips. The orbicularis oris, once felt to be a series of complete ellipses of striated muscle surrounding the buccal orifice and functioning as a sphincter, is now understood to consist of four independent quadrants (right, left, upper, and lower) of striated muscle, each containing a pars peripheralis and a pars marginalis. These two right and left anatomic parts (right and left partes peripheralis and right and left partes marginalis) are juxtaposed to each other respectively, and roughly correspond to the exterior anatomic delineations of the free or unattached portion of the lip. The smaller pars marginalis corresponds to the vermillion of the lip and the larger pars peripheralis corresponds to the remainder of the free unattached portion of the lip that is encompassed by glabrous skin. Consequently, the orbicularis oris is perceived as being composed of eight segments, each resembling a fan, whose apex begins at the modiolus, one set on top of the other (Figure 5.5). Most of the muscle fibers in the pars peripheralis are thought to originate within the modiolus, as a direct continuation of the many modiolar muscles. A considerable number of these muscle fibers also originate from the buccinator, an accessory muscle of mastication, which reinforces the complex of deeper intrinsic muscle fibers of the orbicularis oris. Muscle fibers of the buccinator pass anteriorly and decussate at the angles of the mouth, crisscrossing each other as they continue on to their insertions in the upper and lower lips. Those fibers that arise from the maxilla pass inferiorly around the angle of the mouth and insert into the lower lip. Those fibers that arise from the

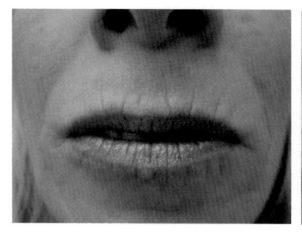

At rest before

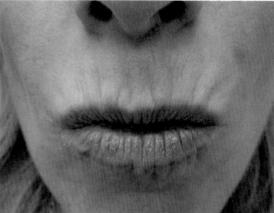

Puckering before

Figure 5.4a   This 53-year-old with deep peribuccal rhytides and severe solar elastosis of the face and lips is shown at rest and with puckering before a treatment with BOTOX®. Note that rhytides intensify with puckering

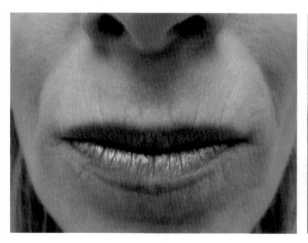

At rest 3 weeks after

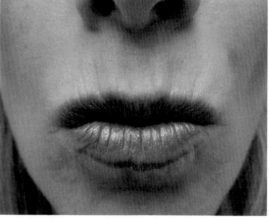

Puckering 3 weeks after

Figure 5.4b   Same patient at rest and 3 weeks after her first treatment of BOTOX®. Note the rhytides at this early post-treatment time have only partially effaced. Note also the fullness and eversion of the vermillion after BOTOX®

mandible travel around the angle of the mouth and insert into the upper lip. The uppermost and lowermost muscle fibers of the buccinator, however, traverse across the lips from side to side in a pursestring fashion without decussating (Figure 5.6).

Superficial to those deep intrinsic muscle fibers is another stratum of muscle fibers formed on either side of the mouth by the levator anguli oris and the depressor anguli oris. The fibers of both the depressor and levator crisscross each other at the corners of the mouth and continue away from each other. The muscle fibers of the levator anguli oris continue inferiorly into the lower lip and insert into the skin near the midline of the lower lip. The muscle fibers of the depressor anguli oris follow the same pattern in the upper lip, inserting into the skin at the

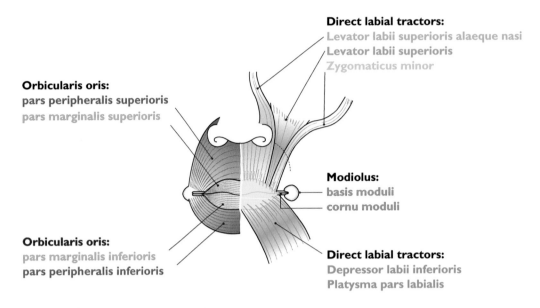

Direct labial tractors:
Levator labii superioris alaeque nasi
Levator labii superioris
Zygomaticus minor

Orbicularis oris:
pars peripheralis superioris
pars marginalis superioris

Modiolus:
basis moduli
cornu moduli

Orbicularis oris:
pars marginalis inferioris
pars peripheralis inferioris

Direct labial tractors:
Depressor labii inferioris
Platysma pars labialis

Figure 5.5   The orbicularis oris. Courtesy of *Gray's Anatomy*

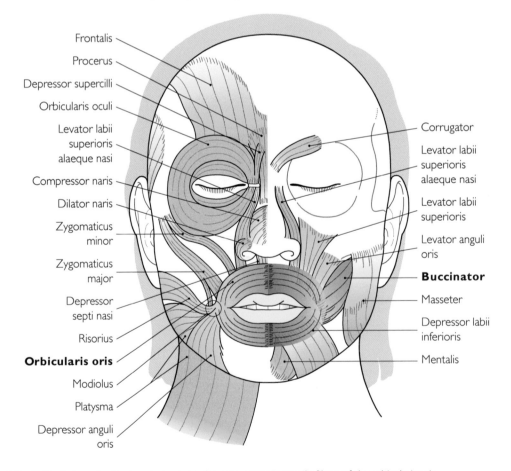

Frontalis
Procerus
Depressor supercilli
Orbicularis oculi
Levator labii superioris alaeque nasi
Compressor naris
Dilator naris
Zygomaticus minor
Zygomaticus major
Depressor septi nasi
Risorius
Orbicularis oris
Modiolus
Platysma
Depressor anguli oris

Corrugator
Levator labii superioris alaeque nasi
Levator labii superioris
Levator anguli oris
Buccinator
Masseter
Depressor labii inferioris
Mentalis

Figure 5.6   Orbicularis oculi – the buccinator helps form the intrinsic muscle fibers of the orbicularis oris

midline. Reinforcing these superficial transverse fibers of the upper and lower lips are interdigitating oblique muscle fibers from the levator labii superioris, the zygomaticus major, and the depressor labii inferioris. In addition, there are the intrinsic muscle fibers of the lips, which run in an oblique direction and pass from the undersurface of the skin through the thickness of the lip and into the mucous membrane. Finally, there are additional slips of muscle fibers of the orbicularis oris which attach to the alveolar process of the maxilla, the nasolabial sulcus, and the nasal ala and septum superiorly and the alveolar process of the mandible inferiorly, anchoring the orbicularis oris in place as low as the mentolabial sulcus. All of these fibers decussate with the other muscle fibers at the angles of the mouth. Most muscle fibers also continue toward the midline, crossing it at least 5 mm into the opposite side of the lip. It is these interlacing and crisscrossing intrinsic fibers in the center of the upper lip that play a role in forming the lateral ridges of the philtrum with its central depression on the skin surface found at the base of the nose in the midline. These interlacing, crisscrossing intrinsic fibers also help form the depression found in the lower lip at the mentolabial sulcus. The pars marginalis of the orbicularis oris is unique to human lips and is crucial in the production of sound and speech (see Appendix 4).

The function of the orbicularis oris is to close the mouth by approximating the lips. By contracting the deep fibers and the superficial oblique ones, the orbicularis oris can apply the lips closely to the alveolar arch. The superficial interdigitating muscle fibers of the orbicularis oris, on the other hand, shape the lips in different configurations and either bring the lips together against the teeth or protrude the lips and the corners of the mouth forward to produce the maneuver of pursing or puckering the lips for certain functions such as whistling or kissing. Because of its mouth-closing function, the orbicularis oris can be considered, in part, an antagonist to the lip levators and depressors.

Direct labial retractors are those levators and depressors that enter directly into the tissue of the lips without passing through and interlacing with the modiolus (Figure 5.5). For the most part, when these muscles contract, they exert a vertical pull at right angles on the buccal aperture. That is, they either elevate or evert in part or entirely the upper lip; and they depress or evert in part or entirely the lower lip (Figure 5.6). The direct lip retractors are from medial to lateral: the lateral labial portion of the levator labii superioris alaeque nasi, levator labii superioris, and zygomaticus minor in the upper lip, and the depressor labii inferioris and platysma (pars labialis) in the lower lip (Figure 5.5). The pars labialis of the platysma is in the same plane as the depressor anguli oris and depressor labii inferioris and interdigitates its fibers with them, occupying any vacant space between them (Figure 5.7). In both the upper and lower lips the direct retractors interlace their fibers into a continuous sheet of muscle superficial to the intrinsic fibers of the pars peripheralis and pars marginalis of the orbicularis oris as they travel through the substance of the free lip and sequentially attach to the undersurface of the dermis and mucous membrane.

The buccinator, on the other hand, is not a typical facial muscle. It is a deep, thin, quadrilateral muscle that spans the void between the maxilla and mandible and forms the deep muscular boundaries of the cheek. It originates from the posterior portion of the alveolar process of the maxilla, from the upper medial surface of the mandible at the junction of the body and ramus, just posteromedial to the last molar and from the pterygomandibular raphe or ligament. This raphe stretches from the medial pterygoid process to the inner surface of the mandible, and represents the line of juncture between the buccinator and the superior constrictor of the pharynx. The muscle fibers of the buccinator traverse forward toward the

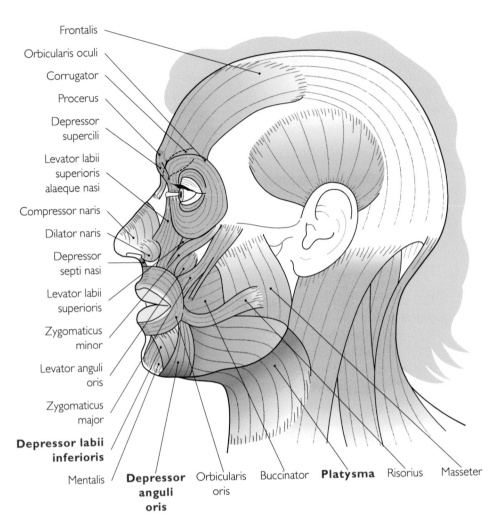

Frontalis
Orbicularis oculi
Corrugator
Procerus
Depressor supercili
Levator labii superioris alaeque nasi
Compressor naris
Dilator naris
Depressor septi nasi
Levator labii superioris
Zygomaticus minor
Levator anguli oris
Zygomaticus major
Depressor labii inferioris
Mentalis
Depressor anguli oris
Orbicularis oris
Buccinator
Platysma
Risorius
Masseter

Figure 5.7   The depressor labii inferioris, depressor anguli oris, and the platysma

modiolus near the angle of the mouth to become continuous with the intrinsic fibers of the orbicularis oris. The upper fibers of the buccinator continue as muscle fibers of the lower lip and the lower fibers of the buccinator merge with those of the upper lip without decussating and insert into the mucous membrane and skin of the upper and lower lips. The buccinator's function is to keep the cheek against the gums and teeth during mastication, holding food between the teeth and preventing it from becoming lodged between the teeth and cheek. It also assists the tongue in directing and maintaining the food between the teeth while chewing. As the mouth closes, the teeth glide over the buccolabial mucosa, which must be continuously and progressively retracted away from the opposing surface of the teeth, otherwise a person would inadvertently bite down on the inner surface of the buccal mucosa consistently.

Contraction of the buccinator also prevents the cheeks from becoming overly distended by positive air pressure when air fills the oral cavity. The buccinator also assists in gradually expelling from inbetween the lips accumulated air within the oral cavity, as when playing a wind instrument or blowing up a balloon (*buccinator* is Latin for trumpet player).

On either side of and just lateral to the oral commissures, a number of mimetic facial muscles converge toward a centralized anatomic location where they interlace their muscle fibers to form a dense, compact, mobile fibromuscular mass called the modiolus (Figure 5.8). As many as seven facial muscles, divided in different bundles within various anatomic planes, converge in a spiraling configuration into the modiolus, interlacing and attaching to it, each in their own distinctive way. Each person's modiolus is subject to individual variation, predicated upon their age, sex, ethnic, and genetic background. The modiolus has no precisely delineated anatomic boundaries, nor does it have uniformly recognizable histologic features. The modiolus has the overall configuration of a blunt kidney-shaped cone (Figure 5.5). Its base (basis moduli) is adjacent and adherent to the buccal mucosa. It is located approximately 2 cm lateral to the center of the oral commissure and measures about 2 cm above and below an imaginary horizontal line that passes through the center of the oral commissure. From mucosa to dermis, its vertical thickness is approximately 1 cm. The facial artery passes through an oblique fibrous cleft through its center. The cone-shaped modiolus is extended by two rounded edges or cornua which give it its kidney shape and which extend into the lateral tissue margin of the free lip, above and below the angle of the mouth (Figure 5.5).

The subtle, three-dimensional movements of a modiolus, either bilaterally and symmetrically or unilaterally and asymmetrically, enable one to integrate common, routine movements of the cheeks, lips, jaws, oral aperture and vestibule into the daily activites of biting, chewing, drinking, sucking, swallowing, and controlling changes in oral vestibular contents and pressure. The innumerable subtle variations in movement involved in speech, the generation and modulation of sounds and musical tones or the harsh sounds used in shouting, screaming, crying, and all the permutations of facial expression, ranging from mere hints to exaggerated distortions, be they symmetric or asymmetric, are enabled by the intricately synergistic and subtle displacements of the modiolus.

Many of the major movements of the modiolus seem to involve most, if not all, of its associated muscles, whose actions are predicated upon the amount of separation between the upper and lower teeth (i.e. the gape of the mouth). The principal modiolar muscles include the zygomaticus major, levator anguli oris, depressor anguli oris, platysma pars modiolus, risorius, and the main functional sphincteric effectors, the buccinator and orbicularis oris (Figure 5.8). As the interlabial and interdental distances approach their maximum separation of about 4 cm, the modiolus occupies the interdental space, moves anteriorly 1 cm closer to the oral commissure, and becomes immobile. With the mouth wide open, the nasolabial sulci elongate, becoming straighter and more vertical, and the inferior buccolabial sulci (marionette lines) are less deep and curved. With the lips in contact and the teeth in tight approximation, the modiolus can move only a few millimeters in all directions. The mobility of the modiolus is maximized when the upper and lower teeth are separated by 2–3 mm, similar to its position when speaking. The muscular modiolar activities are enhanced by the partial separation of the jaws, integrating buccal functional movements with the direct labial retractors (levators of the upper lip and depressors of the lower lip). All of the delicate but complex movements of the lips and mouth can be consciously and many times involuntarily set into motion from moment to moment by subtle and intricate contractions of the multifariously complex mimetic muscles of the perioral area. (See Appendix 4).

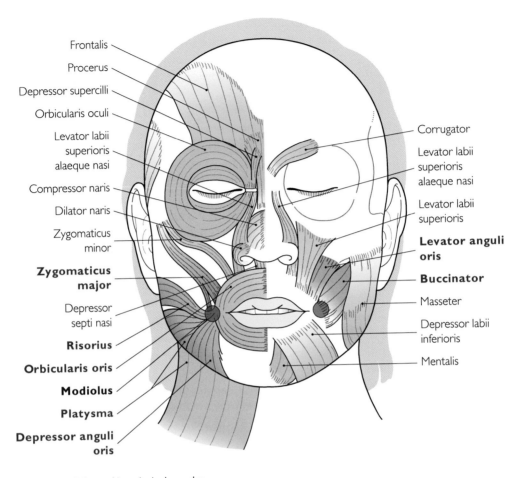

Frontalis
Procerus
Depressor supercilli
Orbicularis oculi
Levator labii superioris alaeque nasi
Compressor naris
Dilator naris
Zygomaticus minor
Zygomaticus major
Depressor septi nasi
Risorius
Orbicularis oris
Modiolus
Platysma
Depressor anguli oris

Corrugator
Levator labii superioris alaeque nasi
Levator labii superioris
Levator anguli oris
Buccinator
Masseter
Depressor labii inferioris
Mentalis

Figure 5.8   The modiolus and its principal muscles

Dilution

When injecting BOTOX® into the orbicularis oris, minimal dosage must be used[2]. Because there may be a multitude of vertical lines across the lips, concentrated BOTOX® will not spread readily across the expanse of the surface of the superficial fibers of the orbicularis oris. In order to have the BOTOX® spread evenly and extensively over the superficial fibers of the orbicularis oris, one can reconstitute a 100 U vial of BOTOX® with anywhere from 1 to 4 ml of normal saline. In this way, dilute, large volumes of BOTOX® can be allowed to spread across the expanse of the superficial fibers of the orbicularis oris when only 1 or 2 U are injected in each quadrant of the pars peripheralis of the upper and lower lips. Applying BOTOX® superficially and in low dosages will avoid any compromise in the sphincteric function of the deeper muscle fibers of the orbicularis oris[3,4] (see Appendix 1).

Dosing: how to correct the problem (what to do and what not to do)

Because of the complex nature of the orbicularis oris and the way it functions, injections of BOTOX® in the perioral area should be performed only by an experienced physician injector. Each patient should be evaluated and treated individually, and standard injection points should not necessarily be adhered to in this area or any other area of the face for that matter. BOTOX® or any botulinum toxin should be injected into an area of maximal muscle contraction. This is particularly important in the lips where the vertical lip lines may not be exactly symmetrical and do not always appear at the same depth or location, because they are dependent upon the particular strength of the various superficial fibers of the orbicularis oris at that location along the lip, which are different in every patient.

In properly selected patients in the upright sitting or semirecumbent position, 1–2 U of BOTOX® can be injected into each pars peripheralis of the upper and lower lips at the level of the lower dermis and no deeper than the dermo-subcutaneous junction. At this level the superficial fibers of the orbicularis oris can be found. Injection points can be either into the border between the pars peripheralis and pars marginalis (Figure 5.9), or 3 and no more than 5 mm superior to the vermillion border into the pars peripheralis of the orbicularis oris (Figure 5.10). It is recommended that, at the initial treatment session, quadrants of the pars peripheralis of both the upper and lower lips be treated with no more than 2 U of BOTOX® injected into each site, applied symmetrically. BOTOX® should not be injected directly into the center of the philtrum, for risk of flattening its lateral edges. If the lower lip does not possess very deep rhytides, then it should be treated with only minimal amounts of BOTOX®, i.e. no more than 1 unit in each quadrant, especially at the initial treatment session, for risk of weakening the overall sphincteric action of the lips. It is best to treat the lips symmetrically, injecting the four quadrants of the pars peripheralis so as to weaken the orbicularis oris in a relatively proportional and symmetric manner, but the dose in each quadrant can vary depending on the number and depth of rhytides present. Since only the superficial fibers of the orbicularis oris should be treated, then only 1–2 U of BOTOX®, injected subdermally, will suffice to produce the desired effect[2–4]. In patients who have had repeated treatments of BOTOX® over many years and, therefore, are well known to the physician injector, slightly higher doses, but not more than 3–4 U of BOTOX®, can be injected into each lip quadrant (Figure 5.11a–e).

Some physicians use different patterns to inject the lips that include as many as 10 or 11 injection sites between the upper and lower lips, usually at the points of maximal muscle

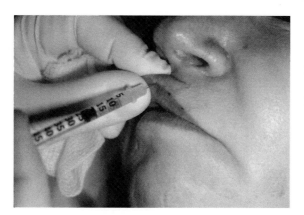

Figure 5.9   Injections of BOTOX® at the junction of the upper pars marginalis and pars peripheralis of the orbicularis oris in this 59-year-old patient were painful

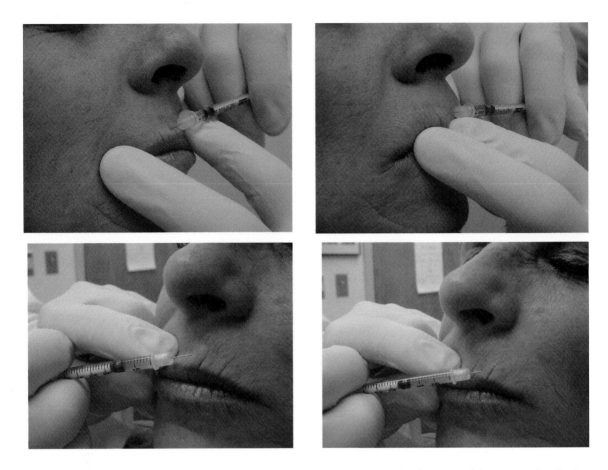

Figure 5.10   Injections of BOTOX® placed 3 to 5 mm above the vermillion border within the center of the pars peripheralis of the orbicularis oris were less painful for this 53-year-old patient

contraction[4] (Figure 5.12). It is important that the patient return 2 to 3 weeks after a treatment session with BOTOX® so that the physician can assess the patient for any asymmetry or aberration in lip function[4].

For those patients who also have their lips injected with soft tissue fillers, it has been found that injections of BOTOX® may prolong the effects of the fillers, since the constant muscle contraction and stress on the filler material by normal, routine lip movement is reduced by the effects of the BOTOX®[5]. When other cosmetic procedures are performed during the same treatment session in which BOTOX® needs to be injected, the BOTOX® treatment should be given last.

The total dose for BOTOX® injected into the upper lip should not exceed 6 U, and that for the lower lip should not exceed 4 U, unless the physician knows the patient very well and has

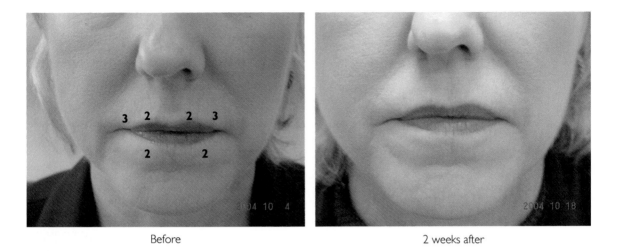

Before   2 weeks after

Figure 5.11a   This 47-year-old is shown at rest before and 2 weeks after her third BOTOX® treatment of perioral vertical rhytides. Note the subtle fullness of the vermillion and eversion of its border

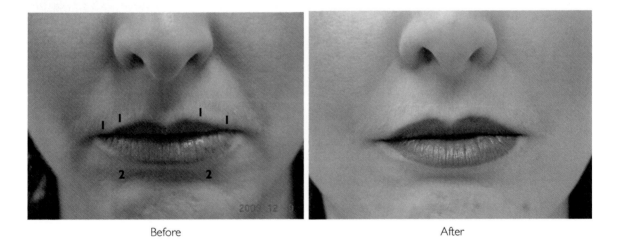

Before   After

Figure 5.11b   This patient is shown at rest before and 3 weeks after a treatment of perioral vertical rhytides. Note the subtle fullness of the vermillion and eversion of its border

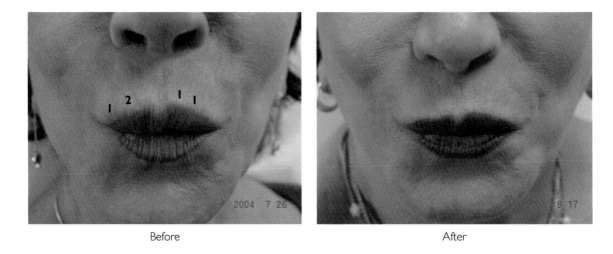

Before   After

Figure 5.11c   This 56-year-old is shown puckering before and 3 weeks after a treatment of perioral vertical rhytides

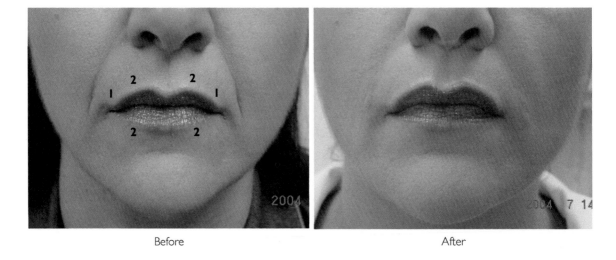

Before   After

Figure 5.11d   This 39-year-old is shown at rest before and 2 weeks after a treatment of perioral vertical rhytides. Note the subtle fullness of the vermillion and eversion of its border

treated the patient successfully without complications in the past with higher doses of BOTOX® (Figure 5.11a) (see Appendix 2).

Outcomes (results)

Of all the areas of the face that are treated for wrinkling, the perioral area is the least predictable and responsive no matter what invasive or non-invasive modality is used, including injections of BOTOX®. Even so, the perioral area is high on the treatment list when patients request cosmetic rejuvenation of the face.

When BOTOX® injections of the lips are effective as intended, a pleasing effacement of the depth of the vertical lip lines occurs, which can dramatically improve the overall physical

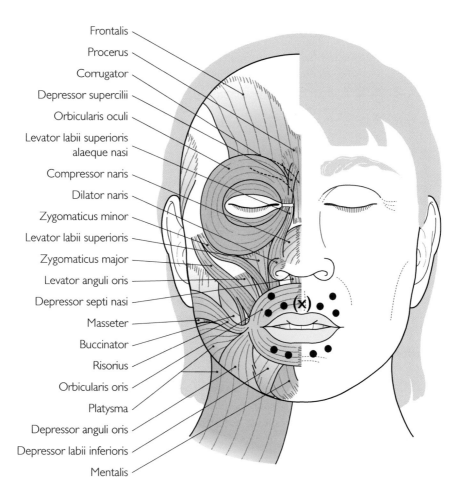

Frontalis
Procerus
Corrugator
Depressor supercilii
Orbicularis oculi
Levator labii superioris
alaeque nasi
Compressor naris
Dilator naris
Zygomaticus minor
Levator labii superioris
Zygomaticus major
Levator anguli oris
Depressor septi nasi
Masseter
Buccinator
Risorius
Orbicularis oris
Platysma
Depressor anguli oris
Depressor labii inferioris
Mentalis

Figure 5.12   Point (X) should only be injected in extreme cases of excessively deep rhytides in the center of the lip (philtrum). Adapted from Smychyshyn N, Sengelmann R. Botulinum toxin A treatment of perioral rhytides. *Dermatol Surg* 2003;29:490–5

appearance and emotional status of the patient. In addition to relaxing the superficial fibers of the orbicularis oris and producing a smoothening of the cutaneous surface of the lip, there also can be a widening of the philtrum and a slight eversion of the vermillion, producing an attractive 'pseudo' augmentation of the lips3,4,6 (Figure 5.11). Many feel that this pseudoaugmentation and eversion of the lips are best realized when BOTOX® is injected directly into the cutaneo-vermillion border (Figure 5.9), but similar lip fullness and eversion can be seen when BOTOX® is injected a few millimeters above the vermillion line (Figures 5.10 and 5.11a-d).

Only dynamic perioral wrinkles can be attenuated by BOTOX®, not the static rhytides that result from photodamage and age (Figure 5.3). For correction of static wrinkles and solar elastosis, various soft tissue fillers and different resurfacing procedures with adjunctive treatments of BOTOX® when appropriate will give the best results. Because low doses are used to efface perioral rhytides, the usual duration of effect from injections of BOTOX® in the lips is sometimes 2 and generally no more than 3 months (see Appendix 3).

Complications (adverse sequelae) (see Appendix 5)

The perioral area of the face is probably the most difficult to treat with BOTOX® without the frequent occurrence of adverse sequelae. This is because, unlike the sphincteric action of the orbicularis oculi which has only one opposing levator muscle (frontalis) and a few co-depressor muscles (corrugator supercilii, procerus, and depressor supercilii), the orbicularis oris is interlaced with muscle fibers from the different groups of upper and lower lip levators and depressors, making it easy for the injected BOTOX® to diffuse readily into an adjacent interdigitating muscle or group of muscles that produce a different set of facial movements. Consequently, adverse sequelae or, at the very least, annoying side effects are bound to occur.

Using a higher dosing range ($\geq$ 5–6 U per upper lip and $\geq$ 3–4 U per lower lip) of BOTOX® will subject the patient to difficulties with lip puckering when attempting to whistle or kiss. A slightly asymmetric smile is relatively common in the general population (see Chapter 4). It also can be created or accentuated by unequal dosing and asymmetric injections of BOTOX®. In the case of overdosing, many different adverse functional changes can occur, which can include, but are not limited to, the inability to form certain letters (e.g. b, p, f, w, o, and u), to articulate different sounds, and to pronounce various words. Involuntary tongue, inner cheek, and lip biting may result, along with flattening of the philtrum, or even lip paresthesias. There can be a disturbance in proprioception of the lips which makes it difficult to apply lipstick, whistle, kiss or there can be a concomitant inability to approximate the lips tightly which can lead to fluid or even food incontinence, causing one to drool or actively dribble liquid out of the mouth while drinking from a glass or cup, or sipping from a straw, or eating from a spoon[7–9]. The inability to purse or pucker the lips can last up to one month or even longer after a treatment of BOTOX®. One should not be tempted to inject higher doses of BOTOX® into the lips similar to the way one can increase the injection dose in the periorbital area. Doing so will definitely lead to any number of the adverse sequelae as identified above. It is important to understand that there is only a very narrow margin for the successful treatment of the orbicularis oris with BOTOX®. If 2 U of BOTOX® can be injected effectively and safely into a patient's lip, as

Treatment implications when injecting perioral rhytides

1. Only dynamic wrinkles in the lips are reducible by BOTOX® treatments. Accurate patient assessment is the key to a successful outcome.
2. Treating hyperkinetic superficial fibers of the orbicularis oris with BOTOX® will relax surface rhytides, evert the vermillion, and create the appearance of fullness in the lips.
3. Inject low doses of high-volume BOTOX® superficially in the lips, and see the patient 2–3 weeks after each treatment.
4. Treat the lips with symmetrically placed injections of BOTOX®. Each individual injection site can be dosed differently.
5. Inject the lower lip conservatively and with a lower dose of BOTOX® than in the upper lip to avoid functional aberrations.
6. Avoid injecting BOTOX® into the base of the philtrum.
7. Avoid treating close to the corners of the mouth, for risk of creating incompetent commissures, eklabion, an asymmetric smile, drooling, and even dribbling.

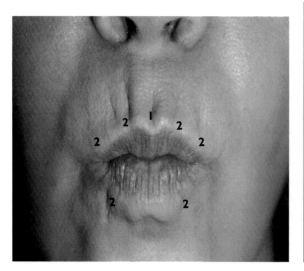

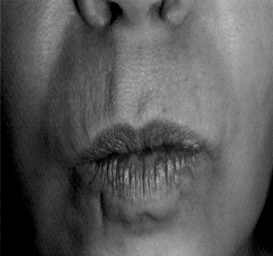

Figure 5.13a   This 59-year-old is accentuating her dynamic perioral rhytides by puckering. She has had at least four BOTOX® treatments in the past

Figure 5.13b   Same patient puckering 5 weeks after a BOTOX® treatment. Note the subtle fullness of the lips and the eversion of the vermillion border

little as 3 or 4 U of BOTOX® in that same individual may result in some or all of the adverse sequelae of an asymmetric smile and lack of sphincter control, causing food and liquid incontinence, and difficulty with speech and sound articulation as described above. So the temptation to inject even 1 U more in an upper or lower lip to improve the results or extend the duration of BOTOX® treatment must be overcome, unless visible ineffectiveness of a particular dosage of a BOTOX® treatment already has been experienced by the patient. Then a gradual increase in dose and number of injection sites can be attempted with each subsequent BOTOX® treatment session.

Melomental folds

Introduction

Patients who have a chronic downward projection of the corners of the mouth commonly also will possess pronounced melomental folds. These superfluous folds of skin are created by deep furrows in the skin emanating away and generally downward from the oral commissures and are identified as inferior melolabial sulci, 'drool grooves', or 'marionette lines'. When these lines are present, they usually impart to others the negative expressions of sadness, disapproval, unpleasantness, and melancholia. When these 'marionette lines' extend downward along lateral sides of the mentum they reinforce the downward turn of the corners of the mouth creating an inverted smile or 'Chinese moustache' and evoke the outward appearance of someone who is old and senile, no matter how young they might be chronologically. Marionette lines can be a source of frustration and embarrassment, particularly for women during social interactions, or for those who maintain a prominent position in the work force. Until recently the only way to efface these lines was either by invasive surgical procedures such as rhytidectomies and resurfacing, or injections of soft tissue fillers which would produce results that were mediocre and temporary at best. Injections of BOTOX® have enhanced these results, bringing them a little closer to a more satisfactory outcome.

Functional anatomy

Formation of an inverted smile because of the downward projection of the corners of the mouth is produced by the hyperkinetic activity of the depressor anguli oris pulling on the lateral oral commissures (Figure 5.14). The depressor anguli oris is a small triangular muscle (also known as the triangularis) whose wide base originates at the mental tubercle and along the external oblique line of the body of the mandible below the canine premolar and first molar, lateral and superficial to the larger depressor labii inferioris (Figure 5.15). The muscle fibers of the depressor anguli oris narrow as they travel upward and converge onto the angle of the mouth, where some muscle fibers insert directly into the undersurface of the skin while other fibers insert into the modiolus and interdigitate with muscle fibers of the risorius and orbicularis oris in the area of the upper lip. The lower posterior fibers of the depressor anguli oris interdigitate with those muscle fibers of the upper platysma (pars labialis) and cervical fascia that converge toward the lateral oral commissures. There are still some other deeper muscle fibers of the depressor anguli oris that interdigitate with muscle fibers of the levator anguli oris. In some individuals the depressor labii

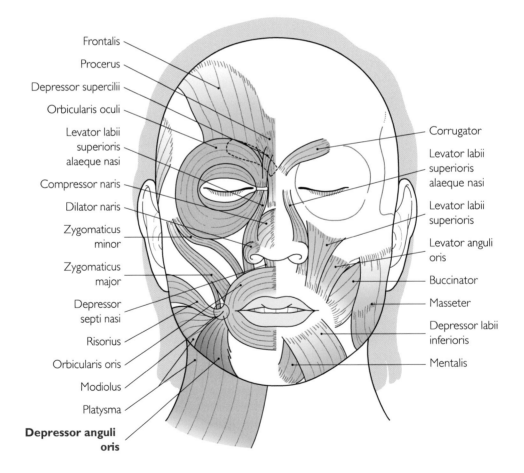

Figure 5.14   Depressor anguli oris pulls the corners of the mouth downward

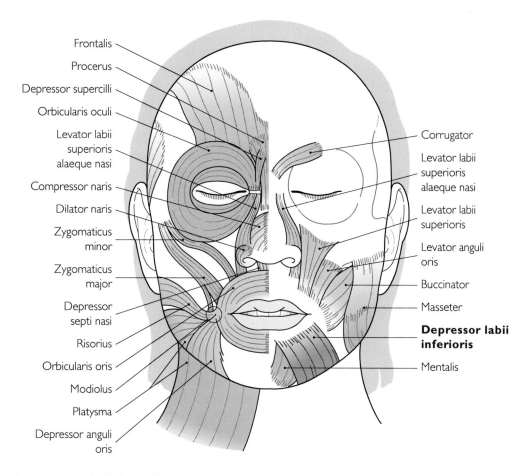

Frontalis

Procerus

Depressor supercilli

Orbicularis oculi

Levator labii
superioris
alaeque nasi

Compressor naris

Dilator naris

Zygomaticus
minor

Zygomaticus
major

Depressor
septi nasi

Risorius

Orbicularis oris

Modiolus

Platysma

Depressor anguli
oris

Corrugator

Levator labii
superioris
alaeque nasi

Levator labii
superioris

Levator anguli
oris

Buccinator

Masseter

**Depressor labii
inferioris**

Mentalis

Figure 5.15   Depressor labii inferioris depresses the lateral aspect of the lower lip

inferioris will traverse the midline inferior to the mental tubercle and decussate with fibers of its paired muscle of the opposite side, creating the transversus menti or the 'mental sling'.

The function of the depressor anguli oris is to depress the oral commissures slightly laterally and downward when opening the mouth. The depressor anguli oris is an antagonist to the levator anguli oris and zygomaticus major, displacing the corners of the mouth downward and slightly laterally when it contracts in an expression of grief, sorrow, and sadness. Upon opening the mouth, the mentolabial sulcus becomes more horizontal and deeper in its center (see Appendix 4).

Dilution

When treating the depressor anguli oris and the perioral area, BOTOX® should not be allowed to diffuse beyond the targeted muscle, otherwise, cosmetic aberrations such as an asymmetric smile, and functional disturbances such as drooling, dribbling, or even dysarthria are sure to follow. Therefore, the highest volume of diluent that should be used to reconstitute a 100 U vial of BOTOX® is 1 ml of normal saline. Any volume of diluent higher than 1 ml is sure to invite adverse sequelae (see Appendix 1).

Dosing: how to correct problem (what to do and what not to do)

The downward angling of the 'marionette lines' can be improved by injecting 2–5 U of BOTOX® intramuscularly at the border of the mandible at a point that is most inferior to an imaginary vertical line that passes through the nasolabial sulcus (Figure 5.16). This point should be approximately 8 to 10 mm lateral to the oral commissure and 8 to 15 mm inferior to this point, depending on the idiosyncratic shape of the patient's face. The appropriate injection point can be identified by palpating someone who is actively contracting the corners of the mouth downward while they are pronouncing the letter 'e' in an exaggerated fashion[9,10]. Another maneuver to assist in the localization of the depressor anguli oris is to have the patient bite down, forcibly contracting the jaw muscles. This will contract and enlarge the belly of the masseter, which is a muscle very easily identified by palpation (Figure 5.17). In the majority of individuals, the depressor anguli oris lies approximately 1–2 mm anterior to the masseter. After the patient clenches their teeth and the anterior border of the masseter is identified, have them exaggerate the pronunciation of the letter 'e'. The location of a hypertrophic depressor anguli oris should be easily palpated along the anterior border of the masseter along the body of the mandible. At times the depressor anguli oris can be detected more easily by palpating it intraorally along the inferior alveololabial sulcus. At the point at which the enlarged belly of the depressor anguli oris can be felt, 3–5 U of BOTOX® can be injected with the patient in the upright sitting or semirecumbent position (Figure 5.18). If the depressor anguli oris cannot be palpated, then it should not be treated. Be precise and accurate when injecting BOTOX® into the depressor anguli oris, since the orbicularis oris and depressor labii inferioris are immediately adjacent to it, and unsightly and dysfunctional perioral changes can result if either one of these two muscles is inadvertently weakened along with the depressor anguli oris. Care should be taken not to inject into the marginal mandibular nerve and facial artery and vein that lie in this general vicinity in a bony groove just anterior to the masseter (Figures 5.16 and 5.17). If the depressor anguli oris is palpated over this bony groove, lift the skin and muscle with the non-dominant hand before injecting BOTOX®. With this technique BOTOX® can be injected directly

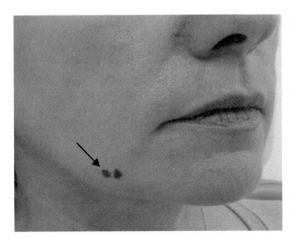 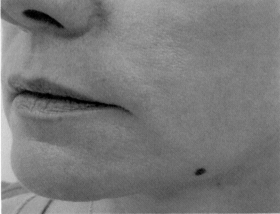

Figure 5.16   The correct point of injection for the depressor anguli oris is not at the inferior extent of the melomental crease, but slightly more posteriorly at the most inferior point of an imaginary line that passes through the nasolabial sulcus

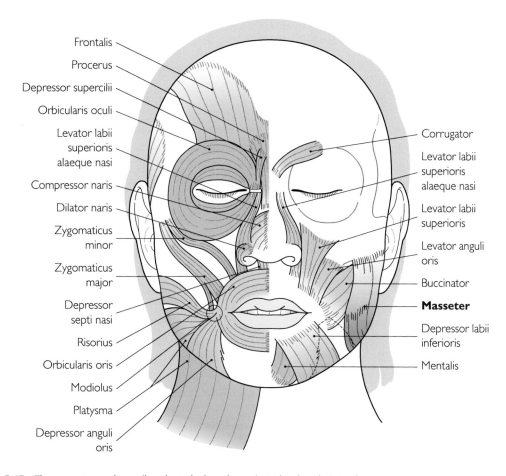

Figure 5.17 The masseter can be easily palpated when the patient clenches their teeth

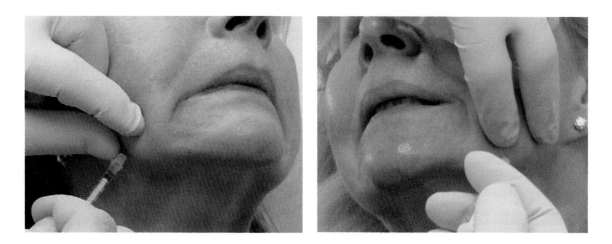

Figure 5.18 Injecting the depressor anguli oris at the most inferior point of the nasolabial sulcus at the lower border of the body of the mandible, approximately 1 cm lateral and 1 cm inferior to the corner of the mouth. During the injection the patient pronounces the letter 'e' in an exaggerated manner

into the fibers of the depressor anguli oris, while avoiding injecting the neurovascular structures of that area[11–13] (See Appendix 2).

Outcomes (results)

Injections of BOTOX® will relax the depressor anguli oris and allow the unopposed elevation of the corners of the mouth to occur by the upward pull of the risorius, levator anguli oris, and the zygomaticus major and minor. When the corners of the mouth are relaxed and elevated with BOTOX® a person appears younger and naturally relaxed and pleasant (Figure 5.19 and 5.20a,b).

Depending on the intensity of the marionette lines present, this area is best treated in combination with soft tissue fillers and some form of resurfacing. BOTOX® then will usually prolong the beneficial effect of such rejuvenation procedures. The beneficial effects from injections of BOTOX® can last from 4 to 6 months (see Appendix 3).

Complications (adverse sequelae) (see Appendix 5)

It is extremely important to inject inferior to and far enough away from the orbicularis oris when treating the depressor anguli oris. Otherwise, BOTOX® can diffuse focally into the muscle fibers of the orbicularis oris and produce a localized area of inadequate sphincteric closure of the oral cavity and a segmental inability to pucker the lips, resulting in a localized area of eklabion, an asymmetric smile, drooling and even dribbling, and a change in speech and word pronunciation. Injections given too medially also can weaken the depressor labii inferioris, causing a flattening of the contour of the lower lip and an inability to purse or even pucker the lips, contain fluid in the mouth or drink from a glass, sip from a straw, or eat from a spoon. Pronunciation of certain sounds can be hampered and the articulation of words will be difficult. Also, an annoying adynamic smile, with only the upper lip moving, is likely to occur. Overzealous injections with doses over 6–8 U of BOTOX® will also place patients at risk for developing the adverse sequelae as described above. Even when the appropriate dose is precisely injected, intense massaging of

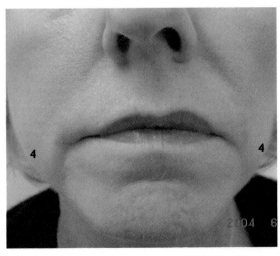
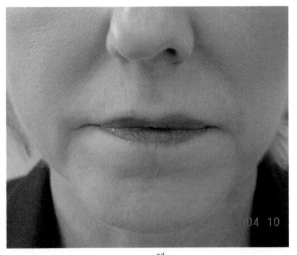

Before   4 months after 2nd treatment

Figure 5.19   This 47-year-old possesses a deep labiomental furrow and downward projecting corners of the mouth before injection of BOTOX®.

the area after the injection can displace the BOTOX® and cause similar adverse events as described. For the first-time patient, treatment in this area can produce similar but transient side effects that may be disconcerting to the uninformed and unprepared patient so pretreatment warning of these potential side effects is advisable.

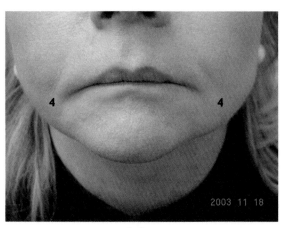
Before

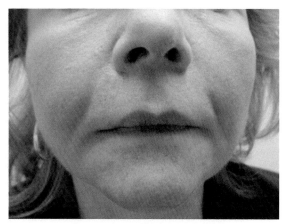
3 weeks after treatment

Figure 5.20a   This 52-year-old is shown at rest before and 3 weeks after a BOTOX® treatment of her depressor anguli oris

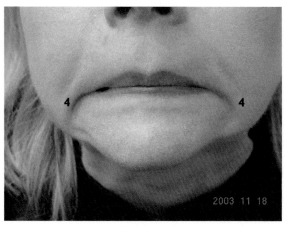
Before

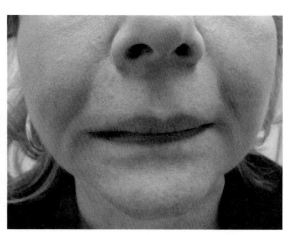
After

Figure 5.20b   Same patient frowning before and 3 weeks after a BOTOX® treatment of her depressor anguli oris. Note the slightly asymmetric smile with forced frowning, which lasted approximately 2–3 weeks after the initial BOTOX® treatment, and was of no concern to the patient. No other adverse sequelae were experienced by the patient

Treatment implications when injecting marionette lines

1. Inject BOTOX® only when the depressor anguli oris can be precisely palpated and securely identified.
2. The depressor anguli oris usually can be identified at the inferior end of the nasolabial sulcus and anterior to the masseter.
3. Avoid injecting BOTOX® into the marginal mandibular nerve and facial artery and vein by lifting the soft tissue before injecting.
4. Avoid injecting BOTOX® into the depressor labii inferioris and orbicularis oris by remaining at least 1 cm lateral and 1–1.5 cm inferior to the lateral oral commissure and injecting minimal volumes.
5. Always inject minimal volumes of highly concentrated BOTOX® in the perioral area.

Deep mental crease and chin puckering

Introduction: problem assessment and patient selection

For some men and especially women, a hyperkinetic mentalis produces an accentuated, deep transverse labiomental crease between the lower lip and the prominence of the chin that amplifies the forward projection of the apex of the mentum (Figure 5.21a,b). This is viewed as a sign of dotage or senility by the casual observer, because with age the tip of the chin can elevate and project forward, producing the so-called 'wicked witch's chin'. Men are not as frequently bothered by similar changes and even less often do they seek relief from them.

In other individuals, a hyperkinetic mentalis can produce an involuntary puckering of the chin, creating convolutions of deep ridges and furrows while they speak or convey a particular facial expression. For most individuals who voluntarily or involuntarily crinkle their chin during animation or even at rest, these changes generally go undetected by the person producing them unless disclosed by others. Once identified, chin puckering can then be verified by the patient by personally viewing these chin corrugations with a mirror while animating or speaking (Figure 5.21). In still another group of people, chin puckering can be a frustrating annoyance when it occurs post-operatively as a secondary dysfunction of augmentation mentoplasty[14]. Because not all of the bony attachments of the muscle fibers of the mentalis can be repositioned and reapproximated exactly as they were prior to the implantation of a chin implant, the contracting fibers of the mentalis then become anomalously positioned, producing an irregular crimping of the skin surface, either at rest or with each movement of the mentalis (Figure 5.22a,b). This can be an unexpected and frustrating substitution for the correction of an inadequately projecting chin.

Functional anatomy

The deep concavity of a (labio)mental crease or the wrinkled, convoluted skin of the surface of the chin is produced by a hyperkinetic mentalis. The mentalis is a short, stout, conical, two bellied muscle that originates deep to the depressor labii inferioris on the anterior aspect of the mandible on either side of the midline at the level of the incisive fossa and root of the lower lateral incisors (Figure 5.23). It travels downward, converging its two muscle bellies toward the midline to insert into the skin of the apex of the chin on either side of the frenulum of the lower lip. The mentalis elevates the skin of the lower lip upward, helping to force the lower lip

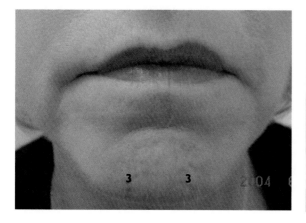

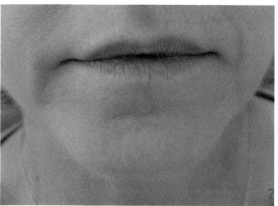

Figure 5.21a   This 47-year-old women is shown at rest before a treatment of BOTOX® to her mentalis. Note the crimping of the chin and deep mental crease

Figure 5.21b   Same patient at rest 3 weeks after a BOTOX® treatment. Note the reduction of chin crimping and effacement of the mental crease

against the gums. This maneuver intensifies the indentation of the mentolabial crease. The mentalis also protrudes and everts the lower lip during drinking. It also wrinkles the skin of the chin in pouting to produce an expression of doubt, displeasure, sadness, or disdain. With age, the loss of collagen, soft tissue support, and subcutaneous fat along with a hyperkinetic response of the mentalis can enhance the appearance of uncontrollable chin dimpling. In most individuals, when frowning in displeasure or projecting an expression of sadness, doubt, or disdain, the depressor anguli oris contracts simultaneously with the mentalis, so the melomental or marionette lines are also accentuated. This is why, for some patients, it is advisable to treat the presence of marionette lines at the same time that a hyperkinetic mentalis is treated. (See Appendix 4).

Dilution

When treating the mentalis, lateral diffusion of the BOTOX® runs the risk of weakening the depressor labii inferioris and producing sphincter and motor movement incompetence of the mouth, causing an inability to depress the lower lip when smiling, laughing, speaking, drinking and eating. Therefore, low volumes of concentrated BOTOX® must be accurately injected when treating the mentalis. The preferred way to accomplish this is to reconstitute a 100 U vial of BOTOX® with only 1 ml of normal saline (see Appendix 1).

Dosing: how to correct the problem (what to do and what not to do)

A hyperactive mentalis can be relaxed by injecting 3–5 U of BOTOX® subcutaneously or intramuscularly at one point on both sides of the midline at the apex of the mentum just above the lower edge of the body of the mandible, especially if the patient has a vertical mental cleft or a widely shaped, square chin (Figures 5.22a,b and 5.24a,b). Injections are best done with the patient in the upright sitting or semirecumbent position. If the patient has a narrower, rounded or pointed chin, the insertion of the mentalis into the undersurface of the skin probably is more

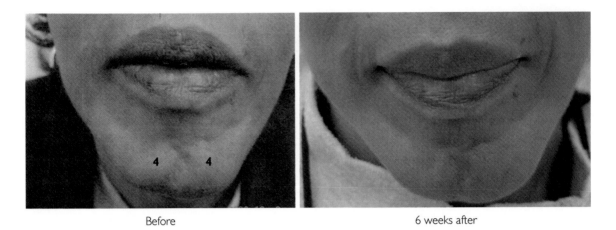

Before   6 weeks after

Figure 5.22a   This 67-year-old is shown before and 6 weeks after her third BOTOX® treatments for a dysfunctionally hyperkinetic mentalis caused by an augmentation mentoplasty 2–3 years previously. Note the difference in the pattern of chin crimping before and after a treatment with BOTOX®

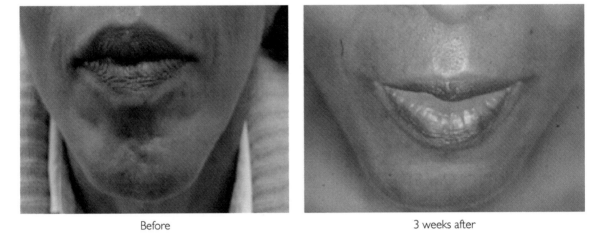

Before   3 weeks after

Figure 5.22b   The same patient is plagued with the appearance of chin crimping both at rest and during animation, seen here before and 3 weeks after her fourth treatment of BOTOX®

centrally located. Therefore, for these patients, an alternative technique is to inject 4–8 U of BOTOX® into one point only in the center of the mentum at the apex of the chin close to the inferior border of the body of mandible (Figure 5.25).

It is imperative to avoid inadvertent diffusion of BOTOX® into any of the muscle fibers of the orbicularis oris, which can result in sphincter and motor movement aberrations. This can be accomplished by injecting BOTOX® inferior to the transverse mental crease and as close as possible to the lower edge of the body of the mandible. Light massage will relieve the pain of injection. Vigorous massage will displace the BOTOX® laterally, particularly if the two injection point technique is used, and cause the BOTOX® to diffuse into the fibers of the depressor labii inferioris and unintentionally weaken it (see Appendix 2).

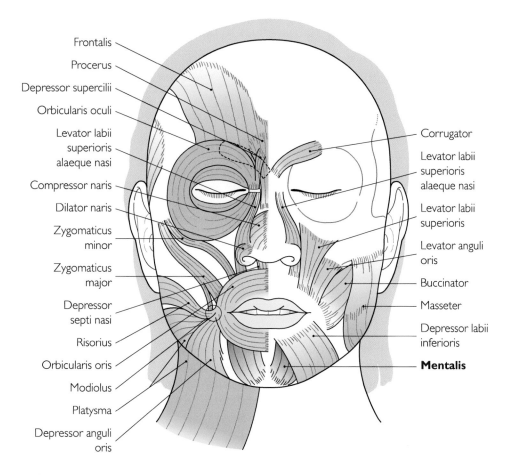

Frontalis
Procerus
Depressor supercilii
Orbicularis oculi
Levator labii superioris alaeque nasi
Compressor naris
Dilator naris
Zygomaticus minor
Zygomaticus major
Depressor septi nasi
Risorius
Orbicularis oris
Modiolus
Platysma
Depressor anguli oris

Corrugator
Levator labii superioris alaeque nasi
Levator labii superioris
Levator anguli oris
Buccinator
Masseter
Depressor labii inferioris
Mentalis

Figure 5.23   The mentalis elevates the lower lip, indents the mentolabial furrow, and creates surface convolutions over the mentum

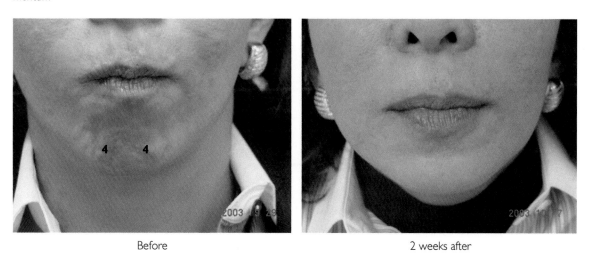

Before

2 weeks after

Figure 5.24a,b   This 50-year-old was unaware that her chin puckered when she was animated or spoke. Forced contraction of her mentalis produced multidirectional corrugations before BOTOX®, which disappeared 2 weeks after BOTOX®

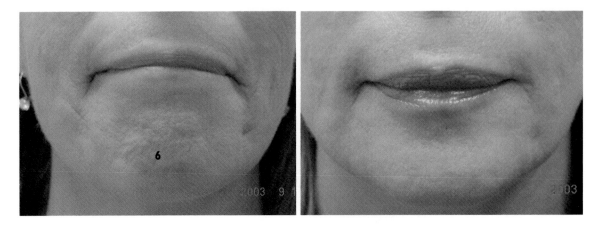

Figure 5.25   This 53-year-old, with chin puckering at rest that was exacerbated with animation, is seen before and 2 weeks after a BOTOX® treatment. Note the narrowness of the apex of the mentum and the location of the single injection point

Outcomes (results)

Relaxing the hyperkinetic muscle fibers of the mentalis can reduce or eliminate the involuntary convolutions and crinkling of the chin when one is performing such mundane activities as speaking or emotionally expressing oneself (Figures 5.24 and 5.25). A weakening of the mentalis also can drop the anterior projection of the skin of the chin slightly downward, effacing a deep transverse labiomental crease and possibly rotating the lower lip slightly upward (Figure 5.26). When the transverse labiomental crease is exceptionally deep and resistant to treatment with BOTOX®, elevating and effacing it with soft tissue fillers is a viable alternative. However, depending on the fillers used, visible beading and an overall less than optimal outcome can result. For those patients who have a distorted convoluted chin apex as a result of a previous augmentation genioplasty with a chin implant, injections of BOTOX® can

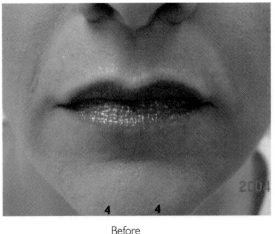

Before

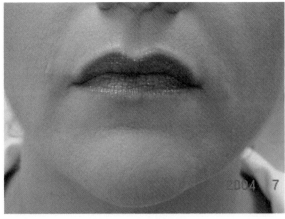

3 weeks after

Figure 5.26   This 38-year-old is shown at rest with a deep transverse mental crease before and 3 weeks after a treatment of BOTOX®. Note the effacement of the mental crease and upward rotation of lower lip vermillion

produce a softening and a relaxation of the chin that is much appreciated by those who are vexed by these anxiety provoking wrinkles and convolutions of the mentum (Figure 5.22). The beneficial effects from injections of BOTOX® can last anywhere from 4 to 6 months (see Appendix 3).

Complications (adverse sequelae) (see Appendix 5)

When injections of BOTOX® are placed too high on the lower lip, i.e. above the transverse mental crease, the orbicularis oris and even the depressor labii inferioris can certainly be weakened, particularly when using the two point technique. Diffusion of BOTOX® into the depressor labii inferioris and orbicularis oris also can occur when vigorous massaging is performed immediately after injection. If either the orbicularis oris or the depressor labii inferioris is inadvertently affected by BOTOX®, a relaxation of a tight oral sphincter, a reduction in lip competence, and a diminution in buccal motor movements will occur. This can cause a patient to form certain letters, such as b, p, w, f, o, and u, and articulate certain sounds and words with embarrassing difficulty. Also, an asymmetric smile can be produced as a result of an adynamic lower lip. An overzealous treatment of the mentalis with too high a dose of BOTOX® that virtually immobilizes the mentalis will cause an inability to approximate the lower lip tightly against the teeth, or a glass, or cup, producing involuntary dribbling from the lower lip when drinking, or drooling from the corners of the mouth when at rest.

Treatment implications when injecting the mentalis

1. Inject BOTOX® below the transverse mental crease and as close as possible to the lower border of the body of the mandible.
2. Injections can be placed in one site centrally or in two sites separately on either side of the midline depending on the width of the mentum.
3. High-volume injections or improper technique can cause diffusion of BOTOX® into the orbicularis oris, or depressor labii inferioris, or both, and produce motor dysfunction of the lower lip and sphincter incompetence of the buccal aperture.
4. Immobilizing the mentalis with a high dose of low-volume BOTOX® can prevent the lower lip from approximating tightly against the teeth or a drinking vessel, resulting in dribbling while drinking and drooling while at rest. Inability to articulate words and sounds distinctly also can occur.
5. Injections of BOTOX® can correct post-operative chin puckering secondary to augmentation mentoplasty.

Horizontal lines and vertical bands of the neck

Introduction: problem assessment and patient selection

Frequently, the neck can be a more accurate gauge of a person's chronologic age than the overall appearance of his or her face. This is especially true in those individuals who have spent a lot of time outdoors and who have taken advantage of various cosmetic procedures available for facial rejuvenation. The neck as well as the perioral region have remained the bane of esthetic rejuvenation for most age-conscious individuals seeking relief from the ravages of time and from the innumerable hours spent outdoors, whether for work or pleasure. None of the available invasive surgical procedures (i.e. cervicoplasties or rhytidectomies), chemical or ablative laser resurfacing and non-ablative laser or intense pulsed light procedures, along with soft tissue fillers and implants or topical medical treatments, have yet to satisfactorily and safely eliminate horizontal necklace lines, vertical platysmal bands and cords nor the usual superficial skin surface alterations of solar elastosis, pigmentary and textural changes that are so characteristic of photodamage.

Upon animation with different neck movements, vertical bands and cords may become prominent at an early age (in the fourth or fifth decade) in predisposed individuals or eventually in the sixth or seventh decade for many others (Figure 5.27). With age, the skin of the neck progressively develops loss of elasticity, increased laxity, and redundancy. There is a diminution of soft tissue support, causing the skin of the neck to be susceptible to continuous horizontal creasing which leads to persistent transverse wrinkles that are perpendicular to the normal vertical contractions of the platysma. These horizontal lines traverse the anterolateral aspect of the neck between the anterior borders of the right and left sternocleidomastoid from the submandibular area down to the clavicles like multiple parallel rings around the neck (Figure 5.27).

When the platysma becomes less elastic with age, it separates anteriorly and can be appreciated clinically as two or more divergent bands or folds of skin that extend from the lower margin of the mandible to the medial aspect of the clavicles. These anterior neck bands often tighten and become more visible, especially when the patient turns the head from side to side as

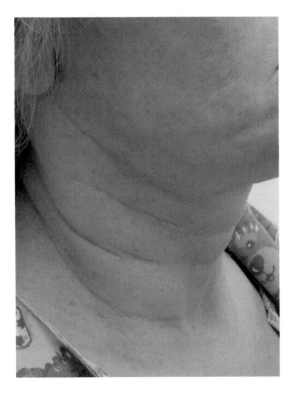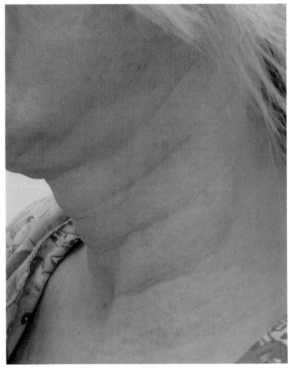

Figure 5.27   This 55-year-old began to notice deep horizontal wrinkles of the anterior neck at age 40

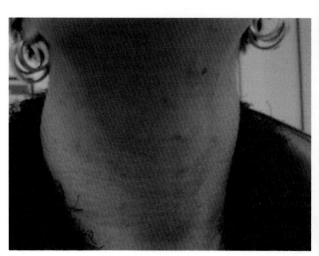
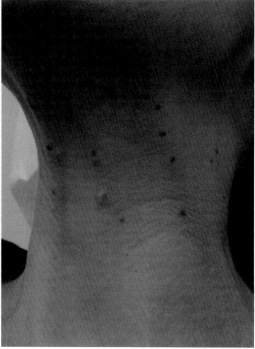

Figure 5.28   This 49-year-old developed vertical platysmal bands at the age of 40 as seen before and immediately after injections of BOTOX®

they speak or gesticulate (Figure 5.28)[15]. Vertical bands and cords develop as the result of a hyperactive platysma attempting to support the ptotic structural changes so characteristic of a senescent neck. The anterior edges of the fibers eventually lose muscle tone, separate over time, and protrude anteriorly, creating the cords and bands that are sometimes referred to as the 'turkey neck' deformity (Figure 5.29). For some carefully selected individuals who are unable for medical or unwilling for other reasons to undergo the rigors and post-operative morbidity of an invasive surgical procedure such as a cervicoplasty or rhytidectomy, injections of BOTOX® have become a viable and frequently sought alternative solution to their problem.

Functional anatomy

The platysma is composed of two separate broad, thin sheets of muscle running up the front and lateral aspects of the neck from the upper chest to the mandible, fusing and blending its muscle fibers with the superficial muscular aponeurotic system (SMAS) superiorly in the face. It can vary considerably in thickness and extent and in some individuals the platysma may even be absent. The platysma originates from the superficial fascia of the upper part of the thorax over the pectoralis major and deltoid. It ascends in a superomedial direction across the clavicle and acromion of the scapula and up the lateral neck. Its anterior fibers from both sheets of muscle on either side of the neck interdigitate with each other in various patterns at or near the symphysis menti of the mandible. The posterior fibers pass over the lower border of the body of the mandible superficial to the marginal mandibular branch of the facial nerve, artery, and vein. The upper fibers of the platysma (pars mandibularis) then insert onto the lower border of the body of the mandible below the oblique line and into the skin and subcutaneous tissue of the

Figure 5.29 The pendulous 'turkey neck' deformity is apparent in this 73-year-old woman

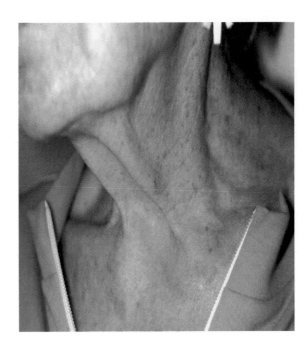

lower part of the face. Some platysmal fibers (pars labialis) also interdigitate and blend into the muscles around the angle of the mouth (orbicularis oris and risorius), the chin (mentalis), and the depressors of the lower lip, especially the depressor anguli oris (Figure 5.30). Occasionally, fibers of the platysma may be present as low as the fourth to sixth intercostal space in the chest and as high as the ear or zygoma (i.e. near the origin of the zygomaticus major or up to the margin of the orbicularis oculi), participating in the formation of the SMAS in the lower and lateral face. With maximum contraction the platysma pulls the skin lying over the clavicle upward and wrinkles the skin of the neck in an oblique direction increasing the diameter of the neck, as one does when relieving the pressure of a tight collar. Its anterior portion and thickest fibers can pull the lower lip and corners of the mouth downward and laterally, widening the buccal aperture at the corners of the mouth as in an expression of horror. The platysma also slightly depresses the mandible, partially opening the mouth during an expression of surprise. The platysma also is active during sudden, rapid, and deep inspiration. Contracting the platysma can increase negative pressure in the superficial jugular veins of the neck, facilitating venous circulation. Electromyographic studies have demonstrated that the platysma is not actively contracting during laughing, opening the mouth, or moving the head[16].

Some authors like to emphasize the different anatomic variations of the platysma based on the pattern of decussation of its interlacing fibers as they approach the submental region[17,18]. The most common variant seen in approximately 75 per cent of patients identified as type I is where the fibers of the platysma interdigitate with its counterpart on the opposite side of the neck 1–2 cm below the chin. In patients with the type II variant, seen approximately 15 per cent of the time, the decussation of the fibers occurs at the level of the thyroid cartilage and becomes a unified sheet of muscle from there on up over the entire submental region. Approximately 10 per cent of patients have the type III variant, which is seen as two separate straps of platysma that run parallel to each other up the neck, attaching to the mandible and skin without decussating its fibers[18,19] (Figure 5.31).

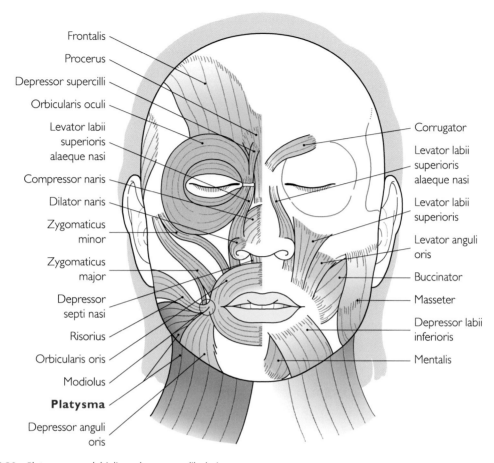

Frontalis
Procerus
Depressor supercilli
Orbicularis oculi
Levator labii superioris alaeque nasi
Compressor naris
Dilator naris
Zygomaticus minor
Zygomaticus major
Depressor septi nasi
Risorius
Orbicularis oris
Modiolus
Platysma
Depressor anguli oris

Corrugator
Levator labii superioris alaeque nasi
Levator labii superioris
Levator anguli oris
Buccinator
Masseter
Depressor labii inferioris
Mentalis

Figure 5.30   Platysma, pars labialis and pars mandibularis

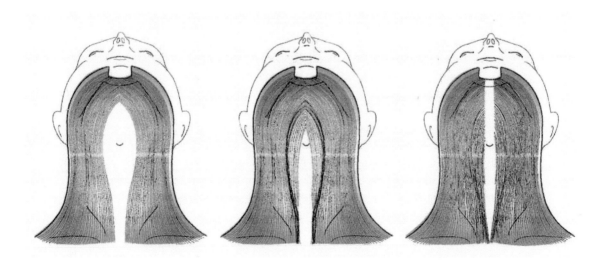

Figure 5.31   Three types of decussating platysma. (Reproduced from Bendetto. Commentary: botulinum toxin in clinical medicine. *Clin Dermatol* 2003;21(6):465–8 with permission from Elsevier)

195

There are two distinctly separate depots of fat in the submental region of the neck that must be taken into consideration when planning rejuvenation procedures for the aging neck. The more superficial one of the two is the submental or submandibular fat pad, which lies directly anterior to the platysma in the subcutaneous plane. The other, the subplatysmal fat pad, lies more deeply in the neck, residing behind and posterior to the platysma. Herniation and protrusion of the subplatysmal fat pad in the aging neck are predicated upon the type of anatomic variant of the platysma present in an individual and whether or not there is a significantly wide enough separation of the two muscle sheets inferior to the mentum. In those individuals with excessive amounts of submental fat in the subplatysmal layer, the loss of platysmal muscle tone permits the subplatysmal fat pad to herniate through the free borders of the platysma and establish a central fullness of submental fat in between vertical columns of neck bands, the so-called 'turkey neck' deformity (Figure 5.29). (See Appendix 4).

Dilution

Because the platysma is a large sheet of muscle that drapes over the anterolateral aspect of the neck, injections of large volumes of dilute BOTOX® may be more expedient when the entire neck needs to be treated. Therefore, reconstituting a 100 U vial of BOTOX® with 2–4 ml of normal saline is more practical than reconstituting it with a smaller volume when injecting the platysma (see Appendix 1).

Dosing: how to correct the problem (what to do and what not to do)

To eliminate most of the dynamic horizontal lines of the neck, inject approximately 1–2 U of BOTOX® above and below the main horizontal line at points 2–3 cm apart into the deep dermis, rather than the subcutaneous plane, using dilute volumes of BOTOX®. This is performed with the patient sitting upright and forcibly contracting their platysma by clenching their teeth (Figure 5.32). Depending on the size of the patient's neck, no more than 25–50 U of BOTOX® should be given per treatment session.

In the properly selected patient, BOTOX® also can be used to reduce the appearance of vertical neck bands and cords[10–15]. In those patients with extensive cutaneous laxity and flaccid platysmal cords, injections of BOTOX® can actually cause the patient to appear worse, and therefore should not be attempted.

With the patient sitting upright or in a semirecumbent position and contracting their platysma, grasp the platysmal band between the thumb and index finger of the non-dominant hand (Figure 5.33). Inject 2–4 U of BOTOX® into the lower dermis per injection site along the vertical extent of the band, starting approximately 2 cm below the inferior border of the mandible. Repeat each injection at intervals of 1.5–2 cm from each other, descending down the neck toward the border of the clavicle[18]. Raising a visible wheal with each injection attests to the appropriately superficial position of the injected BOTOX® (Figure 5.34). Keeping the injections as superficial as possible will avoid post-injection ecchymoses that result from puncturing superficial muscular vasculature. Gentle massage of the area after injecting BOTOX® helps to alleviate some of the pain that accompanies an intracutaneous injection, and it also may help reduce the potential for bruising. Most patients require three to five injection points to treat a

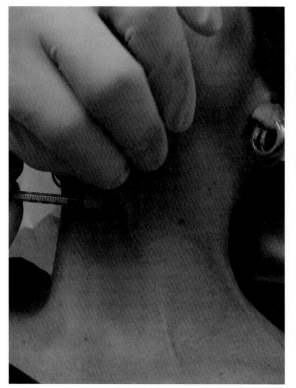 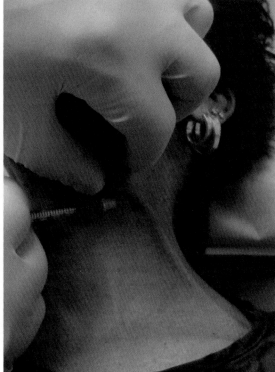

Figure 5.32   Contracting the platysma makes the injecting of BOTOX® into the lower dermis easier

Figure 5.33   Grasping the platysmal band with the non-dominant hand makes it easier to inject BOTOX® into the lower dermis of the thin skin of the neck

platysmal band adequately, and some may require even more, depending on the length of their neck. It is advisable to inject no more than 20–25 U of BOTOX® along the vertical extent of each cervical platysmal band for a total of 40 to 50 U per treatment session when two or three neck bands are treated[20]. When more than two platysmal bands are present in the neck, i.e. two bands or more on each side of the neck, the other two or more platysmal bands should be treated at another treatment session 2 to 4 weeks later, especially when more than 50 U of BOTOX® have already been injected. When the neck bands present as thick cords and a hypertrophic platysma can be palpated, an additional 1 or 2 units of BOTOX® can be applied at each injection point. Some authors have injected as much as 200 U per treatment session, a practice that does not seem to be necessary in most cases[21]. There are others who use electromyographic guidance to accurately place a minimum amount of BOTOX® in a platysmal band when treating the neck. They typically use less than a total of 20 U of BOTOX® in any given treatment session[22] (see Appendix 2).

Outcomes (results)

Relaxation of a hypertrophic platysma with diminution of horizontal neck lines and vertical bands will occur 5–7 days after a treatment with BOTOX®. The effects can last anywhere from 3 to 5 or more months, depending on the precision of the injections and the strength of the

Figure 5.34 Raising a wheal while injecting BOTOX® in the neck attests to the superficial placement of the BOTOX®

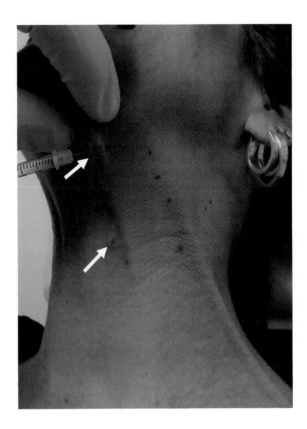

platysma and the patient's neck movement habits. Usually patients who are too young for rhytidectomies or older patients who have had rhytidectomies will have the best results when there is minimal ptosis of subplatysmal fat and soft tissue. It is advisable to have the patient return 2–3 weeks after a treatment session with BOTOX® to assess their response to the treatment and their satisfaction with the overall results. Touch-up injections always can be done to correct any asymmetry or lack of a response along a particular neck band or cord.

Treatment with BOTOX® has been beneficial in preparing a patient for submental liposuction because, by relaxing the neck bands, a more even draping of the anterior neck skin can be achieved in the post-operative period after liposuction. When there is a significant amount of fat herniation from in between the two lateral sheets of platysma in certain patients, and not only submandibular but also subplatysmal fat protruding in the submental area, both submandibular and subplatysmal liposuction with or without a platysmaplasty, and possibly a rhytidectomy, are the only treatments that will be corrective. Injections of BOTOX® in these patients are marginally helpful. On the other hand, when there is no herniation or protrusion of subplatysmal fat and the presence of submental fat is negligible, injections of BOTOX® will be effective in reducing the vertical neck bands and cords created by a hypertrophic platysma. In some authors' experience the anatomic type of platysmal decussation (Figure 5.31) does not necessarily prove to be predictive of whether or not a treatment of BOTOX® will be successful[19]. It is the length of the platysma, the extent of muscle flaccidity, and the degree of muscle hypertrophy that seem to be the predictive factors that mostly influence the success rate of a treatment of BOTOX® in the neck, and not the anatomic configuration or type of platysmal decussation in the submental area. In fact, flaccid neck bands that are heavy and loose can be made worse with injections of BOTOX®.

In patients who experience suboptimal results with residual banding and asymmetric draping of the anterior neck skin after rhytidectomy, injections of BOTOX® can help normalize these types of unwanted outcomes. The additional benefit of a slight elevation of the lower lip and buccal commissures and a tightening of lower cheek jowels has been observed when BOTOX® diffuses from the fibers of the upper platysma (pars mandibularis) and into decussating fibers of the depressor anguli oris (pars labialis), immediately subjacent to the mandibular ramus during injections of the platysmal bands[21–23.] For some, electromyographic guidance when treating the platysma is a necessity[22] (see Appendix 3).

Complications (adverse sequelae) (see Appendix 5)

Treatment of horizontal rhytides and vertical bands in the neck with BOTOX® usually is very safe, and untoward sequelae occur at a very low rate. When they do occur, however, they usually are the result of improper technique.

Since the underlying nine muscles of deglutition, phonation, and neck flexion are also cholinergic in origin, overdosing with BOTOX® when treating the neck can result in xerostomia (dry mouth), dysphagia, dysarthria, and neck weakness[24,25]. The static wrinkles caused by solar elastosis and age usually are not affected by BOTOX®.

An injection of more than 50 U of BOTOX® in the neck increases the risk for temporary dysphagia (i.e. difficulty with swallowing) and hoarseness. Older patients are more at risk for complications, because they present with more wrinkling and banding of their necks and commonly require higher doses of BOTOX® overall for satisfactory results. They also have a diminution in the soft tissue support of the neck, making it easier for the BOTOX® to diffuse to other deeper muscles of the neck (e.g. sternocleidomastoid and other strap muscles of the neck), which will affect deglutition, speech, and the overall strength of the neck in keeping it erect. Similar complications can be produced in younger patients when BOTOX® is injected too deeply, because it can affect the deeper musculature of the neck.

In patients treated for cervical dystonia in whom over ≥200 U of BOTOX® are injected into the strap muscles of the neck during one treatment session, dysphagia, hoarseness, dry mouth, and flu-like syndromes have been observed[26,27].

When BOTOX® is injected in the neck only to reduce platysmal banding and transverse rhytides, mild and transient neck discomfort can occur 2–5 days after treatment, with only a rare occurrence of neck weakness experienced with head elevation and flexion[19]. Only one patient out of 1500 in the multiple center treatment study experienced clinically significant dysphagia, which resolved spontaneously within 2 weeks. Profound dysphasia was reported when more than 75–100 U of BOTOX® were used to treat platysmal bands during one treatment session[28]. A naso-gastric tube was temporarily required to feed the patient until she was able to swallow without assistance.

Commonly observed and expected side effects include transient edema and erythema, both of which usually resolve within 1–2 days. Post-injection ecchymoses may last a few days longer. Other less commonly occurring adverse sequelae can include muscle soreness or neck discomfort and mild headache. A few patients complain of either a difficulty or, in extreme cases, an inability to lift the head from the supine position and then to keep it still and erect.

Treatment implications when injecting the neck

1. Superficial injections of BOTOX® can diminish horizontal wrinkles and vertical bands of the neck.
2. The platysma lies superficial to the muscles of deglutition and neck flexion and deep injections of large amounts of BOTOX® can cause varying degrees of dysphagia and an inability to raise the head and keep it erect.
3. Injecting the superior, mandibular fibers of the platysma can affect the corners of the mouth, lower lip and chin, because of the interdigitation of platysmal fibers into the mimetic muscles of the lower face.
4. In older patients with lax, redundant skin and attenuated platysma fibers that are separated and form flaccid neck bands and cords, injections of BOTOX® may enhance rather than diminish the appearance of those neck bands.
5. Injections of BOTOX® cannot correct the herniation of subplatysmal fat or reduce the fullness of excessive amounts of submental or submandibular fat.

Upper chest wrinkling

Introduction: problem assessment and patient selection

When the fashion of women's clothing becomes more revealing, the décolleté takes on an entirely new significance, revealing the tell-tale skin surface changes caused by the innumerable amount of hours one has spent in the sun, either at leisure or at work. The youthful appearance of resurfaced and redraped inelastic, sagging facial skin that has been rejuvenated with soft tissue fillers and implants is now only flawed by the appearance of the crepe paper-like wrinkling of the 'V' of the upper chest. On the upper chest both static and dynamic wrinkling also can co-exist. When they do, the person exhibiting them appears deceptively older than their stated age, spoiling the youthful impression that is portrayed by a wrinkle-free face and neck. Recently, superficial and mid-depth wrinkles on the upper anterior chest wall have been successfully treated with BOTOX®[2,29].

There have been reports describing the use of BOTOX® to relax post-surgical myospasm of the fibers of the pectoralis complex after breast implantation surgery[30,31.] Subsequently, there appeared a report describing the use of injections of another type of botulinum toxin serotype A (Dysport® – Ipsen Limited; INAMED Distributor's 5540 Ekwill Street Santa Barbara, California 93111, USA) to reduce wrinkles of the lower anterior neck and upper chest wall attributed to the excessive contractions of the platysma[31].

Functional anatomy (see above pp 193–196)

The platysma is a very thin, superficial, broad sheet of muscle of varying prominence that originates from the fascia covering part of the upper pectoralis major and deltoid. Apparently, in certain patients the platysma can originate lower than the second, and as far down as the fourth to the sixth, intercostal space. If contraction of the platysma in these patients is hyperkinetic and constant, excessive horizontal and vertical wrinkling of the central, mid to the lower décolleté can occur[29]. (See Appendix 4)

Dilution

Because of the large surface area of the upper chest, a more extensive coverage of BOTOX® is necessary and widespread diffusion is encouraged. Therefore, a 100 U vial of BOTOX® can be reconstituted with 2–5 ml of normal saline (see Appendix 1).

Dosing: how to correct the problem (what to do and what not to do)

The patient can be treated more comfortably in the semirecumbent rather than in the erect, upright position. Approximately 2–8 U of BOTOX® can be injected into each site on the anterior chest wall in several different treatment patterns. The key to a successful outcome is to have the BOTOX® diffuse throughout the entire anterior expanse of the upper chest wall[29]. Injections should be applied superficially into the deep dermis or at the dermo-subcutaneous junction. The pattern of injection depends on the particular shape of an individual's upper chest wall. Accordingly, the area to be treated is outlined as either an upside down isosceles or equilateral triangle, whose apex is at a point over the middle of the xiphoid process of the sternum and whose base is an imaginary line that connects two points placed over the middle of both clavicles (Figure 5.35)[29]. This triangle corresponds to the points of interdigitation of the clavicular portion and the sternocostal portion of the platysma and pectoralis major. Approximately 2–5 U of BOTOX® are injected into the dermo-subcutaneous plane at multiple sites that are roughly

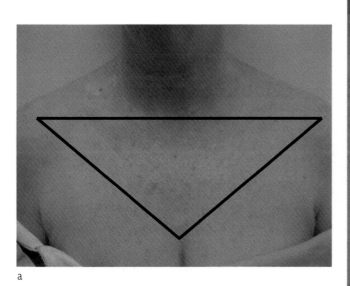

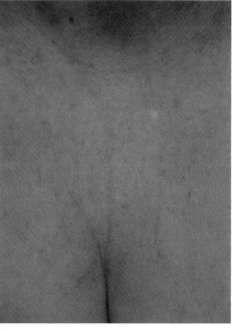

a

b

Figure 5.35   An upside down triangle represents the area where BOTOX® can be injected to reduce wrinkling (a). Note fine wrinkling on chest in close up (b)

1.5–2.0 cm apart from each other within the triangle. The total dose injected should range from 50 to 100 U (average is 75 U) of BOTOX®, depending on the overall strength of the platysma, the number and depth of the wrinkling, and the size and expanse of the anterior chest wall of the patient being treated. Some chests will require anywhere from 4 to 15 injection sites to be successful.

Gentle massage and point pressure to the area injected can prevent post-injection bleeding and ecchymoses (see Appendix 2).

Outcomes (results)

A smoothening of the surface of the central mid to lower décolleté usually occurs within 1–3 weeks of a treatment session (Figures 5.36 to 5.38). The diminution of chest wrinkling

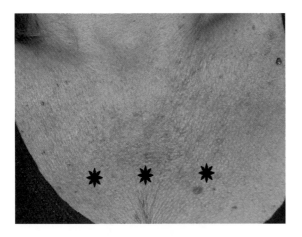 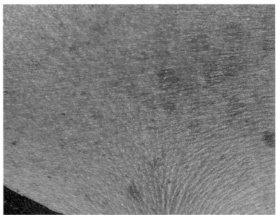

Figure 5.36   Asterixes represent points where 5 U of BOTOX® were injected. (Courtesy of Dr Francisco Atamoros-Pérez)

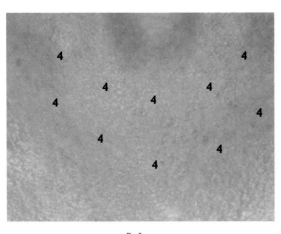 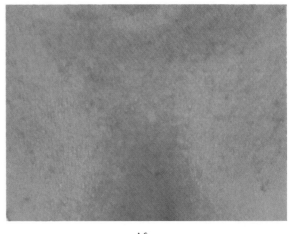

Before   After

Figure 5.37   Area of the central upper chest of a 56-year-old treated with BOTOX® before and 5 weeks after. (Courtesy of Dr Francisco Atamoros-Pérez)

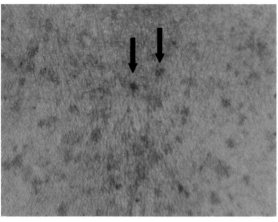
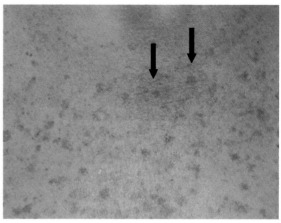

Before   After

Figure 5.38   Area of the central upper chest of a 49-year-old treated with BOTOX® before and 6 weeks after 42 U of BOTOX® were injected. (Courtesy of Dr Francisco Atamoros-Pérez)

usually commences more slowly than when BOTOX® is injected in the face, and it may be effective for only 2–3 months. Widespread diffusion of the injected BOTOX®is necessary to achieve total coverage and complete reduction in the wrinkling of the skin surface of the upper chest wall. Therefore, injections in the upper chest wall are preferably performed with high volumes of low concentration BOTOX®2 (see Appendix 3).

Complications (adverse sequelae) (see Appendix 5)

The most common side effect reported is inadequate clinical results because of insufficient dosing. Additional adverse sequelae include a reduction in upper extremity muscle strength, especially upon adduction and internal rotation as when performing a hugging motion. If BOTOX® is injected too deeply and at higher doses, exceeding 100 U per treatment session, unintended weakening of the intercostal musculature can occur which may interfere with deep respiration. The clinical results of pectoral platysma weakening can take up to 15 days or longer to occur, a much slower onset of effect compared to that which occurs after BOTOX® injections of facial muscles[29].

Treatment implications when injecting the upper chest

1. Injections of high-volume, low concentration BOTOX® in the upper 'V' of the anterior chest wall can suppress the fine surface wrinkling of the skin of that area.
2. Induction of effect in the upper chest takes longer and lasts for a shorter amount of time compared to BOTOX® injections in the face.
3. Overdosing can cause difficulty with deep inspiration or with adducting the upper extremities, as is done when one performs a hug.

References

1. Standernig S (ed.). *Gray's Anatomy. The Anatomical Basis of Clinical Practice*, 39th edn. Elsevier, Churchill, Livingstone, 2005

2. Atamoros FP. Botulinum toxin in the lower one third of the face. *Clinics in Dermatol: Botulinum Toxin in Clinical Medicine (Part I)*, ed. Anthony V. Benedetto2003: 21;505–12

3. Fagien S. BOTOX® for the treatment of dynamic and hyperkinetic facial lines and furrows: adjunctive use in facial aesthic surgery. *Plast Reconstr Surg* 1999;103:701–13

4. Smychyshyn N, Sengelmann R. Botulinum toxin a treatment of perioral rhytides. *Dermatol Surg* 2003;29:490–5

5. Carruthers J, Carruthers A. A prospective, randomized, parallel group study analyzing the effect of BTX-A (Botox) and nonanimal sourced hyaluronic acid (NASHA, Restylane) in combination compared with NASHA (Restylane) alone in severe glabellar rhytides in adult female subjects: treatment of severe glabellar rhytides with a hyaluronic acid derivative compared with the derivative and BTX-A. *Dermatol Surg* 2003;29:802–9

6. Carruthers J, Carruthers A. Aesthetic botulinum A toxin in the mid and lower face and neck. Dermatol Surg 2003;29:468–76

7. Klein AW. Complications and adverse reactions with the use of botulinum toxin. *Seminars Cut Med Surg* 2001;20:109–20

8. Alam M, Dover JS, Klein AW *et al*. Botulinum A exotoxin for hyperfunctional facial lines. Where not to inject. *Arch Dermatol* 2002;138;1180–5

9. Mazzuco R. Perioral wrinkles. In: Hexel D, Almeida AT de (eds) *Cosmetic Use of Botulinum Toxin*. Porto Allegre, Brazil: AGE Editora, 2002:158–63.

10. Biglan AW, Burnstine RA, Rogers GL *et al*. Management of strabismus with botulinum toxin A. *Ophthalmol* 1989;96:935–43

11. Blitzer A, Brin MF, Green PE *et al*. Botulinum toxin injection for the treatment of oromandibular dystonia. *Ann Otol Rhinol Laryngol* 1987;98:93–7

12. Carruthers J, Carruthers A. Botulinum toxin (BOTOX®) chemodenervation for facial rejuvenation. *Facial Plast Surg Clin N Am* 2001;9(2):197–204

13. Loos BM, Mass CS. Relevant anatomy for botulinum toxin in facial rejuventation. *Facial Plast Surg Clin N Am* 2003;11:439–43

14. Papel ID, Capone RB. Botulinum toxin A for mentalis muscle dysfunction. *Arch Facial Plast Surg* 2001;3:268–9

15. Hoefflin SM. The platysma aponeurosis. *Plast Reconstr Surg* 1996;97:1080–8

16. Janfaza P, Nadol JB, Galla HJ *et al. Surgical Anatomy of the Head and Neck*. Philadelphia, PA: Lippincott Williams and Wilkins, 2001:520

17. Cardoso de Castro C. The changing role of platysma in face lifting. *Plast Reconstr Surg* 2000;105:764–75

18. Brandt FS, Boker A. Botulinum toxin for rejuvenation of the neck. *Clin Dermatol* 2003;21:513–20

19. Matarasso A, Matarasso SL, Brandt FS *et al*. Botulinum A exotoxin for the management of platysma bands. *Plast Reconstr Surg* 1999;103:645–52

20. Carruthers A, Carruthers J. Clinical indications and injection technique for the cosmetic use of botulinum A exotoxin. *Dermatol Surg* 1998;24:1189–94

21. Brandt FS, Bellman B. Cosmetic use of botulinum A exotoxin for the aging neck. *Dermatol Surg* 1999;24:1232–4

22. Blitzer A, Binder WJ. Cosmetic uses of botulinum neurotoxin type A. *Arch Facial Plast Surg* 2002;4:212–20

23. Hoefflin SM. Anatomy of the platysma and lip depressor muscles. A simplified mnemonic approach. *Dermatol Surg* 1998;24:1225–31

24. Klein AW. Complications and adverse reactions with the use of botulinum toxin. *Seminars Cut Med Surg* 2001;20:109–20

25. Blitzer A, Binder WJ, Aviv JE. The management of hyperfunctional facial lines with botulinum toxin: a collaborative study of 210 injection sites in 162 patients. *Arch Otolaryngol Head Neck Surg* 1997;123:389–92

26. Dayan S. *Facial Plastic Surgery Clinics of North America; Botox*. Philadelphia, PA: WB Saunders Company, 2003:488–92

27. Thiers B. *Dermatologic Clinics; The Clinical Use of Botulinum Toxin*. Philadelphia, PA: WB Saunders Company, 2004: Volume 22

28. Carruthers J, Fagien S, Matarasso S and the BOTOX® Consensus Group. Consensus recommendations on the use of botulinum toxin type A in facial aesthetics. *Plast Reconstr Surg* 2004;114(Suppl):15–225

29. Isaac C, Gimenez R, Ruiz R de O. Breast wrinkles (décolleté folds). In: Hexel D, Almeida At de (eds). *Cosmetic Use of Botulinum Toxin*. Porto Allegre, Brazil: AGE Editora, 2002:178–81

30. Richards A, Ritz M, Donahoe S *et al*. BOTOX® for contraction of pectoral muscles. *Plast Reconstr Surg* 2001;108:270–1

31. Becker-Wegerich PM, Rauch L, Ruzicka T. Botulinum toxin A: successful décolleté rejuvenation. *Dermatol Surg* 2002;28:168–71

MUSCLE CONTOURING WITH BOTULINUM TOXIN

Michael S Lehrer

Muscle contouring

Introduction

In the majority of cosmetic indications for botulinum toxin discussed thus far, objectionable rhytides and asymmetries are created by the activity of superficial skeletal muscles upon the overlying skin. Partial paralysis of carefully selected muscles may result in the reversal of these undesirable features, creating a more relaxed, youthful appearance.

The cosmetic significance of muscles is not, however, limited to their functional activity. In men, large biceps brachii, pectoralis, quadriceps, and gastrocnemius muscles project an image of strength and vitality and are often seen as desirable. Firm but gently curving quadriceps and gluteal muscles are more frequently seen as the female ideal. With increasing regularity, both men and women exercise aerobically and with weights to shape and contour their visible muscle groups. More often than not, this ritual may be explained by vanity as opposed to a true need for increased strength.

Similarly, the muscles of mastication help to mold the face and its cosmetic appearance. The masseter overlies the angle of the mandible and gives shape to the inferolateral cheek. A large masseter portrays a 'strong' jaw in men, but may be less desirable in women. At the opposite extreme, atrophy of the temporalis is common in the elderly and infirm, and may create a sunken temple and a frail appearance.

Recently, botulinum toxin has been used to selectively atrophy 'hypertrophic' muscles, thereby decreasing their size and recontouring cosmetically unacceptable large areas. In this chapter, jawline recontouring by masseteric atrophy and calf reduction with injections into the gastrocnemius are reviewed.

Jawline recontouring

Introduction: problem assessment and patient selection

In most cultures, the ideal female face is perceived as delicate and smoothly contoured. Asian women in particular prefer an almond-shaped or oval appearance. A square jawline, on the other hand, widens the lower face and is considered masculine[1].

In many patients, the square lower jawline is created by idiopathically enlarged masseters. In others, the masseters may become hypertrophied by asymmetric chewing due to dental problems, congenital arteriovenous fistulae, temporomandibular joint dysfunction, focal dystonia, gum chewing, bruxism, or psychiatric conditions. When an inciting factor for masseteric hypertrophy can be determined, correction of this problem alone may result in aesthetic improvement.

In those patients requiring cosmetic intervention, debulking of the masseter has been attempted with systemic muscle relaxants, antispasmodics, tranquilizers, and antidepressants, as well as with relaxation therapy or occlusal splints. These treatments are, however, limited to those patients in whom overuse of the masseter contributes to its hypertrophy. For the remainder of patients, surgery has become a popular approach. Partial resection of the masseter or bony angle of the mandible may reshape the lower jaw. Surgery may, however, create swelling, hematomas, pain, scars, or facial nerve palsy. The cosmetic benefit of successful surgery also may not be apparent until all post-operative changes resolve.

The use of less invasive botulinum toxin injections for the atrophy and recontouring of the lower face was described simultaneously by two groups in 1994[2,3]. Both reported botulinum toxin A therapy to be effective, safe, and of rapid onset. Numerous refinements have been subsequently published, including a series in which patients recalcitrant to traditional approaches and patients with marked asymmetry were successfully treated with botulinum toxin[4,5].

Functional anatomy

The muscles of mastication include the masseter, temporalis, lateral pterygoid, and medial pterygoid. The most superficial and visible of these, the masseter, provides contour to the inferolateral cheek at the angle of the jaw (Figure 6.1).

The masseter originates at the inferior border and medial surface of the zygomatic arch. This quadrangular muscle then inserts on the lateral surface of the ramus of the mandible and its coronoid process. When contracted, the masseter shortens and thickens, elevating and protruding the mandible and closing the jaws.

While the masseter remains one of the strongest muscles of mastication, it is assisted by both the temporalis and medial pterygoid. The temporalis originates in the temporal fossa and inserts deep to the masseter on the coronoid process of the mandible. The medial pterygoid originates on the pterygoid plate, palatine bone, and tuberosity of the maxilla and inserts on the mandible deep and anterior to the masseter. These redundant masticatory muscles are sufficiently separated to allow injection into the masseter without inadvertently injecting additional muscles.

In some patients, the jawline appears square despite a small or normally sized masseter. In these patients, the wide inferolateral silhouette of the lower face is caused by the large bony prominence at the angle of the mandible. Nevertheless, a thinner masseter overlying this bony prominence would result in a narrower jawline.

Intimate knowledge of the surrounding anatomy is also critical for any practitioner planning to inject the masseter. Perhaps most at risk are the superficial mimetic muscles of the face. These are located just below the skin overlying the masseter. From superior to inferior, they include the zygomaticus major, risorius, buccinator, and depressor anguli oris. Above the masseter and just below these muscles lie their motor nerves. Four of the five branches of the facial nerve – the zygomatic, buccal, marginal mandibular, and cervical – cross above the masseter. Overlying the masseter posteriorly is the parotid gland; the parotid duct traverses the masseter posteriorly to anteriorly at approximately two-thirds its vertical height. Finally, the facial artery and vein cross the masseter at its anteroinferior corner and then course superiorly and anteriorly. Deep to the masseter, however, lies the much less delicate bony ramus of the mandible.

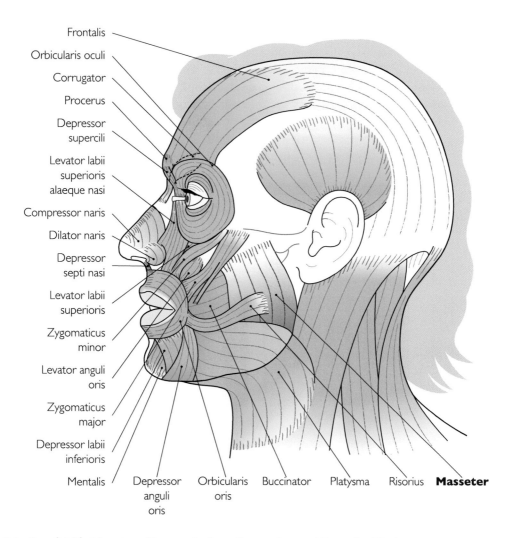

Frontalis
Orbicularis oculi
Corrugator
Procerus
Depressor supercili
Levator labii superioris alaeque nasi
Compressor naris
Dilator naris
Depressor septi nasi
Levator labii superioris
Zygomaticus minor
Levator anguli oris
Zygomaticus major
Depressor labii inferioris
Mentalis
Depressor anguli oris
Orbicularis oris
Buccinator
Platysma
Risorius
Masseter

Figure 6.1   Superficial facial anatomy. The masseter forms the prominence at the angle of the jaw

Dilution

Because the mimetic muscles of the lower face overly the masseter, limiting the diffusion of botulinum toxin following injection is imperative. For this reason, preferably 1 ml and no more than 2 ml of saline should be used to reconstitute a 100 U vial of BOTOX®.

Dosing: how to correct the problem (what to do and what not to do)

Though no standard treatment regimen has been universally accepted, the majority of authors follow quite similar protocols. In a well-lit room with adequate crosslighting, the patient should first be asked to strongly clench the teeth. This will accentuate the contours of the masseter at the angle of the jaw. Next, the most visible two to six bulges of the masseter should be marked with ink. Using a 1-inch long 25- to 30-gauge needle, these prominent portions should be injected intramuscularly for a total dose of 25–30 units of BOTOX® per side.

Because the surrounding facial musculature, nerves, vessels, and ducts lie superficial to the masseter, injection of the deeper portions of the muscle is recommended[6]. The needle should be inserted until the bony ramus of the mandible is struck. This marks the deep fascia of the masseter. The needle tip should then be withdrawn 2–5 mm to guarantee its placement within the muscular body of the masseter. Despite this careful technique, it is wise to withdraw gently on the barrel of the syringe to rule out the intravascular placement of the needle before injecting the botulinum toxin.

For physicians comfortable with intraoral injections, the masseter may also be approached through the buccal mucosa laterally and superiorly to the posterior molars. Those favoring electromyographic localization during injection may be assisted with this technique. Two groups, however, obtained equally acceptable results both with and without electromyographic assistance[1,5].

Following injection, the patient is asked to apply ice to the area several times daily for 2 days. This may reduce post-injection aching or swelling. Although most authors have found it

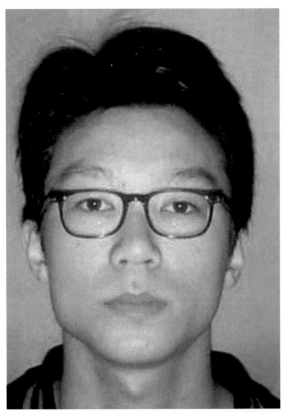

Before

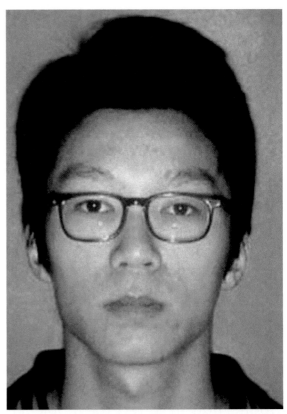

After

Figure 6.2a   Prominent jaw angle in a man due to masseteric hypertrophy

Figure 6.2b   Same patient 3 months following treatment. Reprinted from To EWH *et al*. A prospective study of the effect of botulinum toxin A on masseteric muscle hypertrophy with ultrasonographic and electromyographic measurement. *Br J Plast Surg* 2001;54:197, copyright 2001, with permission from the British Association of Plastic Surgeons

unnecessary, patients may also be instructed to massage the area regularly or to chew gum vigorously after treatment[7,8].

Outcomes (results)

Following injection with botulinum toxin, a visible decrease in the size of the masseter may be seen in as few as 2 weeks. While the initial benefit may be noted only with the patient's teeth clenched, improvement at rest appears between 3 and 8 weeks. This decreased masseteric girth should produce a gentler, more rounded lower face and jawline. Maximal cosmetic benefit is apparent 6 to 8 weeks following injection, with clinical improvement visible for 5–8 months (Figures 6.2 and 6.3).

In a series of 45 patients, Park *et al.* reported that 80 per cent of patients were either satisfied or very satisfied with their results. Only five patients were dissatisfied[1]. In a smaller trial, Blitzer and colleagues reported that 19 out of 20 patients were satisfied. Peak improvement was noted at 1 to 2 months, with results lasting 6 to 8 months[6].

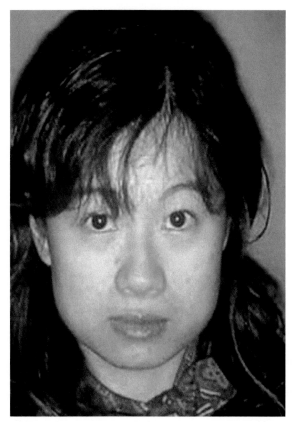

Before

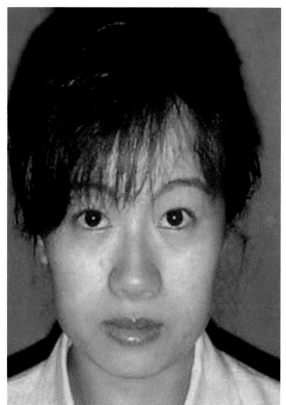

After

Figure 6.3a   Prominent jaw angle in a woman due to masseteric hypertrophy

Figure 6.3b   Same patient 3 months following treatment. Reprinted from To EWH *et al*. A prospective study of the effect of botulinum toxin A on masseteric muscle hypertrophy with ultrasonographic and electromyographic measurement. *Br J Plast Surg* 2001;54:197, copyright 2001, with permission from the British Association of Plastic Surgeons

Several authors have attempted to more precisely quantify the response of the masseter to botulinum toxin. Kim *et al.* assessed the volume of the masseter with computerized tomography both prior to injection and 3 months following injection with BOTOX®. An average volume decrease of 22 per cent (range 8.1–35.4 per cent) was reported[8]. To *et al.*[7] used ultrasound to measure the volume of patients' masseters before injection with Dysport®, as well as at 1, 2, 3, and 4 weeks, and 3, 6, and 12 months later. They noted a reduction in volume of 7.1 per cent as early as 1 week following therapy, and a peak reduction of 30.9 per cent at 3 months. This maximal effect persisted until 6 months, then slowly fell to a 13.4 per cent reduction in volume at 1 year. Park et al used either computerized tomography or ultrasound to measure changes in the thickness, rather than volume, of the masseter[1]. Three months following injection with BOTOX®, they reported a mean decrease in thickness of 2.9 mm, or 20 per cent.

Complications (adverse sequelae) (see Appendix 5)

While most studies report no adverse events following botulinum toxin injection into the masseter, side effects nevertheless occur. First, many patients describe an aching discomfort in the masseter for the first 48 hours after treatment. Post-injection compression with ice may alleviate this result. In addition, masseter fatigue or difficulty chewing hard foods may be noted in 10–44 per cent of patients[1,6]. This side effect is, however, tolerable and resolves in 4 to 8 weeks. Because of the large size of the masseter, and the redundancy afforded to the masticatory system by the temporalis and medial ptyerygoid muscles, it is unlikely that extreme difficulty with chewing will occur.

Speech disturbances or changes in facial expression may be more disconcerting. Park *et al.* noted speech changes lasting no more than 1 month in 7 of 45 patients treated[1]. In another study, 3 of 11 patients noted changes in facial expressions while smiling[8]. These changes lasted for up to 2 months. It is likely that each of these side effects was due to the accidental weakening of the zygomaticus major or depressor anguli oris muscles. The injector must remember that the mimetic muscles of the face lie superficially; to avoid their accidental weakening, all injections should be directed toward the deeper portions of the masseter.

Finally, two patients have complained of sunken cheeks following injection[8]. This complication was attributed to atrophy of the superior portion of the masseter in patients with prominent zygomatic arches. Because the superior portion of the masseter lies just below the bony prominence of the cheekbone, thinning the masseter may result in a sharp drop-off between the zygomatic arch and cheek. The authors therefore recommend that treatment of the upper portions of the masseter be avoided in Asians and other patients with prominent zygomatic arches.

Treatment implications

1. For many patients, a soft rounded jawline is preferred over a wide, square jawline.
2. Much of the shape at the angle of the jaw is created by the bulk of the masseter muscle.
3. The muscles of mastication are somewhat redundant, allowing for weakening and atrophy of the masseter without significant adverse effects.
4. Following injection of the masseter with BOTOX®, a significant softening of the jawline may appear within weeks, maximize by 3 months, and persist for 6 months to 1 year.
5. Overly superficial injection of the masseter may result in inadvertent weakening of the mimetic muscles of the face, resulting in temporary difficulty with phonation or smiling.

Calf recontouring

Introduction: problem assessment and patient selection

With both short skirts and shorts becoming more acceptable around the world, the lower leg has become recognized as an area of esthetic significance. In Asian women in particular, shapeless legs with thick calves are considered a cosmetic problem. Of singular concern may be a bulging prominence on the medial calf, approximately two-thirds the vertical height from the ankle to the knee. This protrusion is created by a hypertrophic medial head of the gastrocnemius muscle, and is most apparent when standing on the toes or wearing high-heeled shoes.

In the past, aggressive therapy was pursued by patients bothered by large calves. The medial head of the gastrocnemius could be resected surgically or atrophied via selective denervation[9–11]. These procedures were invasive and fraught with both potential and real complications. Although frequently used for recontouring in other body areas, liposuction is not effective in this setting, as the excess bulk is created not by fat but by muscle.

Botulinum toxin has been used therapeutically in the gastrocnemius to correct the gait of idiopathic toe walkers, to relieve spasticity in cerebral palsy patients and quadriplegics, and to alleviate spastic foot drop following cerebral vascular accidents[12–14]. In these cases, intramuscularly injected botulinum toxin causes temporary muscle paralysis and eventual muscle atrophy. Recently, this atrophic feature of botulinum toxin has been exploited to correct asymptomatic but cosmetically disfiguring calf hypertrophy[15,16].

Functional anatomy

The muscles of the lower leg may be divided into the anterior, lateral, and posterior compartments. The small anterior and lateral muscles dorsiflex, stabilize, and evert the foot, but add little contour to the leg. The shape of the calf is created predominantly by the powerful superficial muscles of the posterior compartment – gastrocnemius, soleus, and plantaris (Figure 6.4).

The gastrocnemius is the largest and most superficial of these muscles. Proximally, it may be divided into two bellies. The stronger medial component originates at the popliteal surface of the femur, superior to the medial condyle, while the lateral head originates at the lateral aspect of the lateral condyle of the femur. These two portions fuse into a single muscle more distally, and insert into the posterior calcaneous via the tendo calcaneus or Achilles tendon. When contracted, the gastrocnemius becomes shorter and wider, plantarflexes the foot, raises the heel while walking, and flexes the knee joint.

Cosmetically, the gastrocnemius appears to form the majority of the calf prominence. It is the largest and most superficial muscle of the lower leg. In addition, its two bellies may project significantly more laterally and medially than the deeper calf muscles. Finally, gastrocnemius may extend more superiorly than both soleus and plantaris, and therefore produce the entire superomedial and superolateral contour of the calf.

In most cases, enlargement of the gastrocnemius is idiopathic and does not create functional impairment. Rarely, however, the oversized gastrocnemius may be caused by muscular dystrophy, peripheral nerve lesions, chronic spinal atrophy, chronic recurrent polyneuropathy, or poliomyelitis[17–20].

When considering cosmetic alteration of the calf, the redundancy of the posterior compartment muscles cannot be overly emphasized. First, the gastrocnemius is composed of

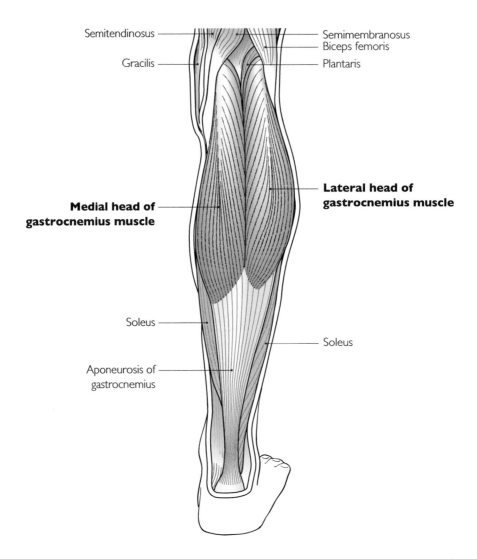

Semitendinosus

Semimembranosus
Biceps femoris

Gracilis

Plantaris

**Lateral head of
gastrocnemius muscle**

**Medial head of
gastrocnemius muscle**

Soleus

Soleus

Aponeurosis of
gastrocnemius

Figure 6.4   Anatomy of the posterior compartment of the leg, highlighting the prominent gastrocnemius muscles

two independent bellies. Next, like the gastrocnemius, the much smaller plantaris originates at the femur and inserts on the calcaneus. When contracted, it weakly assists the gastrocnemius in plantarflexing the foot and flexing the knee joint. Finally, the broad, powerful soleus lies deep to the gastrocnemius. It originates on the posterior tibia and fibula and inserts with the gastrocnemius on the tendo calcaneus, assisting the gastrocnemius in plantarflexing the foot and steadying the leg. Should one of these muscles become injured or impaired, the gait is generally undisturbed and the lower leg and ankle are supported by the remaining posterior compartment muscles.

Dilution

Because diffusion throughout the large medial head of the gastrocnemius is desired, approximately 4.0 ml of saline should be added to each 100 unit vial of BOTOX®. Any inadvertent diffusion into the neighboring soleus and plantaris would likely be of insufficient quantity to result in functional weakening of these powerful skeletal muscles. Using a dilute solution of botulinum toxin may also create less waste. Because a relatively large-bore needle is needed to inject the gastrocnemius, any drops of solution 'lost' during treatment will be larger than those lost when injecting with the usual 30-gauge needle. Working with a less concentrated preparation of botulinum toxin may, therefore, result in fewer wasted botulinum toxin units.

Dosing: how to correct the problem (what to do and what not to do)

Before injecting, the medial head of the gastrocnemius should be identified by having the patient stand in tiptoe position. The contracted, protruding area should then be marked for three to six injections at 1.5–2 cm intervals. The patient may then be placed in a prone position for injection. In order to allow for adequate penetration and drug delivery into this bulky muscle belly, a 1-inch needle, 23- to 27-gauge, is recommended.

Total doses varying between 32 and 100 units of BOTOX® per calf have been reported effective[15,16]. Until a larger dose-finding study is completed, it would be prudent for injectors to select a dose within this range based upon the size of the contracted gastrocnemius muscle.

Outcomes (results)

Because the esthetic effect of botulinum toxin in calf reduction is a function of both muscle weakening and atrophy, improvement following injection is more gradual than seen in many other body areas. Recontouring of the leg will first be evidenced by a smaller medial calf bulge with contraction of the gastrocnemius in the tiptoe position; this may be noted within 1–2 weeks. As atrophy occurs over the next 1–2 months, smoother contours at rest will follow. (Figure 6.5).

In their series of six patients, Lee et al observed that leg circumference decreased by between 5 and 20 mm following treatment with BOTOX®[16]. This improvement was maintained for at least 6 months. In the one patient available for long-term follow-up, a modest reduction in girth remained at 12 months. In addition to a decrease in width, the most prominent point in the contour of the medial calf moved upward to a more cosmetically elegant position near the knee. Finally, patients subjectively reported a softening of the medial calf following injection.

Complications (adverse sequelae) (see Appendix 5)

Because of the previously described muscle redundancy in the posterior compartment of the leg, patients remain functionally normal following injection of botulinum toxin. No changes in ankle mobility or gait have been reported to date in the literature.

Patients do, however, experience mild tenderness at the injection sites for several days after treatment. Bruising also may be evident. These complications may be attributed to the relatively larger gauge needle than is usually used in botulinum toxin treatments in other body areas.

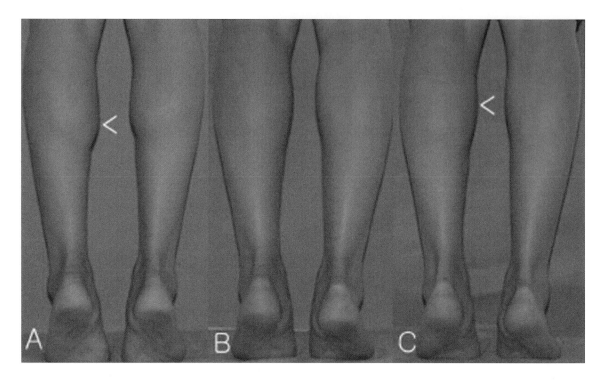

Figure 6.5 A Angulated, masculine bulging of the medial gastrocnemius in a young woman. B Same patient 1 month following injection of 48 U of botulinum toxin A in each medial gastrocnemius muscle. C Same patient 6 months after injection. Bulging of the medial gastrocnemius muscle has disappeared after the botulinum toxin A treatment with an upward movement of the most prominent point (indicated by the pointer) of the leg contour. Reprinted from Lee HJ *et al*. Botulinum toxin A for aesthetic contouring of enlarged medial gastrocnemius muscle. *Dermatol Surg* 2004;30:867, copyright 2004, with permission

Finally, one patient with frequent leg swelling and pitting edema following treatment has been described[16]. This complication persisted for at least 2 months. Stasis following weakening of the gastrocnemius is likely secondary to temporary weakening of the venous calf-pump mechanism.

Treatment implications

1. Poorly contoured lower legs may constitute a significant esthetic problem.
2. A common complaint among women, particularly in Asian countries, is a central bulge created by the medial head of the gastrocnemius muscle.
3. The muscles of the calf are redundant and therefore may be selectively weakened or atrophied without significant disturbances in function.
4. Following botulinum toxin A injection to the medial head of the gastrocnemius, improvements in contour may be seen as early as 1 week, but are not maximized for at least 1 month. Results may last 6–12 months.
5. Because of the size and depth of the gastrocnemius muscle, a 1-inch 23- to 27-gauge needle should be used.
6. Complications are generally mild and self-limited.

References

1. Park MY, Ahn KY, Jung DS. Botulinum toxin type A treatment for contouring of the lower face. *Dermatol Surg* 2003;29:477–83

2. Moore AP, Wood GD. The medical management of masseteric hypertrophy with botulinum toxin type A. *Br J Oral Maxillofacial Surg* 1994;32:26–8

3. Smyth AG. Botulinum toxin treatment of bilateral masseteric hypertrophy. *Br J Oral Maxillofacial Surg* 1994;32:29–33

4. Mandel L, Tharakan M. Treatment of unilateral masseteric hypertrophy with botulinum toxin: case report. *J Oral Maxillofac Surg* 1999;57:1017–19

5. Von Lindern JJ, Niederhagen B, Appel T, Berge S, Reich RH. Type A botulinum toxin for the treatment of hypertrophy of the masseter and temporal muscles: an alternative treatment. *Plast Reconstr Surg* 2001:107:327–32

6. Ahn J, Horn C, Blitzer A. Botulinum toxin for masster reduction in Asian patients. *Arch Facial Plast Surg* 2004;6:188–91

7. To EWH, Ahuja AT, Ho WS *et al.* A prospective study of the effect of botulinum toxin A on masseteric muscle hypertrophy with ultrasonographic and electromyographic measurement. *Br J Plast Surg* 2001;54:197–200

8. Kim HJ, Yum KW, Lee SS, Heo MS, Seo K. Effects of botulinum toxin type A on bilateral masseteric hypertrophy evaluated with computed tomographic measurement. *Dermatol Surg* 2003;29:484–9

9. Kim IG, Hwang SH, Lw JM, Lee HY. Endoscope-assisted calf reduction in Orientals. Plast Reconstr Surg 2000;106:713–20

10. Tsai CC, Lee SS, Lai CS, Lin SD, Chiou CS. Aesthetic resection of the gastrocnemius muscle in postpoliomyelitis calf hypertrophy: an uncommon case report. *Aesthetic Plast Surg* 2001;25:111–13

11. Lemperle G, Exner K. The resection of gastrocnemius muscles in aesthetically disturbing calf hypertrophy. *Plast Reconstr Surg* 1998;102:2230–6

12. Glanzman AM, Kim H, Swaminithan K, Beck T. Efficacy of botulinum toxin A, serial casting, and combined treatment for spastic equinus: a retrospective analysis. *Dev Med Child Neurol* 2004;46:807–11

13. Brunt D, Woo R, Kim HD *et al.* Effect of botulinum toxin type A on gait of children who are idiopathic toe-walkers. *J Surg Orthop Adv* 2004;13:149–55

14. Johnson CA, Burridge JH, Strike PW, Wood DE, Swain ID. The effect of combined use of botulinum toxin type A and functional electric stimulation in the treatment of spastic drop foot after stroke: a preliminary investigation. *Arch Phys Med Rehabil* 2004;85:902–9

15. Park MY, Ahn KY. Botulinum toxin A for the treatment of hyperkinetic wrinkle lines. *Plast Reconstr Surg* 2003;112:148–50S

16. Lee HJ, Lee DW, Park YH *et al.* Botulinum toxin A for aesthetic contouring of enlarged medial gastrocnemius muscle. *Dermatol Surg* 2004;30:867–71

17. Korczyn AD, Kuritzky A, Sandbank U. Muscle hypertrophy with neuropathy. *J Neurol Sci* 1978;38:399–408

18. Pearn J, Hudgson P. Anterior-horn cell degeneration and gross calf hypertrophy with adolescent onset: a new spinal muscular atrophy syndrome. *Lancet* 1978;1:1059–61

19. Valenstein E, Watson RT, Parker JL. Myokymia, muscle hypertrophy and percussion 'myotonia' in chronic recurrent polyneuropathy. *Neurology* 1978;28:1130–4

20. Bertorini TE, Igarashi M. Postpoliomyelitis muscle pseudohypertrophy. *Muscle Nerve* 1985;8:644–9

7 OTHER DERMATOLOGIC USES OF BOTULINUM TOXIN

Kevin C Smith and Francisco Pérez-Atamoros

Introduction

This chapter will discuss the use of botulinum toxin type A (BTX-A) in dermatology for the treatment of pain, and to improve the appearance and presentation of female breasts.

Since BTX-A was first reported to be useful for the reduction in the pain of spasmodic torticollis in 1985[1], the number of references in Medline™ to 'botulinum' and 'pain' have been growing at an increasing rate (Figure 7.1) – by mid-June 2005 there were over 580 references. The list of painful conditions reported to respond well to BTX-A is also growing, and now includes some dermatologic conditions. This chapter will focus on the treatment of post-herpetic neuralgia (PHN), painful scars, and reflex sympathetic dystrophy.

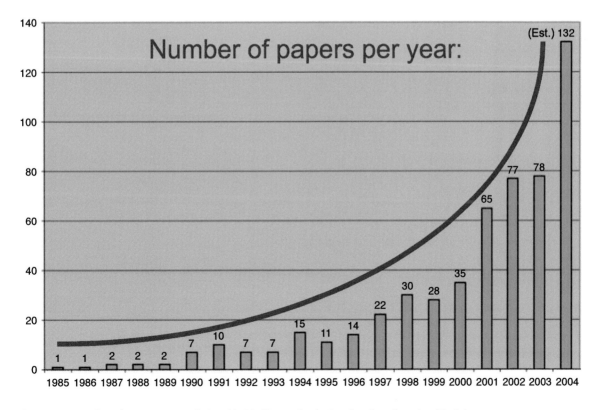

Figure 7.1   Number of papers per year indexed in Medline under the heading 'botulinum' and 'pain'

In addition to its well-known effect of blocking the release of acetylcholine from motor neurons on striated muscle, BTX-A has been shown to block release of the pain-mediating neurotransmitter substance P (SP)[2,3], calcitonin gene-related peptide (CGRP)[4,5,] and glutamate[6] from motor and sensory neurons. Substance P is known to play a role in some cases of post-herpetic neuralgia[7,8]. BTX-A may have additional mechanisms of action for pain relief, apart from those listed above[9,10]. It may act both by blocking peripheral sensitization and by indirectly reducing central sensitization[11].

It is important to note that the BTX-A used by the authors in the management of these conditions was BOTOX®, and the doses described in this paper refer to BOTOX®. Because the diffusion characteristics and other pharmacologic properties of other forms of BTX-A differ from BOTOX® it is not possible to establish a simple ratio for the conversion of BOTOX® doses to other forms of BTX-A, or to other botulinum neurotoxins, for example BOTOX®-B. To reduce the risk of confusion, the trade name of the product actually injected will be used throughout this chapter, and the term BTX-A will be used to refer to the general class of neurotoxin.

BTX-A for post-herpetic neuralgia

Perhaps the first to use BOTOX® for the treatment of PHN were Dr Arnold Klein[12], and later Drs Mariusz Sapijaszko and Richard Glogau (personal communications) who used BOTOX® to treat PHN on the trunk. Their informal oral reports, together with a consideration of the well-

---

Last Name _____ First Name _____ Chart # _____ Date _____

Patient's rating scale:

Please circle the number which best describes the amount of pain you are having today in the involved area:
When you are not touching the area:

NO Pain   0   1   2   3   4   5   6   7   8   9   10   WORST possible pain

When the area is touched or rubbed:

NO Pain   0   1   2   3   4   5   6   7   8   9   10   WORST possible pain

---

Please circle the number which best describes your PAIN in the involved area is BETTER or WORSE compared with how it was at your last visit:

BETTER   5   4   3   2   1   0   1   2   3   4   5   WORSE

Please circle the number which best describes your OVERALL impression of how you are doing, compared with the previous visit:

BETTER   5   4   3   2   1   0   1   2   3   4   5   WORSE

Figure 7.2   Visual analog scale used to measure patients' perception of their pain and of their global wellbeing

established role of SP in the pathogenesis of PHN, and considering reports that BTX-A blocked the release of SP from vesicles in nerve terminals, provided the rationale for additional trials of treatment with BTX-A for severe, intractable PHN.

It is important clinically, for communication with other physicians and with third party payers, and in terms of pharmacoeconomics to objectively quantify patient condition at baseline and in response to therapy. The four tools which are helpful include:

1. Likert pain scale and global assessment (Figure 7.2).
2. Physician's global assessment (Figure 7.3).
3. Number of doses of pain medication taken in the 7 days preceding evaluation, and the number of doses taken since the last visit.
4. Marking the boundaries of the area or areas of PHN and then photographing the involved areas at every visit (Figure 7.4).

Patients are advised to continue their usual pain medications, and to only reduce the dose of pain medication as they respond to their BTX-A treatment.

Last Name   First Name   Chart #   Date

Patient's rating scale:

Please circle the number which best describes the amount of pain the patient appears to be having today in the involved area
When the area is not touched

    NO Pain   0   1   2   3   4   5   6   7   8   9   10   WORST possible pain

When the area is touched or rubbed

    NO Pain   0   1   2   3   4   5   6   7   8   9   10   WORST possible pain

---

Please circle the number which best describes whether the patient's pain in the involved area appears to be BETTER or WORSE compared with how it was at the patient's last visit:

    BETTER   5   4   3   2   1   0   1   2   3   4   5   WORSE

Please circle the number which best describes your OVERALL impression of how this patient is doing, compared with the previous visit:

    BETTER   5   4   3   2   1   0   1   2   3   4   5   WORSE

Figure 7.3   Visual analog scale used to measure the physician's assessment of the patient's pain and of the patient's global wellbeing

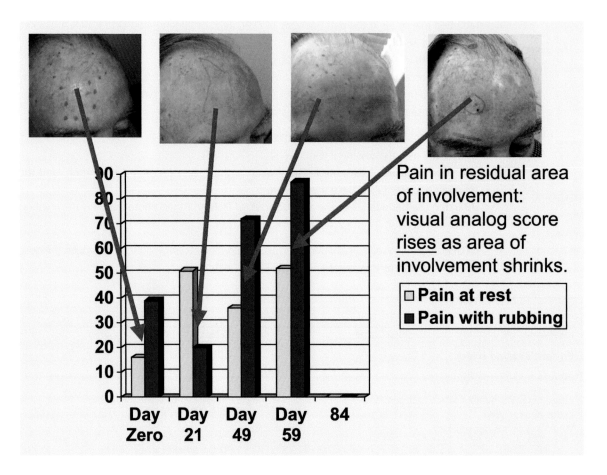

Figure 7.4   The area identified by the patient is marked and photographed, the patient completes a visual analog pain score (Figure 7.2), and then the painful area is injected with BOTOX®

The patient identifies the area or areas of involvement. The boundaries of the area(s) of involvement are marked with washable pink fluorescent marker, photographed (Figure 7.4), then injected with BOTOX® intradermally or subdermally at doses ranging from 2.5 to 5 units per injection, with the injections spaced 2–3 cm apart. The total dose of BOTOX® is generally in the range of 1–2 units per cm or cm².

BTX-A is reconstituted using normal saline with benzyl alcohol preservative (which has local anesthetic properties and reduces injection discomfort). A reconstitution volume of 2.5 ml per 100 units of BOTOX® is generally used, but the reconstitution volume does not seem to influence efficacy – the only thing that matters is how many units of BTX-A are administered. Because there is commonly hyperalgesia in areas of PHN, it is best to use a very fine 31-gauge SteriJect needles mounted on Henke Dose Saver 1 ml syringes (both obtainable from www.air-tite.com). It is not usually necessary to pretreat patients with topical anesthetics like EMLA®, but this could be used in cases where there is a likelihood of intolerable injection discomfort.

Patients should be informed that there will very likely be some unwanted relaxation of muscles in the treated area. Injecting BTX-A intradermally can minimize muscle weakness.

Injections for the pain of PHN seem to be equally effective whether given intradermally, subdermally, or intramuscularly.

The maximum analgesic effect of BTX-A treatment for PHN often occurs at around 3–4 weeks. For this reason, patients are asked to return for reassessment and possibly additional treatment every 3–4 weeks until they are pain free.

While the occasional patient will respond in a dramatic manner to a single session of treatment with BTX-A, it is more typical for patients to improve in a stepwise manner. Patients generally need between one and four treatment sessions to become pain free. Objective quantification of the area of involvement, medication intake, Likert pain score, and patient's and physician's global assessment will help both the patient and the physician to determine whether or not additional treatment is justified.

Usually, serial photographs of the involved area demonstrate progressive reduction of the surface area. Patients find this encouraging. There is often a paradoxical increase in the patient's Likert pain score as the total area of involvement shrinks. The reason for this phenomenon is not well understood. It could be that the mildest areas of PHN resolve first, with the result that because of 'averaging' by the patient the pain score in the residual area of involvement would tend to rise. It is also possible that low-level stimulation from mild areas of involvement or from discomfort traveling down A-alpha or A-beta neurons stimulates the inhibitory interneurons which attenuate the amount of pain signal passing from C neurons and A-delta neurons to the final common pathway leading ultimately to the brain – Melzack and Wall's 'gate control of pain'[13] theory.

As an aside, 'gate control of pain' is also exploited in dermatology when we reduce a patient's discomfort by stroking the skin adjacent to where an injection is being given, or when vibration[14] (this reference includes video demonstrations of vibration being used to reduce the discomfort of a variety of dermatologic procedures) is used to attenuate the discomfort associated with the injection of BOTOX® for palmar or plantar hyperhidrosis (Figure 7.5), to reduce the discomfort when filler materials like hyaluronic acid are injected into the nasolabial folds (Figure 7.6), or when the 1064 nm laser is being used to treat blood vessels on the legs (Figure 7.7)[14].

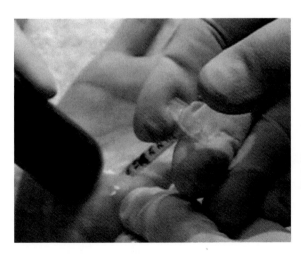

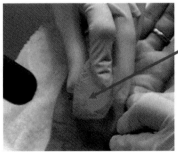

Ice cube wrapped in a single layer of gauze, applied for five seconds before injection

Figure 7.5   Hitachi Magic Wand™ with WonderWand™ vibrating massager applied within 2 cm of the injection site for 3 seconds before insertion of BD-II 31 game needle, and injection of 2.5–4 units of BOTOX® reconstituted using normal saline with preservative, 100 units of BOTOX® in 1 ml

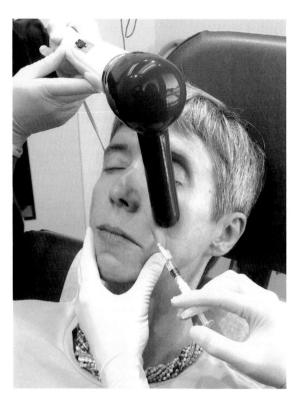

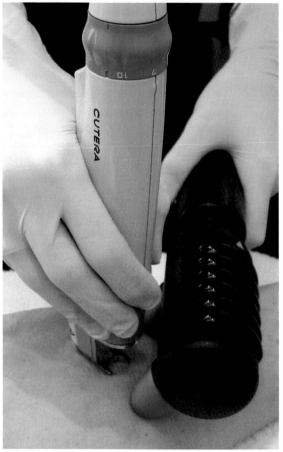

Figure 7.6 Hitachi Magic Wand® vibrating massager with WonderWand® attachment is applied by an assistant within 1–2 cm of where Restylane® will be injected into the nasolabial fold using a 30-gauge MaxFLO® needle (which has the lumen of an ordinary 27-gauge needle, and is so fine that it minimizes injection discomfort and also reduces tissue trauma and reduces the chance of bruising)

Figure 7.7 Conair® Vibrating Massager is applied within several cm of where a Cutera CoolGlide® 1064 nm laser is being used to treat leg veins. This greatly reduces the discomfort of laser treatment, allowing the use of larger spot sizes and higher fluences than would otherwise be intolerable and so contributes to more effective treatment

In these circumstances, mechanoreceptors in the skin detect touch and vibration and send this signal to the CNS along A-alpha and A-beta neurons. This signal acts by way of an inhibitory interneuron to attenuate transmission from the spinal cord to the brain of pain signals which are sent from adjacent skin along afferent C and A-delta neurons to the spinal cord (Figure 7.8).

When the patient with PHN has been rendered pain free by treatment with BTX-A there is usually a long-term drug-free remission of pain. It could be that the same plasticity of the nervous system which led to the development of chronic, intractable pain is now allowing the patient's nervous system to reorganize itself and so escape from the pain loop.

Vibration reduces discomfort in a variety of dermatologic procedures by exploiting "Gate control of pain"

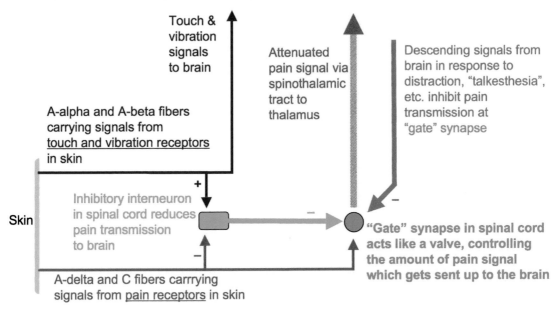

Figure 7.8   Schematic diagram of the neural systems which are thought to play a role in the 'gate contol of pain'

BTX-A in the management of painful scars

Immunohistochemistry has demonstrated substantial numbers of nerves staining for SP and CGRP in some scars[15]. This observation, together with successful experience treating PHN, formed the rationale for offering a trial of treatment with injections of BTX-A to patients suffering from chronic intractable painful scars. Objective quantification of the patient's pain is of great importance in the management of painful scars. Tools which are useful for this purpose are essentially the same as those used in the assessment of patients who have PHN:

1. Likert pain scale and global assessment (Figure 7.2).
2. Physician's global assessment (Figure 7.3).
3. Marking the boundaries of the area or areas of pain and then photographing the involved areas at every visit (Figure 7.9).

Injections are usually performed using a 30-gauge 1-inch needle inserted into the scar. In the case of a thick scar (for example, a keloid on the central chest after thoracotomy, Figure 7.9) the patient may offer advice about whether the pain is deep or superficial and the injection can be adjusted to take this into account. Topical anesthetics like EMLA® cream are generally not necessary, but could be used in a very sensitive patient. One author (KCS) has successfully used injections of BTX-A to treat pain associated with keloid scarring, hypertrophic scarring, and normal scarring.

As is the case when treating PHN, to reduce discomfort BTX-A is reconstituted using normal saline with preservative. The reconstitution volume does not seem to affect efficacy, but to

Week Zero   Week Zero   Week 4

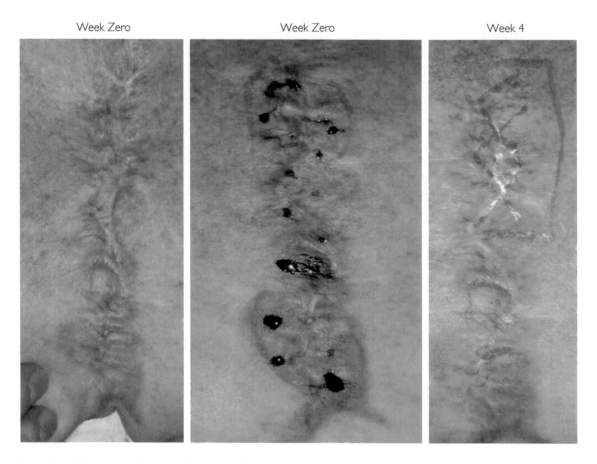

Figure 7.9   Keloid scar on the chest of a woman who had, 8 years previously, had a coronary artery bypass grafting procedure, and whose pain had not responded adequately for surgical resection of the keloid, or to injections of triamcinolone acetonide, or to the application of silicone gel

minimize injection discomfort into hypertrophic or keloid scars the smallest possible volume is preferred, so the author (KCS) uses a reconstitution of 1 ml in 100 units of BOTOX®. In cases where the tissue was very tight and there was unacceptable discomfort, 100 units of BOTOX® could be reconstituted with as little as 0.5 ml of normal saline. The amount of BOTOX® administered in each treatment has ranged from 10 to 50 units per ml of scar tissue.

As with the treatment of PHN, the antinociceptive effect of BTX-A for painful scars seems to reach a maximum at around 3 weeks, so it is the author's (KCS) practice to have patients return for re-assessment and re-treatment every 3–4 weeks until the patient is pain free. The required number of treatments has ranged from one to four. As with PHN, the visual analog or Likert pain score may rise in residual areas of involvement even as the patient globally improves (Figure 7.10), and patients typically remain pain free long term once they have been rendered pain free by treatment with BTX-A. In one case there have been partial relapses at 6–12 month intervals, and these have responded within 5–10 days to additional injections of BTX-A.

There has been no clinically significant improvement in the appearance (assessed by serial photography) of the scars injected by the author (KCS) with BOTOX®, but one hypertrophic

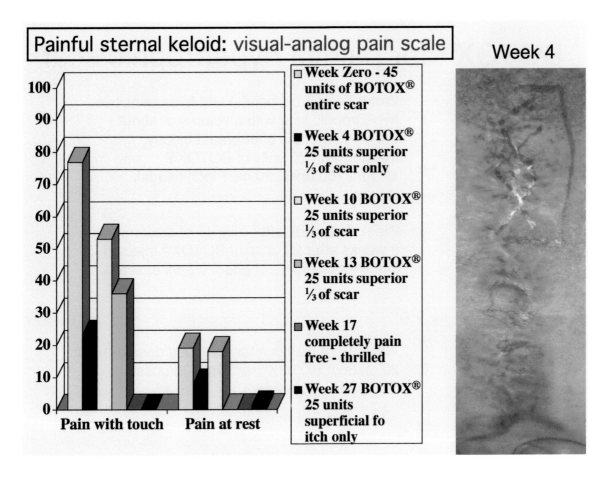

Figure 7.10 Chart illustrating gradual reduction in visual analog pain scores in response to injection of painful areas in the keloid scar with BOTOX®

scar on the breast (Figure 7.11) seemed much softer 6 months after two injections with BOTOX®. Because SP and CGRP interact with some of the cytokines involved in collagen remodeling and collagen deposition[16–18] it is conceivable that treatment with BTX-A could affect the physical properties of some scars, perhaps with repeated treatments or after longer follow-up.

BTX-A in the management of reflex sympathetic dystrophy (complex regional pain syndrome)

Reflex sympathetic dystrophy is characterized by constant burning pain and hyperesthesia in an extremity. Swelling, sweating, vasomotor instability, and sometimes trophic changes often accompany pain. There is often a history of injury or other trauma. Muscle spasms, myoclonus, or focal dystonia may occur. Diffuse pain, loss of function, and autonomic dysfunction are three main criteria suggested for diagnosis. Successful use of BTX-A for this entity has been reported[19,20].

BOTOX® for painful hypertrophic scar

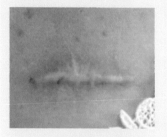

Week Zero: 3 cm painful and hypersensitive hypertrophic scar with a volume of about 0.4 cc 10 months after breast biopsy. Injected with 20 units of BOTOX® @ 1 ml/100 units, 30 ga 1 inch needle.

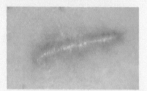

Week 8: 1 week after relapse of discomfort, 8 weeks after 20 units of BOTOX® injected into a total volume of about 0.5 ml of scar.

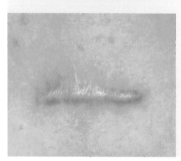

Week 12: 4 weeks after a second dose of 20 units of BOTOX® @ 1 ml/100 units. Completely pain free.

Figure 7.11 Pain in a hypertrophic scar on the upper chest after breast biopsy resolved in response to intralesional injection of BOTOX®

The author (KCS) has treated a 41-year-old woman who had an 8-year history of severe, refractory reflex sympathetic dystrophy rendering her right arm useless since injuries in a motor vehicle accident. Initially injections were exceptionally painful and anxiety provoking. Anxiety was reduced in subsequent injection sessions by pretreating this patient with 80 mg of oxyprenolol (a very lipid-soluble beta blocker which crosses the blood–brain barrier quite well and attenuates the central effects of adrenaline) together with 4 mg of lorazepam, 1–2 hours before injection of BOTOX®. Gradual improvement in the hyperalgesic component of her reflex sympathetic dystrophy has also contributed to improved tolerance of the injections.

The patient characterized her pain as coming predominantly from bone, and deep injections close to bone using a 30-gauge 1-inch needle were of particular benefit. Subcutaneous and intramuscular injections of Botox Therapeutic® (a total of 120–400 units per session, about once a month) into the areas of discomfort in the right hand and arm gave substantial pain relief (for which the patient was very grateful) and also normalized skin color and temperature in the right hand and forearm, but after one year of treatments there has not been any improvement in her ability to use the right hand. Even though the right hand remains useless it is less of an impediment. It should be noted that reduction in pain and sensitivity has allowed this patient to take part in a greater range of activities of daily living and to participate more fully in society, so there has been an overall improvement in general functional ability.

This is consistent with the observations of Cordivari et al[19], who noted that four out of four of their patients with dystonia-complex regional pain syndrome affecting the hand had pain relief after treatment with BTX-A (Dysport®), but only one of the four had functional improvement.

There is less concern now than in the past about the risk that a patient such as this, who is being treated every 4–6 weeks with 400–600 units of BOTOX®, will develop antibodies against the BOTOX® variant of BTX-A. Jankovic et al[21] found that blocking antibodies were detected in 4 of 42 (9.5%) cervical dystonia patients treated only with original BOTOX®, but in none of the 119 patients ($p < 0.004$) treated exclusively with current BOTOX® which has been on the market since late 1997.

BTX-A Overdose reversal

If an acute overdose of BTX-A is recognized (within minutes of the injection), there is limited experimental evidence (K. Smith & D. Schachter, unpublished observations) that immediate reduction in temperature of the injected area to around 4–7°C for 2-4 hours by the application of crushed ice, and the infiltration of the injected area with a fairly large amount (eg. 3 ml) of 2 per cent lidocaine (lignocaine) without epinephrine (adrenaline), may reduce the uptake of BTX-A by cholinergic nerve terminals in the area of the overdose. The scientific rationale for this approach is as follows:

1. Uptake of BTX-A is an energy-requiring process. The rate of most biological reactions declines by about 50 per cent for every 10°C reduction in temperature, so reducing the temperature of the tissue by 30°C might lead to an 8-fold reduction in the rate of uptake of BTX-A.
2. Uptake of BTX-A is greater in cholinergic terminals on muscles which are active, so paralysis of the muscles and reduced metabolic activity of nerves after infiltration with lidocaine could be expected to further reduce BTX-A uptake.
3. BTX-A may be diluted and washed away to some extent by immediate infiltration of the overdosed area with a large volume of 2 per cent lidocaine.
4. Plain lidocaine is a mild vasodilator, so may increase perfusion of the injected area and further contribute to washing away the BTX-A before it has a chance to be taken up by the cholinergic nerve terminals.
5. Application of crushed ice for several hours is uncomfortable, but the discomfort can be considerably reduced by first infiltrating the area with 2 per cent lidocaine.
6. Infiltration with 2 per cent lidocaine alone (without the application of ice) seems to produce some benefit, but less than is seen when both crushed ice and lidocaine infiltration are used.

If more than a couple of hours have passed since the overdose, the effects of BTX-A can be made to wear off more quickly by trying to exercise the affected muscles as much as possible. It has been noted that weightlifters, for example, who make severe facial expressions while exercising, tend to recover faster from BTX-A treatment than similar individuals who do not lift weights. In clinical practice, patients with BTX-A induced brow ptosis or excessive relaxation of

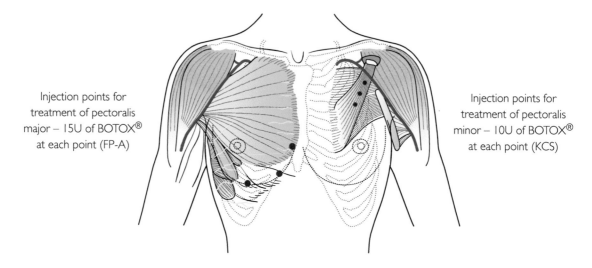

Injection points for treatment of pectoralis major – 15U of BOTOX® at each point (FP-A)

Injection points for treatment of pectoralis minor – 10U of BOTOX® at each point (KCS)

Figure 7.12 Typical injection sites for BOTOX® treatment of the pectoralis minor and pectoralis major muscles

the zygomaticus major and minor seem to recover faster if they attempt to exercise the affected muscles for 5 minutes, 5 times a day for several weeks (K. Smith, unpublished observations).

Formal clinical trials are being prepared to verify and quantify these observations.

BOTOX® 'breast lift'

BTX-A has a long history of being used to improve posture in a variety of conditions[22,23]. The position of the shoulders is determined largely by the balance of forces between the pectoralis minor and pectoralis major muscles (Figure 7.12), which tend to rotate the shoulders medially and to depress the shoulders and the opposing muscles of the back, for example the rhomboids. The pectoralis minor muscles are accessory muscles which assist during strong exhalation. One author (KCS) has noted that three doses of 10 units of BOTOX® injected on each side into of the pectoralis minor muscles in women who are slightly round shouldered can lead to a more erect posture with shoulders back – resulting in what they consider to be a more esthetically pleasing presentation of the breasts (Figure 7.13).

This proposed mechanism of action has been criticized by Dr Otto Wegelin (personal communication, April 2004), who argues that:

1. The muscles (pectoralis minor and rhomboid minor) invoked to carry out the postural changes are far too small to do what is expected of them.
2. The muscles do not in fact rotate the shoulder but rather act primarily to stabilize the scapula – an entirely different function.
3. The muscles are not antagonistic in action, as are the frontalis and the orbicularis oculi, but rather synergistic.
4. There is no way to determine how much, if any, of the BOTOX® is actually acting on the pectoralis minor as the BOTOX® can diffuse widely in a three-dimensional plane unlike the forehead where there is the bony skull limiting diffusion.

Dr Doris Hexsel (personal communication, July 2004), in a study of six women, was not able to obtain satisfactory results, and in two cases noted that the nipples hung lower.

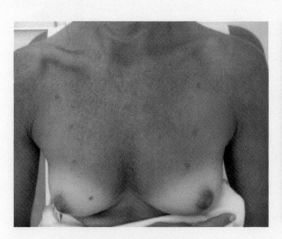 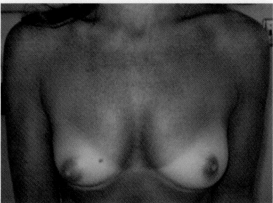

48 year old woman
before BOTOX®
Note shoulders rotated
medio-inferiorly.

3 weeks after BOTOX® 3
doses of 10 units on each side
Note shoulders back and
externally rotated.
Also note erect nipples.

Figure 7.13 Breast presentation before and after treatment of the pectoralis minor muscles with BOTOX®

One of the authors (FP-A) has successfully achieved elevation of the breasts on the side when the nipples are projecting downward by injecting three doses of 15 units of BOTOX® into the part of the pectoralis major which lies medial and inferior to the pectoralis minor (Figure 7.14a). In a series of 100 female patients between 30 and 55 years of age with different degrees of breast ptosis, elevation of the ptotic breast has been achieved, averaging 1.1 cm with the maximum elevation being 1.8 cm. Each patient was injected with BOTOX® on only one side in this pilot study, with the contralateral side as control. 65 of the 100 patients rated the results good to very good, and 73 of the 100 patients would repeat the procedure. Like Dr Smith, Dr Pérez-Atamoros has noted that the best candidates are physically fit women between the ages of 30–55 years, with small or moderate-sized breasts (Figures 7.15, 7.16, and 7.17). The dose recommended per breast is 3 injections ranging from 15U of BOTOX® each. The total dose in one application is 90U to 180U. Approximately 89 per cent of the study patients presented with asymmetry of the breasts before the treatment. The authors have noted that it is important not to correct naturally occurring breast asymmetry by giving higher doses on one side of the chest or the other, but to inject the same total dose of BOTOX® on each side. 5 patients had pain lasting longer than a week. Dr Pérez-Atamoros has suggested that relaxation of the inferior medial portion of the pectoralis major muscle allows the superior portion to lift the ptotic breast

231

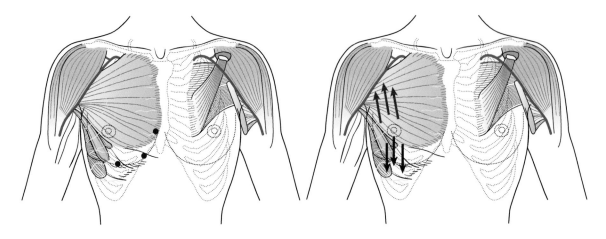

Figure 7.14   Demonstrates the areas in which BOTOX® can be injected in to the lower and medial aspect of the pectoralis major

CUP SIZE 'A'

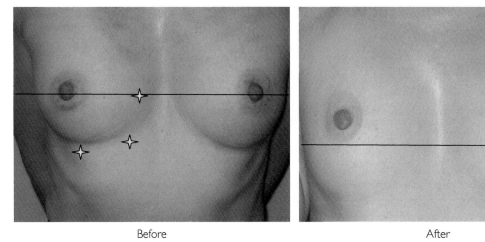

Before

After

Figure 7.15a   A patient in the pilot study with symmetrically positioned breasts and nipples before receiving three injections of 15 units each of BOTOX® into the right lower and medial aspect of the pectoralis major as indicated by the Xs

Figure 7.15b   The same patient one month after the injection BOTOX®; notice the elevation of the right breast and nipple at approximitely 1.1 cm elevation

(personal communications, Botox®, Fillers & More, Vancouver BC, August 2003 and August 2004; American Academy of Dermatology, Washington DC, February 2003 and April 2004). For a comparison of the injection sites used by the authors (FP-A and KCS) see Figure 7.12.

The ideal candidates for this treatment seem to be non-obese women with slightly rounded shoulders or who are slightly stooped forward, with breasts of cup-size A or B. Older

CUP SIZE 'B'

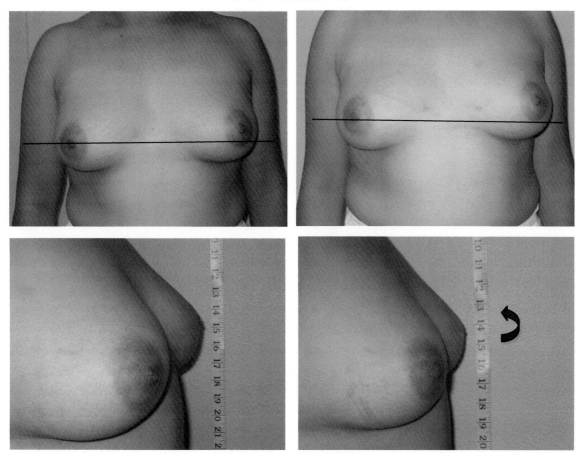

Figure 7.16   In a pilot study the author (FP-A) used several methods to evaluate the elevation of the breast; patients and doctors evaluation; distance from the clavicle to the nipple; a scale to measure elevation with photographic confirmation and assessing consistently at day zero and 1 month post injection

women, and those with larger breasts, tend to respond more slowly and to a lesser extent (Figure 7.18).

The benefits of BOTOX® treatment usually develop over a period of 1–2 weeks, and persist for 3–4 months. The duration of effect is somewhat longer than might be expected considering the relatively low doses of BOTOX® in proportion to the size of the muscles. It may be that improvements in shoulder posture persist for a while once posture has been improved by BOTOX®, altering the balance of forces between the pectoralis minor and/or major muscles and the opposing muscles in the back (Figure 7.14b).

Some women have noted that not only are the breasts and nipples elevated by their more erect posture with shoulders back, but also that there is a pleasing outward projection of the nipples which develops about a week after the BOTOX® treatment that persists for 3–4 weeks.

CUP SIZE 'A'

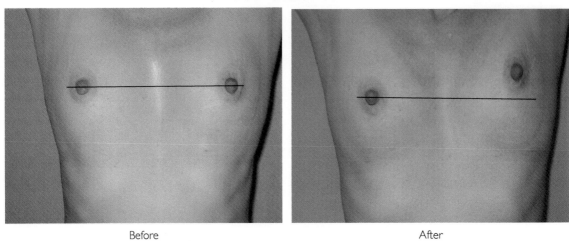

Before   After

Figure 7.17a,b   A patient in the pilot study with symmetrical positioned breasts before receiving 3 injections of 15 units each of BOTOX® in to the left lower and medial aspect of the pectoralis major. She is seen with her arms upwardly extended. The same patient with her arms upwardly extended one month after the injection of BOTOX® showing a 1.3 cm elevation of the left breast

CUP SIZE 'D'

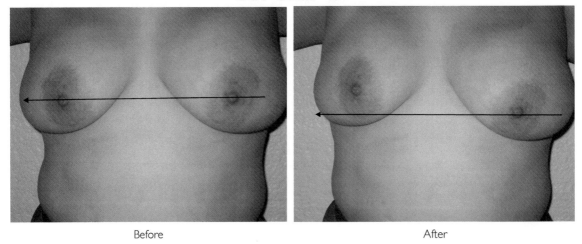

Before   After

Figure 7.18a   A shows a patient in the pilot study with symmetrically positioned breasts but with the right breast slightly rotated laterally. She received 3 injections of 15 units each of BOTOX® in the right lower and medial aspect of the pectoralis major

Figure 7.18b   B shows the same patient one month after the injection of BOTOX®; notice the elevation of the breast and nipple on the right side of approximately 1.3 cm

The reasons for this are not known. Perhaps projection of the breasts as a result of improved shoulder posture leads to increased mechanical stimulation of the nipples under some circumstances. Another, more speculative hypothesis is as follows: SP and CGRP have been demonstrated in neurovascular structures related to the nipple–areolar complex in animals[24] and in humans[25]. BTX-A has been shown to block the release of SP and CGRP from nerve terminals. If some of the injected BOTOX® makes its way from the injection sites to the nipple–areolar complex, it might affect smooth muscle in the nipples by way of its effect on the release of SP and CGRP.

BOTOX® is administered using a 30-gauge 1-inch needle. One author (KCS) usually uses a reconstitution of 100 units of BOTOX® in 2.5 ml of normal saline with benzyl alcohol preservative. The pectoralis minor arises on the third, fourth, and fifth ribs and runs under the clavicle to insert on the coracoid process of the scapula. The pectoralis minor muscles are located by having the patient hold her arms up slightly above shoulder height, pressing the palms together when requested to do so, allowing the examiner to palpate the pectoralis minor starting about 2.5 cm inferior to the lateral third of the clavicle (Figure 7.12). Injection points are generally about 2.5, 5, and 7.5 cm inferior to the lateral third of the clavicle. Injections are done at a depth of less than 2 cm. Occasionally there is muscle or fascial tenderness for several days after injection of BTX-A. In one case where there was excellent improvement in posture and breast presentation, the patient developed low back pain concurrent with the improvement in her upper thoracic posture and she attributed the lower back discomfort to the change in her posture. The lower back pain resolved without treatment after about 8 weeks, perhaps as she adapted to the postural change and perhaps as the effects of the BTX-A waned. In particular, pneumothorax or bleeding has not been seen, and would not be expected with a 30-gauge needle. The risk of entering the pleural space can be reduced by limiting needle insertion depth to less than 2 cm.

Issues which remain to be resolved include optimization of patient selection, BOTOX® dosing, and the placement of BOTOX® doses, and the issue of placebo effect versus biomechanical effect, and elucidation of the mechanism of action if indeed there is a biomechanical effect from BOTOX® treatment of the pectoralis minor and/or pectoralis major muscles with BOTOX®. T–2 weighted magnetic resonance imaging (MRI) before and immediately after exercise is being evaluated as a technique to visualize and perhaps partially quantify the degree of flaccid paralysis induced by BOTOX® treatment[26].

References

1. Tsui JK, Eisen A, Mak E et al. A pilot study on the use of botulinum toxin in spasmodic torticollis. *Can J Neurol Sci* 1985;12(4):314–6

2. Purkiss J, Welch M, Doward S et al. Capsaicin-stimulated release of substance P from cultured dorsal root ganglion neurons: involvement of two distinct mechanisms. *Biochem Pharmacol* 2000;59(11):1403–6

3. Welch MJ, Purkiss JR, Foster KA. Sensitivity of embryonic rat dorsal root ganglia neurons to *Clostridium botulinum* neurotoxins. *Toxicon* 2000;38(2):245–58

4. Durham PL, Cady R, Cady R. Regulation of calcitonin gene-related peptide secretion from trigeminal nerve cells by botulinum toxin type A: implications for migraine therapy. *Headache* 2004;44(1):35–42; discussion 42–3

5. Sala C, Andreose JS, Fumagalli G et al. Calcitonin gene-related peptide: possible role in formation and maintenance of neuromuscular junctions. *J Neurosci* 1995;15(1 Pt 2):520–8

6. Cui M, Khanijou S, Rubino J et al. Subcutaneous administration of botulinum toxin A reduces formalin-induced pain. *Pain* 2004;107(1–2):125–33

7. Bernstein JE, Bickers DR, Dahl MV et al. Treatment of chronic postherpetic neuralgia with topical capsaicin. A preliminary study. *J Am Acad Dermatol* 1987;17(1):93–6

8. Rumsfield JA, West DP. Topical capsaicin in dermatologic and peripheral pain disorders. *DICP* 1991;25(4):381–7

9. Argoff CE. A focused review on the use of botulinum toxins for neuropathic pain. *Clin J Pain* 2002;18(6 Suppl):S177–81

10. Arezzo JC. Possible mechanisms for the effects of botulinum toxin on pain. *Clin J Pain* 2002;18(6 Suppl):S125–32

11. Aoki RK. Evidence for antinociceptive activity of botulinum toxin type A in pain management. *Headache* 2003;43(Suppl 1):S9–S15

12. Klein AW. The therapeutic potential of botulinum toxin. *Dermatol Surg* 2004;30(3):452–5

13. Melzack R, Wall PD. Pain mechanisms: a new theory. *Science* 1965;150(699):971–9

14. Smith KC, Comite SL, Balasubramanian S *et al*. Vibration anesthesia: a non-invasive method of reducing discomfort prior to dermatologic procedures *Dermatology Online Journal* 10(2):1, http://dermatology.cdlib.org/102/therapy/anesthesia/comite.html/August 2004)

15. Crowe R, Parkhouse N, McGrouther D. Neuropeptide-containing nerves in painful hypertrophic human scar tissue. *Br J Dermatol* 1994;130(4):444–52

16. Takeba Y, Suzuki N, Kaneko A *et al*. Evidence for neural regulation of inflammatory synovial cell functions by secreting calcitonin gene-related peptide and vasoactive intestinal peptide in patients with rheumatoid arthritis. *Arthritis Rheum* 1999;42(11):2418–29

17. Hart DA, Reno C. Pregnancy alters the in vitro responsiveness of the rabbit medial collateral ligament to neuropeptides: effect on mRNA levels for growth factors, cytokines, iNOS, COX-2, metalloproteinases and TIMPs. *Biochim Biophys Acta* 1998;1408(1):35–43

18. Jorgensen C, Sany J. Modulation of the immune response by the neuro-endocrine axis in rheumatoid arthritis. *Clin Exp Rheumatol* 1994;12(4):435–41

19. Cordivari C, Misra VP, Catania S *et al*. Treatment of dystonic clenched fist with botulinum toxin. *Mov Disord* 2001;16(5):907–13

20. Saenz A, Avellanet M, Garreta R. Use of botulinum toxin type A on orthopedics: a case report. *Arch Phys Med Rehabil* 2003;84(7):1085–6

21. Jankovic J, Vuong KD, Ahsan J. Comparison of efficacy and immunogenicity of original versus current botulinum toxin in cervical dystonia. *Neurology* 2003;60(7):1186–8

22. Traba Lopez A, Esteban A. Botulinum toxin in motor disorders: practical considerations with emphasis on interventional neurophysiology. *Neurophysiol Clin* 2001;31(4):220–9

23. Gallien P, Nicolas B, Petrilli S *et al*. Role for botulinum toxin in back pain treatment in adults with cerebral palsy: report of a case. *Joint Bone Spine* 2004;71(1):76–8

24. Thulesen J, Rasmussen TN, Schmidt P *et al*. Calcitonin gene-related peptide (CGRP) in the nipple of the rat mammary gland. *Histochemistry* 1994;102(6):437–44

25. Eriksson M, Lindh B, Uvnas-Moberg K *et al*. Distribution and origin of peptide-containing nerve fibres in the rat and human mammary gland. *Neuroscience* 1996;70(1):227–45

26. Smith KC, Ludwig D, Price T; unpublished observations August 2005

8

DYSPORT®: A EUROPEAN BOTULINUM TYPE A NEUROTOXIN

Gary D Monheit

Botulinum type A neurotoxin is available in the United States and Europe to treat a variety of neuromuscular disorders of spasm, spasticity, and muscular rigidity. While BOTOX® has been manufactured and studied in the US since 1985, Dysport® has been studied in Europe since 1988. Manufactured by Ipsen Pharmaceutical in the United Kingdom, the toxin is produced from incubator vats of *Clostridium botulinum* separated from the North American product. The final *Clostridium botulinum* toxin type A hemagglutinin complex from European vats – Dysport® – thus has distinct attributes and characteristics different from that of its North American cousin, BOTOX®[1]. (Table 8.1) The molecular weight of the toxin is the same (150 kDa) as well as the bulk active substrate of the hemagglutinin complex. However, the pharmacologic composition differs in that Dysport® is accompanied by 125 µg human serum albumin with 2.5 mg lactose, while BOTOX® has 500 µg human serum albumin in 0.9 mg sodium chloride[2]. Dysport® is currently registered in 60 countries worldwide, including all European Union countries, and is currently under investigation in the United States.

In 1990 the toxin was approved for treatment of blepharospasm and hemifacial spasm, and in 1992 for spasmodic tortocolis. Treatment of leg and arm spasticity was subsequently approved in 2000 and 2001 respectively, with approval as well for cerebral palsy[3]. Approval for cosmetic indications was first granted for glabellar frown lines in 2002 (Argentina, Brazil, Colombia, and Uruguay). Further clinical cosmetic studies for glabella, forehead and periorbital rhytids have been performed in Europe and the United States during the last few years. Efficacy and dose ranging studies will be summarized.

TABLE 8.1   PRODUCT COMPARISON

	Dysport®	Botox® Cosmetic
Vial size	500 Unit	100 Unit
Composition	*Clostridium botulinum* toxin type A hemagglutinin 125 µg (0.125 mg) Human serum albumin 2.5 mg Lactose	*Clostridium botulinum* toxin type A hemagglutinin 500 µg (0.5 mg) Human serum albumin 0.9 mg Sodium chloride
Molecular weight (neurotoxin)	150 kDa	150 kDa
Bulk active substance	~5 ng	~5 ng
Storage (post-reconstitution)	2–8°C (2–8°C/use within 8 hours)	2–8°C (2–8°C/use within 4 hours)
Final formulation	Lyophilization	Vacuum extraction

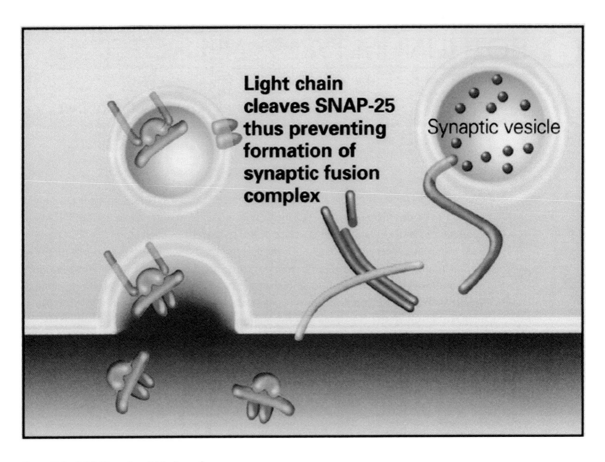

Figure 8.1   Inhibition of acetylcholine release

Dysport® is a botulinum A hemaglutinin neurotoxin and its action is similar to that of BOTOX®. The toxin is a heterodimeric molecule comprised of two chains, a light and heavy chain. The heavy chain targets the linking molecule to the cholinergic nerve ending while the light chain cleaves SNAP-25, inhibiting exocytosis of acetylcholine (Figure 8.1)

Botulinum toxin type A (BTX-A) is measured in units of physiologic action, as either BOTOX® or Dysport® units. Although the units are not interchangeable, various published reports support a conversion ratio from 1:5 to 1:3[4]. Units of potency and thus dilution should be evaluated independently of the BOTOX® product.

The standard dilution of 500 Dysport® units is performed with 2.5 ml saline solution. Dose ranging studies for cosmetic usage have varied this dilution ratio to both a higher and lower concentration. Ascher performed a multicenter, randomized, double-blind, placebo-controlled study of efficacy and safety of each dilutional dose of botulinum toxin A (Dysport®) used for the treatment of glabellar lines. The 119 patients ranged from 18 to 70 years of age, with moderate to severe glabellar frown lines and no prior anesthetic treatment. The dosages used were placebo, 25, 50, and 75 units in a double-blind control. They were injected in five controlled glabellar sites, targeting the obicularis pars frontalis, the corrugators, and the procerus muscle, each with appropriate divided units (Figure 8.2). Outcome measurements were assessed from blinded standardized photographs, investigator assessments, and patient evaluation. These

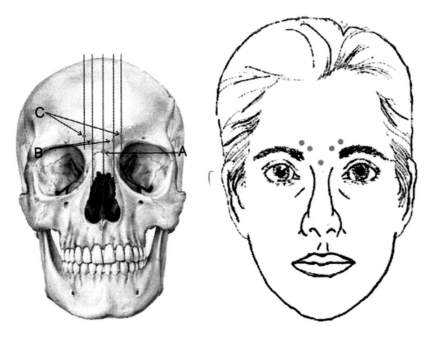

Figure 8.2   French Dysport® – Injection sites, glabella frown line study

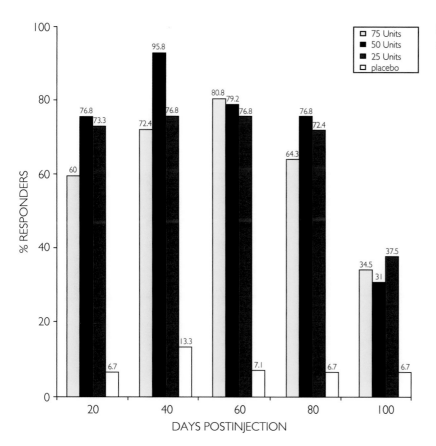

Figure 8.3   French phase II study results

239

were compared to a rating scale 0–3 of glabellar lines as follows: 0 = no lines; 1 = mild lines; 2 = moderate lines; 3 = severe lines (Figure 8.3). A responder was defined as 0:1 on the rating scale. The results indicated that all groups except placebo showed a response at 1 month and at 3 months. At 6 months, approximately two-thirds of the BTX-A treated patients were still responders (Figures 8.4). Although the primary statistical analysis was performed at rest, the assessment at maximal frown was similar up to 3 months, confirming the activity of (Dysport®) BTX-A on the glabellar musculature.

The safety protocol was favorable with a 7.0% rate of adverse events, all mild and reversible. Headache was the most common adverse event, with all resolving within 2 to 10 days. There were no reported cases of blepharoptosis or diplopia. The conclusions indicated that the BTX-A (Dysport®) was an effective cosmetic treatment for glabellar lines as evaluated by

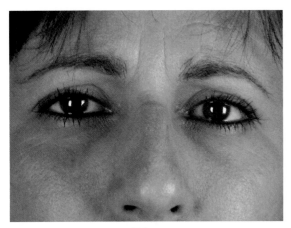

Before

Figure 8.4a   French phase II study results: 25 U Dysport® – Day 0

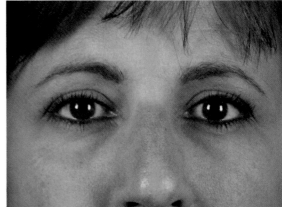

After

Figure 8.4b   25 U Dysport® – 1 month post

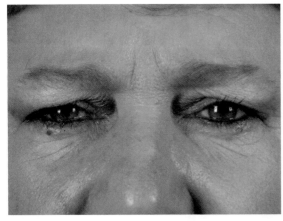

Before

Figure 8.4c   50 U Dysport® – day 0

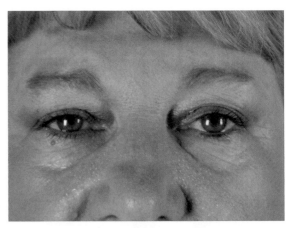

After

Figure 8.4d   50 U Dysport® – 1 month post

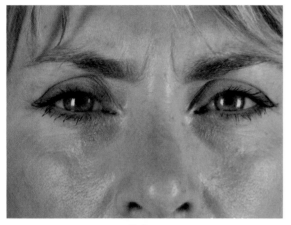

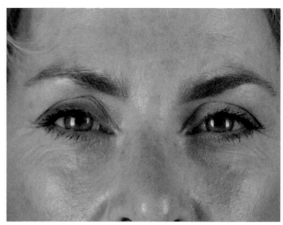

Before

After

Figure 8.4e   75 U Dysport® – day 0   Figure 8.4f   75 U Dysport® – 1 month post

independent photographic analysis and investigator assessment. The result suggested that 50 units were the optimal dosage for the glabella, with 10 units injected into each of five glabellar sites. Most interesting was the long-term result, indicating that one-third of the patients treated were still responders at 6 months[1] (Figure 8.5). Other studies by Asher have indicated similar results of efficacy and safety for BTX-A (Dysport®) in other locations including the forehead and crow's feet[5].

Inamed – Ipsen designed a multicentered North American study to evaluate three doses of BTX-A (Dysport®) to determine the optimal dose, in terms of efficacy and safety, for reducing the severity of hyperfunctional glabellar lines (personal communication – not yet published). In total, 373 patients were tested with the following dosages of Dysport® in a double-blind, placebo-controlled, dose-ranging study: 20, 50, and 75 units. A validated scale was developed both at rest and maximal frown. Each scale was composed of four photographs, grade 0 to 3: 0 = no wrinkles; 1 = mild wrinkles; 2 = moderate wrinkles; 3 = severe wrinkles. Live assessment was used in this study as it was considered to have advantages over photographic evaluations. The assessor was able to note the level of effort being made by the patient in the act of frowning and truly

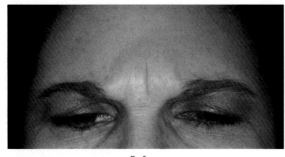

Before

After

Figure 8.5a   Results from North American phase II study: Figure 8.5b   30 days post
Day 0

note the dynamic nature of frowning. Thus – at maximal frown – the dynamic act of frowning is an indicator of pharmacologic activity of the toxin that cannot be truly evaluated by a static photograph. The live assessment of maximal frown proved more objective than photographs, in which factors of lighting and position can blur the accuracy of assessment. An additional assessment at rest was also made on a 0 to 4 scale. The resting phase was felt to represent how the patient appeared in daily life and thus corresponded to treatment efficacy and patient satisfaction. A responder was defined as a patient with a rating of 0 – none or 1 – mild on day 30. However, evaluations were continued until day 120, or 4 months (Figures 6 and 7).

A further language descriptor of glabellar wrinkles was formulated as much confusion has arisen in the literature concerning wrinkles, lines, and grooves. The definitions at maximal frown were as follows:

1. Relaxed skin tension line – no wrinkles.
2. Wrinkle line – a line visualized on the skin no greater than 0.2 mm in diameter and no greater than 2 cm in length – either dynamic or photoaging with no appreciable visible depth.
3. Wrinkle crease – a wider line visible on skin with diameter 0.5–1 mm and 1–3 cm in length with no noticeable depth as perceived by shoulders on either side of the skin-divided crease.
4. Wrinkle furrow – 1–2 mm bulging on either side with deformity of surrounding muscle, creating shortening and dynamic movement (Figure 8.6).

The results indicated that all doses of Dysport® resulted in a statistically better response in the appearance of glabellar frown lines compared with placebo. Twenty units – the smallest dose – were effective at 30 days and remained apparent at 90 days, but not at 120 days. Fifty units of Dysport® were found to be as effective as 75 units in terms of efficacy and duration.

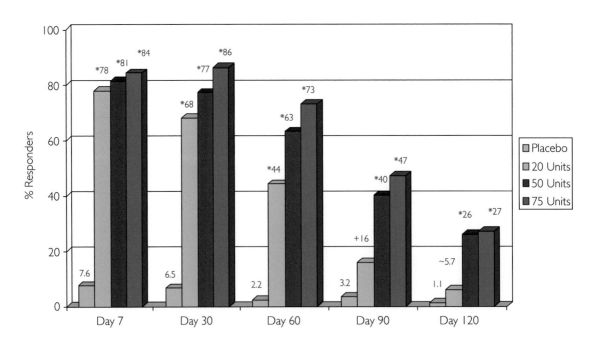

Figure 8.6   Results of North American Phase II Clinical Trials – Percentage of responders at each visit using Investigator's Assessment of Glabellar Lines at maximum frown

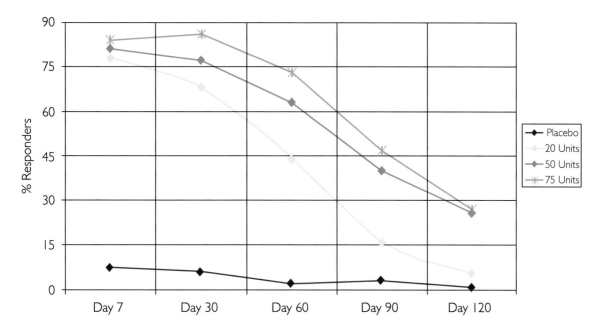

Figure 8.7   Results of North American Phase II Clinical Trials – Proportion of responders at each visit using Investigator's Assessment of Glabellar Lines at maximum frown (ITT Population)

Close to half the patients continued to show an effect at 120 days. In this study, greater benefit was found among women than in men.

All doses were well tolerated with only minor side effects, including headache, needle pricks, and bruising, but blepharoptosis was observed in only three patients. Of those reported cases, only one demonstrated to the investigator a true clinical ptosis. Ptosis had been reported in other product studies, but not in other studies involving Dysport®.[6]

Antibody production has always been of concern with clinical usage of botulinum toxin, but studied only with cervical dystonia[7]. None of the patients in this study showed any evidence of neutralizing antibodies, either at baseline or on follow-up evaluations. From these observations, the 50-unit dosage was recommended as the optimal dose for safety and efficacy.

Dysport® is best injected for cosmetic indications with Diablo or tuberculin syringes, 1.0 ml or 0.5 ml, and using a 30-gauge needle. The standard dilution of 500 units per vial is best performed with 2.5 ml of saline, bacteriostatic. This produces a clinical usage concentration of 10 units Dysport® per 0.05 ml, an easily measured quantity in the 1 ml tuberculin syringe. Thus, for the glabellar injection, aliquots of 10 units per five sites are easily administered (Figures 8 and 9).

The forehead is best treated through five injection sites located in the mid forehead at a distance of at least 2.5 cm above the brow. A dosage of 40 to 60 Dysport® units is effective for forehead wrinkle relaxation. The lateral forehead injection site should be above the highest point of the outer one-third of the brow. This will prevent an undesirable lateral brow elevation, the 'Mephisto look'[8].

Laugh lines or crow's feet are treated with 30 units of Dysport® injected lateral to each orbital rim. The injection sites are 1.0 cm lateral to the orbital rim in the three positions, representing the muscle bulges, superior, mid, and inferior. Care must be taken not to inject the upper or lower lid obicularis muscles as ptosis or ectropion can result (Figure 8.9).

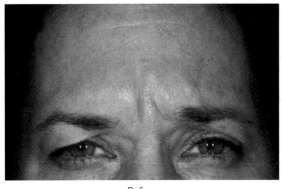

Before

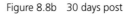

After

Figure 8.8a   Results of North American phase II clinical trials: Figure 8.8b   30 days post
Day 0

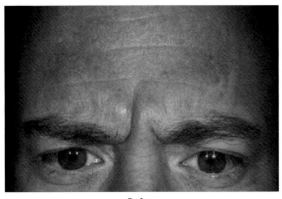

Before

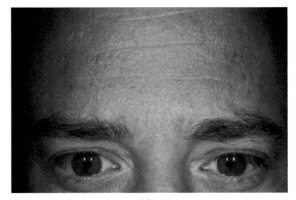

After

Figure 8.9a   Results of North American phase II clinical   Figure 8.9b   30 days post
trials-pre

Lower eyelid wrinkles formed from an overactive or hypertrophic orbicularis muscle can be treated judiciously with 3–4 units Dysport® injected in the lower lid at the mid pupillary line just below the tarsal plate. This will flatten the bulging muscle and create an image of 'open eye.' Overaggressive treatment may, though, create an unwanted ectropion[8].

Areas of the lower face treated with Dysport® have produced results similar to those found with BOTOX®. Treated areas include vertical rhagades of the upper lip, marionette lines at the corners of the mouth, and chin wrinkles. Dosages should be conservative, treatment relying primarily on dermal fillers with chemodenervation only used as a secondary procedure (Table 8.2).

The cosmetic usage of BTX-A has been firmly established in North America with BOTOX®. BTX-A Dysport® is also proving to be an effective cosmetic agent for treatment of glabellar and forehead lines and crow's feet, in carefully controlled studies. More recent studies are expected to highlight differences in the two products in terms of time of onset, longevity, clinical application, and technical usage. The objective evaluations in these studies should yield valuable data on the action of botulinum toxin.

TABLE 8.2 DOSAGE FOR DYSPORT® UNITS

Location	Dosage	Sites	Instructions
Upper lip	8 units	Four sites, 2 units/site	Overcorrection can lead to dysfunction
Marionette lines	20 units	Two sites, origin of depressor anguli oris, 10 units per site	Avoid the obicularis muscle to prevent lip asymmetry
Chin	10 units	Single injection, mid chin	Avoid the orbicular muscle

References

1. Vandenbergh PYK, Lison DF. Dose standardization of botulinum toxin *Adv Neurol* 1998;78:231–5
2. Odengren T, Hjaltason H, Kaakkola S *et al*. A double blind, randomised, parellel group study to investigate the dose equivalence of Dysport® and BOTOX® in the treatment of cervical dystonia. *J Neurol Neurosurgery Psych* 1998;64(1):6–12
3. Marion MH, Sheehy M, Sangla S *et al*. Dose standardisation of botulinum toxin. *J Neural Neurosurg Psych* 1995;59:102–3
4. Ascher B, Zakine B, Kestemont P *et al*. A multicenter randomized, double-blind placebo-controlled study of efficacy and safety of 3 doses of Botulinum toxin A in the treatment of glabellar lines. *J Am Acad Dermatol* 2004;51(2):223–33
5. Ascher B, Klop P, Marion MH. Botulinum toxin in the treatment of frontoglabellar and periorbital wrinkles. *J Med Esthet Dechinergie Dermatol* 1994;21(XX1):161–8
6. Carruthers J, Lowe NJ, Mentor MA, Gibson J. Double-blind placebo-controlled study of the safety and efficacy of Botulinum toxin type A for patients with glabellar lines. *Plastic Reconstr Surg* 2003;112:1089–98
7. Kessler KR, Skutta M, Benecke R *et al*. Long term treatment of cervical dystonia with Botulinum toxin A: efficacy, safety and antibody frequency. German Dystonia Study Group. *J Neurol* 1999;246(4):265–74
8. Rzany B *et al*. Botulinum toxin A in cosmetic dermatology. *Kosmet Med* 2003;24:72–9
9. Ibid 1431

BOTULINUM TOXIN B

Neil S Sadick

Introduction

The formation of glabellar lines is associated with repeated pulling of the skin by the underlying musculature. Movement of the transverse head of the corrugator supercilii muscle produces the vertical glabellar line, while the oblique head of the corrugator supercilii and the depressor supercilii and orbicularis oculi muscles contribute to the formation of the oblique glabellar line[1–3]. Treatments designed to minimize the appearance of glabellar lines include dermabrasion, chemical peel, and injection of collagen, silicone, autologous fat or dermis, or polytetra-fluoroethylene. Surgical options include endoscopy or limited incision to modify function of the corrugator supercilii and procerus muscles, and direct excision of the glabellar line[1,4].

In 1992, the Carruthers', evaluated the use of *Clostridium botulinum* type A purified neurotoxin complex (BTX-A; Botox®, Allergan Inc., Irvine, CA) to chemically denervate the corrugator supercilii to treat glabellar wrinkles[5]. Botulinum toxin blocks the release of acetylcholine from motor nerve endings, producing decrease in muscle tone causing weakness or paralysis depending on dose and subsequent reduction of muscle overactivity. The Carruthers' determined that botulinum toxin provided a safe treatment that addressed the underlying muscle activity contributing to the formation of wrinkle lines. Their results have been corroborated by other studies, and BTX-A is now cleared by the FDA for use in improving the appearance of moderate to severe glabellar lines[6–8].

An antigenically distinct serotype, botulinum toxin type B (BTX-B; Myobloc® in the USA and Neurobloc® in Europe; otherwise identified as Myobloc® henceforth, Solstice Neurosciences, South San Francisco, CA) was cleared in 2000 for treating the abnormal head position and related pain of cervical dystonia. It is currently being investigated in a variety of other disorders as well as in the setting of cosmetic dermatology. BTX-B is available as a ready-to-use liquid formulation (requiring no reconstitution as is necessary with BTX-A)[9–14].

Pharmacology of botulinum toxin B

The BTX-A complex has a total molecular weight of approximately 900 kDa, whereas BTX-B is approximately 700 kDa. These large botulinum toxin complexes are most stable in slightly acidic conditions (pH 5 to 7) and dissociate in alkaline conditions (Table 9.1). Within the large neurotoxin complex, which includes associated proteins (a hemagglutinin and a non-toxic, non-hemagglutinin moiety) the active neurotoxin exists as a 150 kDa dichain molecule consisting of a heavy chain (approximately 100 kDa) and a light chain (approximately 50 kDa) linked by a disulfide bond[15].

The action of botulinum toxin B upon neurons has features which all botulinum toxins share. Cellular intoxication is a three-step process that includes binding, internalization, and

TABLE 9.1 PHARMACOLOGY OF BOTULINUM TOXINS BOTULINUM TOXIN SEROTYPES BY TARGET/CLEAVAGE SIZES

Serotype	Target size	Cleaves at
A	SNAP-25*	Gln^{197}–Arg^{198}
B	VAMP**	Glu^{76}–Phe^{77}
C	Syntaxin	Lys^{253}–Ala^{254}
		Lys^{252}–Ala^{252}
	SNAP-25*	Arg^{198}–Ala^{199}
D	VAMP**	Ala^{67}–Asp^{68}
		Lys^{59}–Leu^{60}
E	SNAP-25*	Arg^{180}–Ile^{181}
F	VAMP**	Gln^{58}–Lys^{59}
G	VAMP**	Ala^{81}–Ala^{82}

*SNAP-25 is soluble NSF attachment protein of 25,000 kilodaltons

** VAMP is vesicle-associated membrane protein (synaptobrevin)

Figure 9.1 Pharmacology of botulinum toxins at the neuromuscular junction. SNAP-25 is the target for the type A toxin (red arrow), synaptobrevin is the target for the type B toxin (black arrow)

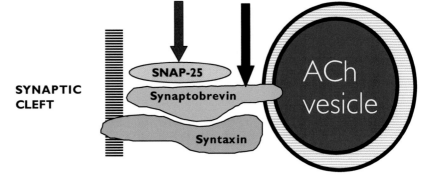

inhibition of acetylcholine release (Figure 9.1). The heavy chain is responsible for irreversible binding of the toxin to serotype specific acceptor sites on the neuronal cell membrane[16]. Next, the toxin is internalized through receptor-mediated endocytosis[17]. Once inside the cell, the light chain of toxin is released and targets a specific protein within the soluble N-ethyl maleimide-sensitive factor attachment protein receptor (SNARE) complex, which is involved in release of acetylcholine-containing vesicles from the presynaptic neuron[18]. Each serotype cleaves a specific residue on one of the soluble N-ethyl maleimide-sensitive factor attachment proteins. BTX-B cleaves vesicle associated membrane protein (VAMP) also known as synaptobrevin. Serotypes F, G, D also cleave VAMP, but at different locations (Table 9.1)[19].

Immunoresistance

As a foreign injected protein, any botulinum toxin is capable of eliciting an immune response[20]. Treated patients can potentially develop neutralizing antibodies that inactivate the toxin's clinical effects. When neutralizing antibodies are formed against either botulinum toxin molecule, the therapeutic effect of botulinum toxin may be considerably or completely reduced. Clinical

TABLE 9.2 PROTEIN IMMUNOGENICITY FACTORS

Myobloc	Botox
Foreign	Foreign
Large	Large
Native	Denatured
Non-aggregated	Aggregated
2–3 months	3–4 months
pH 5.6	Neutral

Cross neutralizing antibodies between the serotypes are not expected based on single exposure. Multiple exposures may lead to cross sensitivity between toxins. Patients who are resistant to BTX-A respond to BTX-B therapy and vice versa

resistance has been reported in 3 to 5 per cent of patients with cervical dystonia who were treated with BTX-A doses of 100 to 1,200 U, based on retrospective studies[21, 22]. Antibody formation to other parts of the complex are not believed to affect clinical performance of these products. The risk of antibody formation is expected to be much lower in patients treated for aesthetic purposes because they require significantly lower doses than do patients with cervical dystonia. Since the botulinum toxin serotypes were not believed to cross-neutralize, patients who become resistant to one serotype may benefit from treatment with another serotype. In studies of patients with cervical dystonia, BTX-A resistant patients have been found to respond to treatment with BTX-B. It should also follow that patients resistant to BTX-B can benefit from BTX-A or any other botulinum toxin serotype. However, recent research has pointed to the possibility of the resistance to one serotype potentiating the development of resistance to the other with a series of injections. The most significant risk factors associated with development of cross-resistant antibodies include injections of high doses of toxin, increased frequency of administration and the amount of neurotoxin protein delivered in each injection[23–27].

A summary of immunogenicity factors associated with botulinum toxin B (Myobloc®) is presented in Table 9.2.

Formulation

BTX B (Myobloc®) is produced as a ready-to-use liquid formulation set at a pH of 5.6 to stabilize the complex. It is available in vials of 2,500, 5,000 and 10,000 U each with a concentration of 5,000 U/ml or 500 U per 0.1 ml (Table 9.3). This preparation can be diluted up to 6-fold without losing any activity[20]. Specifically, one unit is defined as the amount of toxin that is lethal in 50 per cent of female Swiss-Webster mice after intraperitoneal injection (Mouse LD50 bioassay). However, because of variations between products in the sensitivity of different species to each toxin serotype, as well as differences in the potency assays used, different toxin products cannot be directly compared on a unit by unit basis. Individualized dose-ranging studies in humans are necessary for each toxin serotype, for each indication, and dose conversion should not be attempted (see package inserts for both BTX-A and BTX- B).

BTX-B is stored refrigerated at 2°C to 8°C and is stable in this environment for up to 3 years. Studies have also shown that when stored at room temperature (25°C), BTX-B is stable for at least 9 months. In addition, BTX-B has been found to retain activity when stored refrigerated for

TABLE 9.3   BOTULINUM TOXIN B FORMULATION

Parameter	BTX-B (Myobloc®)
Formulation	• Stable liquid
	• Native protein
	• Non-aggregated
	• No reconstitution
	• pH 5.6
Vials	2,500 U, 5,000 U, 10,000 U
Storage	Refrigerator (2–8°C)
Mechanism of action	• Unique receptors for type B
	• Targets synaptobrevin

21 months and then moved to room temperature for 6 months, or then stored at room temperature for 6 months and then moved to 4°C. BTX-B diluted up to 6-fold with either non-preserved or preserved saline remains stable and retains potency for at least 24 hours at room temperature, even though the package insert suggests that it be used within 4 hours.

Aesthetic use of botulinum toxin B

Botulinum toxin B has many proposed therapeutic indications, all of which are off label except for cervical dystonia. The bulk of data and experience resides with BTX-A and has confirmed the effectiveness of this agent for facial wrinkles[28–39]. Recently BTX-B has also been investigated in the treatment for facial wrinkles, with results demonstrating efficacy for this indication. Highlights of some of the key clinical studies with respect to the use of these agents for aesthetic purposes are reviewed herein.

Clinical studies of botulinum toxin B

Despite its relatively recent FDA clearance for cervical dystonia, BTX-B has been evaluated in several small clinical trials for use in aesthetic medicine. Clinical trials in this setting have mostly been dose ranging and open label in terms of study design[40–45].

Ramirez et al evaluated BTX-B in twenty-four subjects with facial wrinkles. Most subjects (82 per cent) had been treated with BTX-A previously, although not within the 6 months before the study[43]. Subjects received 200 to 400 U of BTX-B per unilateral injection site (total dose, 400 to 800 U). Three sites were injected, including the frontalis, the corrugators, and the orbicularis oculi. Improvement in facial wrinkles was assessed using two scales: the Wrinkle Improvement Scale (WIS; 0 indicates no improvement and 3 indicates significant improvement) and the Rated Numeric Kinetic Line Scale (RNKLS). During the study, the RNKLS was added to more objectively characterize wrinkle severity. This scale encompasses a description of wrinkles both at rest and at maximum frown. It ranges from a score of 1, reflecting no wrinkles at rest, which become fine lines with facial animation, to a score of 4, denoting deep lines at rest, which become deep furrows with facial animation. Subjects were evaluated in repose and animation before injection and after injection at weeks 1, 2, 4, 8, and 12. Photographs were also obtained. All subjects had a relatively rapid onset of nearly complete paresis within 72 hours and, in many cases, within 24 hours. Scores on the WIS and RNKLS were moderately to significantly improved by two to three points after BTX-B treatment. However, the duration of effect was suboptimal (mean of 8 weeks). No subjects reported dysphagia, dyspepsia, or dry mouth, which are common side effects seen in treatment of cervical dystonia. Eyelid ptosis, brow ptosis, and dry eye were not measured. This preliminary study showed that BTX-B is effective in treating facial lines of the glabella, forehead, and crow's feet areas, but the authors concluded that doses higher than 400 to 800 U would be necessary for a longer duration of action.

The above study also evaluated the subjects for pain associated with injection, using the McGill Pain Scale. Pain on injection, usually described as a slight stinging sensation, has been reported to occur with botulinum toxin injections. The McGill Pain Scale is a validated scale ranging from 0, signifying no pain to 5, signifying excruciating pain. At the time of treatment, subjects were asked to rate the pain of BTX-B injection and to rate by memory the pain of BTX-A injection. On average, BTX-B was found to be slightly more painful than the memory of BTX-A injection (2.3 vs. 1.6 respectively), although all subjects indicated that the injection pain would not prevent them from undergoing a repeat injection with BTX-B.

A much smaller open-label study investigated preliminary doses of BTX-B and also compared the effects of the drug with those of BTX-A in the treatment of glabellar lines[44]. Subjects received 1,000 U (N = 4) or 2,000 U (N = 4) of BTX-B or 20 U of BTX-A (N = 5), divided equally over five sites (one injection at the procerus muscle and two injections each at the inferior-medial and superior-lateral aspects of the corrugator muscles). Subjects were photographed before and after injection, and glabellar line severity was rated as absent, mild, moderate, or severe, both in the relaxed state and at maximum frowning. Results showed that both BTX-A and BTX-B were both effective in treating glabellar frown lines. However, BTX-B had a more rapid onset of action (by 1 to 2 days) as compared with BTX-A. At the doses used, BTX-A had a longer duration of effect than did BTX-B. The duration of effect of BTX-A 20 U was at least 16 weeks, whereas that of BTX-B was 8 to 10 weeks at the 1,000 U dose and 10 to 12 weeks with the 2,000 U dose. Although the study consisted of a small group of patients, its results suggest that BTX-B's duration of efficacy may be dose dependent. Because limited adverse events were reported at doses used, the investigators concluded that higher doses of BTX-B should be studied.

The author conducted two open-label studies using higher doses of BTX-B for treatment of glabellar wrinkles[45–47]. Both studies were similar in design, but the first study evaluated BTX-B 1,800 U (N = 30), and the second study evaluated 2,400 U (N = 16) and 3,000 U (N = 18). Doses were divided equally among six sites; two in the procerus and two in each corrugator supercilii and orbicularis oculi muscle bilaterally. Most subjects in all treatment groups had not been previously treated with BTX-A. In the first study, efficacy was assessed using photography and a clinical scoring system that was used by both subjects and physicians; 0 denoted marked frowning ability, 1 denoted partial frowning ability, and 2 denoted complete inability to frown because of paralysis. The second study also used the RNKLS. Subjects returned to the office daily post-injection until the effects of BTX-B were observed and then weekly thereafter. Both studies found BTX-B to be effective in treating glabellar frown lines, based on photography, patient satisfaction, and improvements in assessment scores. Overall, BTX-B had a very rapid onset of action. When viewed together, the results of both studies also suggest that the duration of response is dose related. The mean duration of effect was 8.0 weeks with 1,800 U, 9.6 weeks with 2,400 U, and 10.4 weeks with 3,000 U. Lid ptosis was reported in one patient who received 2,400 U and in one patient who received 3,000 U. Headache and mild pain on injection were also reported. Overall, BTX-B was very safe, and there was no increase in adverse effects with the higher doses.

Alster and Lupton chose 20 female patients with vertical glabellar rhytids showing minimal response to BTX-A, which was defined as less than 50 per cent reduction in contraction of the muscles treated with BTX-A. These patients were treated with BTX-B at a total dose of 2,500 U into five standardized intramuscular sites (procerus, inferomedial corrugators and superior medial corrugators). Improvement of wrinkles occurred in all individuals with peak response at 1 month and complete dissolution of effect at month 4[45].

Flynn and Clark showed an increased rate of onset and more widespread diffusion of BTX-B vs BTX-A in a single center study of 24 patients with symmetrical, moderate to severe forehead wrinkles. Subjects received type A (BOTOX®) 5 U on one side and type B (Myobloc®) 500 U on the other side of the forehead. Radius of diffusion and time until full effect were measured. Botulinum toxin type B was found to have a slightly faster rate of onset than type A. A greater radius of diffusion was consistently observed with type B as measured by the greater area of wrinkle reduction at the doses used[46].

Spencer et al in a glabellar and frontalis or forehead dose-response study of 26 patients entered 18 patients to receive botulinum B injections to their frontalis region. Three different dosage schedules, i.e., low-dose (1,875 U), medium-dose (2,500 U) and high-dose (3,125 U) were followed for the glabellar study group for duration of effect. In the frontalis treated group, low-dose regimen (2,250 U), medium-dose group (3,000 U) and a high-dose sub-group (3,750 U) were studied. Results showed that in the glabellar group most subjects showed evidence of paralysis at 2 months. However, only the high dose group showed a continued effect at 3 months after treatment. In the frontalis group, response was often still present at 2 months, however it had totally dissipated by month 3[47].

In a double blinded, randomized, placebo-controlled pilot study of the safety and efficacy of BTX-B for the treatment of crow's feet utilizing 3,000 U in 20 patients, the maximal effect was seen at day 30. Results began to wane by day 60, although the patients were not seen between day 30 and day 60, and most patients had returned to baseline by their day 90 visit. Adverse side effects were reported as flu-like symptoms (55 per cent), dry mouth (45 per cent) and dry eye (25 per cent)[48].

In a type B toxin dosing study, Lowe and co-investigators looked at 13 patients who were injected with BTX-B in two different dose schedules versus BTX-A in the corrugator-procerus complex. One subgroup received a conversion of 50 U of BTX-B (total 1,000) to 1 U of BTX-A, while others received a conversion factor of 100 U of BTX-B (total 2,000) to 1 U BTX-A. Patients treated with BTX-A received a total of 20 U. Both types of botulinum toxins were noted by the author to be effective in improving glabellar frown lines. The onset of action was more rapid (2–3 days) with BTX-B than with BTX-A (3–7 days). Duration of effect with BTX-A was at least 16 weeks. With the 1,000 U BTX-B dose, duration was 6–8 weeks and with the 2,000 U BTX-B dose the duration was 10–12 weeks[41].

Finally, Kim and investigators using an escalating dosage formula of 400 U to 800 U to 1,600 U to 2,000 U and 2,500 U to 3,000 U per site treating the bilateral frontalis, corrugator or orbicularis oculi using a wrinkle improvement scale and rated numerical kinetic line scales, found botulinum toxin type B to be clinically effective for up to 8 weeks in the management of hyperkinetic facial lines and up to week 12 at the higher dosage. In this study, the authors report that patients exhibited excellent skin smoothing which was felt to be secondary to an enhanced diffusion effect of the type B toxin. Reported side effects were headaches (40 per cent), brow ptosis (7 per cent), dry eyes (5 per cent) and dry mouth (13 per cent)[49].

To date, the highest doses of BTX-B to be used for aesthetic purposes are 3,125 U for glabellar lines and 3,750 U for the frontalis region, as reported in an open-label study[47]. Twenty-six subjects received low (1,875 U), medium (2,500 U), or high (3,125 U) doses of BTX-B for glabellar lines. Eighteen subjects received a low (2,250 U), medium (3,000 U), or high (3,750 U) dose of BTX-B in the frontalis. Results were similar to other studies of BTX-B for wrinkles; that is, BTX-B had a very rapid onset of effect and a dose-related duration of effect. At the doses used, there were no reports of lid ptosis. Of note, BTX-B was reported to yield a very uniform paralysis and a smooth aesthetic effect. This effect has also been observed by the author, as well as by others, and may reflect the diffusion characteristics of BTX-B, which may differ from those of BTX-A. Compared with BTX-A, BTX-B appears to diffuse more within the injected muscle.

Taken together, the studies of BTX-B for the treatment of facial wrinkles show that it is effective, has a very rapid onset of effect, and has a dose-related duration of effect. In clinical studies of cervical dystonia, the calculated duration of the effect of BTX-B was 12 to 16 weeks, which is comparable to that seen with BTX-A. These trials demonstrated a dose–response relationship in the duration of effect when treating glabellar lines. It is anticipated that higher doses of BTX-B can be safely and effectively administered to produce an even longer duration of response in the treatment of facial wrinkles. Further studies at higher doses are recommended to determine optimal dosing of BTX-B, with an acceptable level of adverse effects[50,51].

Botulinum toxin B dosing considerations

Preliminary estimates of effective doses of BTX-B based on the studies for the treatment of facial wrinkles are specified in Table 9.4. Results from these studies have clearly shown efficacy at these doses.

For the glabella, the relevant musculature includes the procerus complex and corrugator supercilii. A total of 20 to 30 U of BTX-A may be divided equally and injected into five sites, where BTX-B treatment with 2,000 to 3,000 U divided among only four sites appears to produce similar results (Figure 9.2). For frontalis injection 15 to 30 U of BTX-A divided among five to six injection sites produced adequate results while BTX-B in doses of 1,000 to 2,500 U per side

TABLE 9.4   PROVISIONAL DOSING GUIDELINES FOR BOTULINUM TOXIN B INJECTIONS FOR FACIAL RHYTIDES

Muscle site	BTX-B (Myobloc®)	
	Units	No. of Injections
Glabella	2,000–3,000	3
Frontalis	1,000–2,500	3–6
Brow lift	300–500 per side	1 per side
Periorbital	1,000–1,500 per side	1–2 per side

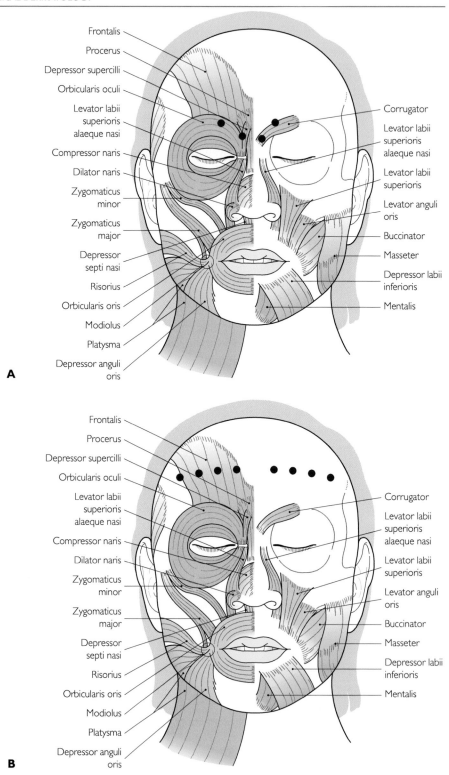

Figure 9.2   Schemata showing the most common sites of botulinum toxin injections in the upper face. (A) Injections in the glabella. (B) Injections in the forehead. (C) Injections in the crow's feet. The author prefers to use the conversion of 150 U of type B toxin for 1 U of type A toxin

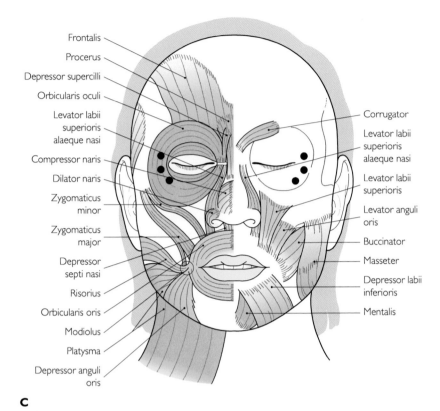

Frontalis
Procerus
Depressor supercilli
Orbicularis oculi
Levator labii superioris alaeque nasi
Compressor naris
Dilator naris
Zygomaticus minor
Zygomaticus major
Depressor septi nasi
Risorius
Orbicularis oris
Modiolus
Platysma
Depressor anguli oris

Corrugator
Levator labii superioris alaeque nasi
Levator labii superioris
Levator anguli oris
Buccinator
Masseter
Depressor labii inferioris
Mentalis

c

produced similar results. Lifting of the brow can be achieved by treatment of the corrugator supercilii, the procerus complex and the medial portion of the orbicularis oculi muscle. In the author's experience, 1,500 U of BTX-B are employed in this setting. For crow's feet, the author injects 10 to 15 U of BTX-A divided into two to three injections per side. Because of the proposed diffusion characteristics of BTX-B, the author employs a single injection of 1,000 to 1,500 U per side to treat the crow's feet. The representative patients treated in the author's dosing studies are presented in Figures 9.3 and 9.4.

Complication profiles

Complication profiles for BTX-A vs. BTX-B are quite similar with eyelid and brow ptosis, mild bruising and asymmetric brow elevation (Figure 9.5).

Conclusion

Facial wrinkles involving the forehead, glabellar, and/or periorbital regions are a common aesthetic problem, and are directly related to overactivity of the underlying facial musculature. Botulinum toxin, which acts by causing flaccid paralysis or weakening of the muscles of facial expression, has become a popular treatment for the management of hyperfunctional facial lines. Two serotypes have been formulated and are currently available for commercial use in the United States: BTX-A (BOTOX®) and BTX-B (Myobloc®). The major differences between the two toxins in terms of pharmacologic mechanism are that each binds to its own serotype-specific acceptors on the neuronal cell membrane, and each targets different specific intracellular

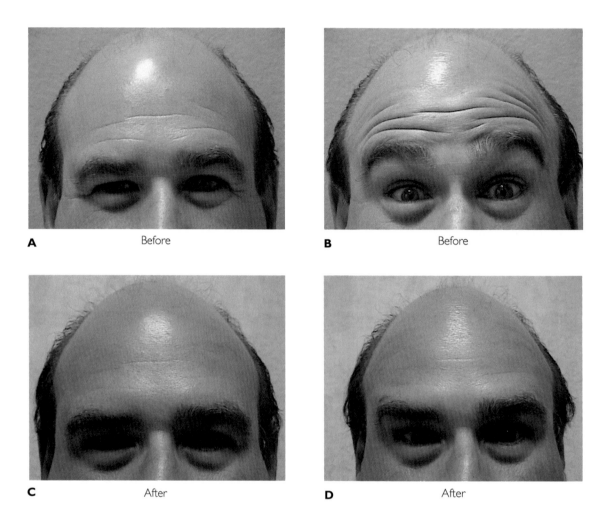

Figure 9.3   Patient (A) at rest and (B) with brows raised before treatment. Same patient, 8 weeks after treatment with 3,000 U of botulinum toxin type B to the frontalis muscle. (C) at rest and (D) with brows raised

proteins. The major differences in formulation are that BTX-A is a vacuum-dried powder that requires reconstitution before use, and BTX-B is a ready-to-use liquid. As bacterial proteins, both toxins can elicit an immune response in treated patients. It is currently unknown whether one toxin is more likely than the other to cause antibody formation and subsequent development of resistance.

The bulk of clinical data exists with BTX-A, due to over 20 years of clinical use in the United States marketplace versus 2 years with BTX-B. These data confirm the effectiveness of BTX-A in the treatment of facial wrinkles. Preliminary data with BTX-B show that it too is effective in this regard. In these preliminary studies, BTX-B, as compared with BTX-A, appears to have a faster onset of effect and potentially a more even, and smoother paralysis (Figure 9.6).

Both botulinum toxins are among the most potent neurotoxins known, and caution in dose escalation is appropriate in any indication and especially in off-label use. At dermatological doses the likelihood of serious adverse events is low with both products. However, as we

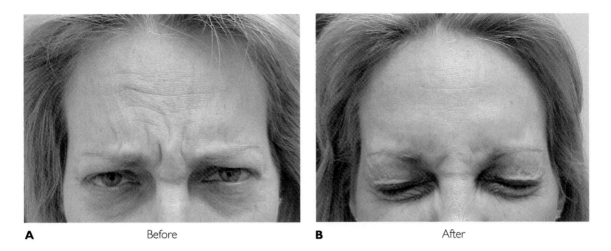

A   Before   **B**   After

Figure 9.4   Patient frowning (A) before, and (B) 12 weeks after treatment with 3,000 U of botulinum toxin type B to the glabella

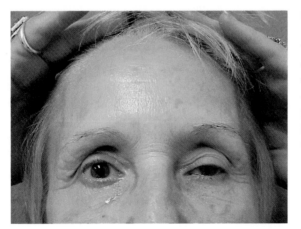

Figure 9.5   Drooping of the left upper eyelid after botulinum toxin type B injection in the glabella. Apraclonidine (0.5 per cent) drops, 3 drops to the affected eye three times a day produces temporary relief of this problem until it completely resolves

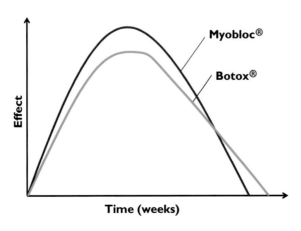

Figure 9.6   A comparison of onset of action and duration of action between botulinum toxin types A and B. Note that the type B toxin has a more rapid onset

become more aggressive with our aesthetic treatments (especially in the lower face), the side effects become more common and more worrisome. In an aesthetic practice, patient safety and satisfaction are paramount. Avoidance of post-treatment complications is crucial.

With further studies and clinical experience, it is likely that each product will have uses for which it is preferable based on its own individual efficacy and safety profile. This may also widen the scope of indications cleared by the FDA, ultimately benefiting a larger group of patients.

References

1. Knize D. Muscles that act on glabellar skin: a closer look. *Plast Recon Surg* 2000;105(1):350–61
2. Kock RJ, Troell RJ, Goode RL. Contemporary management of the aging brow and forehead. *Laryngoscope* 1997;107(6):710–15
3. Pierard GE, Lapiere CM. The microanatomical basis of facial frown lines. *Arch Dermatol* 1989;125:1090–2
4. Vecchione TR. Glabellar frown lines: direct excision, an evaluation of the scars. *Plast Recom Surg* 1990;86(1):46–52
5. Carruthers JDA, Carruthers JA. Treatment of glabellar frown lines with botulinum-A exotoxin. *J Dermatol Surg Oncol* 1992;18:17–21
6. Blitzer A, Brin MF Keen MF, *et al*. Botulinum toxin for the treatment of hyperfunctional lines of the face. *Arch Otolaryngol Head Neck Surg* 1993;119:1018–22
7. Guyron B, Huddleston SW. Aesthetic indications for botulinum toxin injection. *Plast Reconstr Surg* 1994;93:913–8
8. Keen M, Blitzer A, Aviv J *et al*. Botulinum toxin A for hyperkinetic facial lines: results of a double-blind placebo-controlled study. *Plast Reconstr Surg* 1994;94:94–9
9. Brashear A, Lew MF, Dykstra DD, et al. Safety and efficacy of Neurobloc™ (botulinum toxin type B) in type A-responsive cervical dystonia. *Neurology* 1999;53:1439–46
10. Brin M, Lew MF, Adler CH *et al*. Safety and efficacy of Neurobloc™ (botulinum toxin type B) in type A-resistant cervical dystonia. *Neurology* 1999;53:1431–8
11. Sakaguchi G. *Clostridium botulinum* toxins. *Pharmacol Ther* 1983;19:165–94
12. Callaway JE, Arezzo JC, Grethlein AJ. Botulinum toxin type B: an overview of its biochemistry and preclinical pharmacology. *Semin Cutan Med Surg* 2001;20:127–36
13. Simpson LL. Molecular pharmacology of botulinum toxin and tetanus toxin. *Annu Rev Pharmacol Toxicol* 1986;26:427–53
14. Oguma K, Fujinaga Y, Inoue K. Structure and function of *Clostridium botulinum* toxins. *Microbiol Immunol* 1995;39:161–8
15. Olney RK, Aminoff MJ, Gelb DJ, Lowenstein DH. Neuromuscular effects distant from the site of botulinum neurotoxin injection. *Neurology* 1998;38:1780–3
16. Fagien S, Brandt FS. Primary and adjunctive use of botulinum toxin type A (Botox) in facial aesthetic surgery. *Clin Plast Surg* 2001;28:127–48
17. Setler P. The biochemistry of botulinum toxin type B. *Neurology* 2000;55 (Suppl 5):S23–8
18. Greene P, Fahn S, Diamond B. Development of resistance to botulinum toxin type A patients with torticollis. *Mov Disord* 1994;9:213–7
19. Jankovic J, Schwartz KS. Response and immunoresistance to botulinum toxin injections. *Neurology* 1995;45:1743–6
20. Berman B, Seeberger L, Kumar R. Long-term safety, efficacy, dosing, and development of resistance with botulinum toxin type B in cervical dystonia. *Mov Disord* 2005 Feb;20(2):233–7
21. Dressler D, Bigalke H. Botulinum toxin type B de novo therapy of cervical dystonia frequency of antibody induced therapy failure. *J Neurol* 2005;252(8):904–7
22. Dolimbek BZ, Jankovic J, Atassi MZ. Cross reaction of tetanus and botulinum neurotoxins A and B, and the boosting effect of botulinum neurotoxins A and B on a primary anti-tetanus antibody response. *Immunol Invest* 2002;31(3–4):247–62

23. Aoki KR. Pharmacology and immunology of botulinum neurotoxins. *Int Ophthalmol Clin* 2005;45(3):25–37

24. Zuber M, Sebald M, Bathien N *et al*. Botulinum antibodies in dystonic patients treated with type A botulinum toxin: frequency and significance. *Neurology* 1993;43:1715–18

25. Lowe NJ, Maxwell A, Harper H. Botulinum A exotoxin for glabellar folds: a double-blind, placebo-controlled study with an electromyographic injection technique. *J Am Acad Dermatol* 1996;35:569–72

26. Carruthers JA, Lowe NJ, Menter MA *et al*. A multicenter, double-blind, randomized placebo-controlled study of the efficacy and safety of botulinum toxin type A in the treatment of glabellar lines. *J Am Acad Dermatol* 2002;46:840–9

27. Blitzer A, Binder W, Aviv J *et al*. The management of hyperfunctional facial lines with botulinum toxin: a collaborative study of 210 injection sites in 162 patients. *Arch Otolaryngol Head Neck Surg* 1997;123:389–92

28. Brandt F, Bellman B. Cosmetic uses of botulinum A exotoxin for the aging neck. *Dermatol Surg* 1998;24:1232–4

29. Carucci J. Botulinum exotoxin A for rejuvenation of the upper third of the face. *Facial Plast Surg* 2001;17:11–20

30. Carruthers J, Carruthers A. Botox use in the mid and lower face and neck. *Semin Cutan Med Surg* 2001;20:85–92

31. Foster J, Barnhorst D, Papay F *et al*. The use of botulinum A toxin to ameliorate facial kinetic frown lines. *Ophthalmology* 1996;103:618–22

32. Flynn T, Carruthers J, Carruthers A. Botulinum A toxin treatment of the lower eyelid improves infraorbital rhytides and widens the eye. *Dermatol Surg* 2001;27:703–8

33. Hankins C, Strimling R, Rogers G. Botulinum A toxin for glabellar wrinkles, dose and response. *Dermatol Surg* 1998;24:1181–3

34. Huilgol S, Carruthers A, Carruthers J. Raising eyebrows with botulinum toxin. *Dermatol Surg* 1999;25:373–6

35. Matarasso A. Botulinum A exotoxin for the management of platysmal bands. *Plast Reconstr Surg* 1999;103:645–52

36. West T, Alster T. Effect of botulinum toxin type A on movement-associated rhytides following CO_2 laser resurfacing. *Dermatol Surg* 1999;25:260–1

37. Carruthers A, Carruthers JDA. The use of botulinum toxin to treat glabellar frown lines and other facial wrinkles. *Cosmet Dermatol* 1994;7:11–15

38. Lew MF, Adornato BT, Duane DD *et al*. Botulinum toxin type B: a double-blind, placebo-controlled, safety and efficacy study in cervical dystonia. *Neurology* 1997;49:701–7

39. Hexsel DM, De Almeida AT, Rutowitsch M *et al*. e: Hexsel, R *et al*. Multicenter, double-blind study of the efficacy of injections with botulinum toxin type A reconstituted up to 6 consecutive weeks before application. *Dermatol Surg* 2004;30(5):823

40. Ramirez AL, Reeck J, Maas CS. Botulinum toxin type B (Myobloc®) in the management of hyperkinetic facial lines. *Otolaryngol Head Neck Surg* 2002;126:459–67

41. Lowe NJ, Yamauchi PS, Lask GP *et al*. Botulinum toxin types A and B for brow furrows: preliminary experiences with type B toxin dosing. *J Cosmet Laser Ther* 2002;4:15–18

42. Sadick NS. Botulinum toxin type B (Myobloc) for glabellar wrinkles: a prospective open-label response study. *Dermatol Surg* 2002;29:817–21

43. Sadick NS. Prospective open-label study of botulinum toxin type B (Myobloc) at doses of 2,400 and 3,000 units for the treatment of glabellar wrinkles. *Dermatol Surg* 2003;29(5):501–7; discussion 507

44. Sadick NS. Botulinum toxin type B for glabellar wrinkles: a prospective open-label response study. *Dermatol Surg* 2002;28:817–21

45. Alster TS, Lupton JR. Botulinum toxin type B for dynamic glabellar rhytides refractory to botulinum toxin type A. *Dermatol Surg* 2003;29:516–18

46. Flynn TC, Clark RE. Botulinum toxin type B (Myobloc) versus botulinum toxin type A (Botox) frontalis study: rate of onset and radius of diffusion. *Dermatol Surg* 2003;29(5):519–22

47. Spencer JM, Gooden M, Goldberg DJ. Botulinum B treatment of glabellar and frontalis regions: a dose response analysis. *J Cos Laser Ther* 2002;4:19–23

48. Bauman L, Slezinger A, Vujevich J *et al*. A double-blinded randomized placebo-controlled pilot study of the safety and efficacy of Myobloc (botulinum toxin type B).-purified neurotoxin complex for the treatment of crow's feet: a double-blinded placebo-controlled trial. *Dermatol Surg* 2003;29:508–15

49. Kim EJ, Ramirez AL, Reeck JB, Maas CS. The role of botulinum toxin type B (Myobloc) in the treatment of hyperkinetic facial lines. *Plast Reconstr Surg* 2003; 112 (5 Suppl):88S–93S; discussion 94S–97S

50. Jacob CI. Botulinum toxin type B – onset duration and efficacy: comparing dilution with preserved versus un preserved saline. *Cos Dermatol* 2003;16:25–30

51. Jacob CI. Botulinum neurotoxin type B – a rapid wrinkle reducer. *Sem Cutan Med Surg* 2003;22:131–5

10 BOTULINUM TOXIN IN THE MANAGEMENT OF FOCAL HYPERHIDROSIS

Oliver P Kreyden

Hyperhidrosis: definition and different forms

Sweating is an important mechanism in the regulation of body temperature. Hyperhidrosis is defined as the production of excess sweat, beyond the amount required to return elevated body temperature to normal, which is slightly below 37°C[1].

Hyperhidrosis can be divided into primary and secondary forms. Primary, or essential, hyperhidrosis occurs typically in young individuals experiencing mental stress (nervous sweating), without other pathogenetic factors. The sweating is focal and located chiefly in the axillae, the palms of the hands, the soles of the feet, or the forehead. Secondary hyperhidrosis is caused by an underlying neurologic or endocrinologic disease or malignancy. The sweating is usually diffuse (Table 10.1).

Primary or focal hyperhidrosis is caused by the overactivity of normal sweat glands and not by glandular hypertrophy. Focal hyperhidrosis is diagnosed in individuals if the area of excess sweating is visibly focal and excessive for at least 6 months without any apparent cause and is associated with at least two of the following characteristics:

- Bilateral and relatively symmetric sweating
- Impairs daily activities
- Frequency of at least one episode per week
- Age of onset less than 25 years
- Positive family history
- Cessation of focal sweating during sleep.

Histopathologic samples from patients with primary hyperhidrosis do not show an increase in the number or size of sweat glands. Sweating episodes are mediated by escalating sympathetic activity, channeled through sudomotor fibers that innervate the eccrine sweat glands. Patients suffering from focal hyperhidrosis who are exposed to mental stress can demonstrate a greater than 10-fold increase in activity of the sudomotor fibers, compared to non-hyperhidrotic controls exposed to the same level of stress, because the severity of hyperhidrosis is very individualized[2].

There is a genetic predisposition and a family history of focal hyperhidrosis in 30–65 per cent of patients suffering from the disorder[3–5]. About 1–2 per cent of the population suffers from hyperhidrosis. In the United States alone, 2.8 per cent of the population, or 8 million

TABLE 10.1   PATHOGENESIS OF HYPERHIDROSIS (MODIFIED FROM KREYDEN *ET AL*[9])

Causative disorder	Example
Physiologic hyperhidrosis	Acclimatization
	Menopause
	Idiopathic gustatory sweating
Endocrinologic disorders	Hyperpituitarism
	Hyperthyroidosis
Elevated catecholamines	Hypoglycemia
	Shock
	Pheochromocytoma
Neurologic disorders	Cervical rib
	Carpal-tunnel syndrome
	Auriculotemporal syndrome and other types of symptomatic gustatory sweating
	Tabes dorsalis
	Syringomyelia
	Encephalitis
	Diabetic neuropathy
	Hemiplegia
	Plexus lesions
	Sympathetic chain lesions
Compensatory hyperhidrosis in association with widespread anhidrosis	Ross syndrome
	Diabetic neuropathy
	Miliaria
	Sympathetic chain lesions
Axon reflex sweating	Inflammatory skin lesions
Nevoid disorder	Nevus sudoriferus
Idiopathic hyperhidrosis	Hyperhidrosis axillaris
	Hyperhidrosis manuum
	Hyperhidrosis pedis
	Hyperhidrosis cruris
	Hyperhidrosis corpis localis
	Hyperhidrosis faciei

individuals, is affected with hyperhidrosis. The estimated number of unknown cases may be even higher for several reasons:

- Patients are not aware that hyperhidrosis is a disease and have learned to live with their symptoms.
- Patients do not know whom they should approach for advice (family practitioner, dermatologist, neurologist, endocrinologist)

- Patients may be told to live with their hyperhidrosis, because of their physician's lack of knowledge of treatment options.

The subjective grading of the severity of sweating is wide: some patients are hardly disturbed by excessive sweating, whereas others ask for treatment for negligible sweating. Essential hyperhidrosis is the most common skin disease associated with co-morbidity of psychiatric disorders (anxiety, neurosis, depression). The psychopathologic characteristics of patients with essential hyperhidrosis can be divided into three groups:

- Patients with objective hyperhidrosis associated with a psychosomatic disorder.
- Patients with objective hyperhidrosis associated with a secondary psychiatric reaction arising from the chronic skin disease (sociophobia, depression, anxiety).
- Patients with body dysmorphic disorder (BDD – a disturbed body image resulting in a pathologic concern about appearance and an extreme lack of self-confidence and self-identity), without any objective symptoms of essential hyperhidrosis.

While treatment of hyperhidrosis in the first two groups can ameliorate the psychologic distress, patients with BDD must be protected from invasive treatment and should be referred for psychiatric assessment (see prologue)[6].

Anatomy of sweat glands[7]

Sweat glands are found all over the body. Their total number is between 2 and 4 million. There are two types of sweat glands: eccrine sweat glands, forming the majority (Table 10.2), and apocrine sweat glands, which are present only in limited areas such as the axillae, perianal region, areolae, periumbilical region, prepuce, scrotum, mons pubis, and labia majora. The ratio between apocrine and eccrine sweat glands is 1:1 in the axillae, but 1:10 in other regions.

TABLE 10.2   ECCRINE SWEAT GLANDS: AREA AND QUANTITY (AFTER GROSCURTH[7])

Area	Quantity (cm²)
Sole of foot	620
Forehead	360
Palms	300
Axillae	300
Thigh	120
Scrotum	80
Back	65
Lips	None
Nail bed	None
Nipple	None
Inner preputial surface	None
Labia majora	None
Glans penis	None
Glans clitoridis	None

Eccrine sweat glands

Eccrine sweat glands are long-branched, tubular structures with a coiled secretory portion and a straight ductal portion. The secretory coil is situated deep in the dermis; clear and dark cells can be distinguished within its epithelium. Clear cells have a round, large, moderately euchromatic nucleus. The major constituents of sweat – water and electrolytes – are formed by the clear cells. Dark cells have a cuboidal shape and secrete PAS-positive glycoproteins from dense granules within their cytoplasm. These glycoproteins are the most prominent protein constituents of sweat. The function of dark cells is unknown.

Eccrine sweat glands are innervated by sympathetic nerve fibers from the spinal cord. Nerve cells from spinal cord segments T1 to T4 supply the skin of the face (thoracic segment of the spinal cord), from T2 to T8 the skin of the upper limbs; from T4 to T12 the trunk, and from T10 to L2 the lower limbs (lumbar segment of the spinal cord). An understanding of this innervation is important for the surgical treatment of hyperhidrosis with endoscopic thoracic sympathectomy (see below).

Apocrine sweat glands

Apocrine sweat glands consist of a basal secretory coil and a straight duct leading to the skin surface. The secretory region is situated in the deep dermis. The secretory cells are cuboidal, but may be squamous when the gland is distended with secretory product. The ducts of apocrine glands are morphologically similar to the eccrine ducts. The innervation of apocrine glands is similar to that of the eccrine glands – by sympathetic nerve fibers coming from the same spinal segments as those of the eccrine glands. The secretory product of apocrine glands is a sterile, thick, milky, and odorless fluid containing protein, carbohydrate, ammonia, lipids, ferric ions, and fatty acids. The characteristic smell is generated only after bacterial decomposition. Apocrine sweat glands may be a relic of human evolution: in animals, the secretory product contains pheromones that are an important signal for potency and territorial behavior. However, their particular teleonomic function in humans is still not clear.

Pathophysiology of sweating

Thermoregulation

Sweating is one of the physiologic bodily functions that helps provide for constant body temperature. The normal perspiration rate is approximately 0.5–1 ml/min, i.e. 1–2 liters per day. However, in stressful situations up to 10 liters per day can be produced. Other thermoregulatory mechanisms include changing the diameter of peripheral blood vessels and modifying metabolic and muscular activity[8]. Increasing peripheral cutaneous blood circulation achieves heat loss by convection (i.e. heat emanating from a radiator); sweating, on the other hand, generates evaporative heat loss from the body surface. As with all vital homeostatic regulatory systems of the body, sweating is controlled by the autonomic nervous system, located in the hypothalamus. The body is very sensitive to increases in temperature, which should be always slightly below 37°C (98.7°F). An increase of only 0.5°C (to 99.5°F) causes discomfort; an increase of 1°C (to 100.4° F) causes collapse. Several factors modify thermoregulation in the hypothalamic center, including hormones, pyrogens, physical activity, and emotional stimuli. Temperature changes during the menstrual cycle and thermoregulatory imbalances during the climacteric are not well understood. Emotional and physical activity also can influence the thermoregulatory center via the limbic system.

Mechanism of sweat secretion[9]

The secretory activity of the human eccrine sweat gland consists of two major functions: secretion of an ultrafiltrate of a plasma-like precursor fluid by the secretory coil in response to acetylcholine released from the sympathetic nerve endings, and re-absorption of sodium in excess of water by the duct, producing hypertonic sweat on the skin surface.

Sato originated the concept of an ionic mechanism of fluid secretion by the clear cells of the eccrine acini of exocrine glands[10]. Acetylcholine, released from periglandular cholinergic nerve endings in response to nerve impulses, binds to cholinergic receptors in the clear cells of sweat glands. The activation of these receptors stimulates an influx of extracellular calcium into the cytoplasm (Figure 10.1) that stimulates chloride channels in the luminal membrane and potassium channels in the basolateral membrane, causing a net KCl efflux from the cell. The cell volume therefore decreases, because water follows the solutes to maintain iso-osmolarity, and the cell shrinks. The decrease in potassium and chloride concentration provides a favorable chemical potential gradient – probably the driving force for Na–K–2Cl co-transporters located in

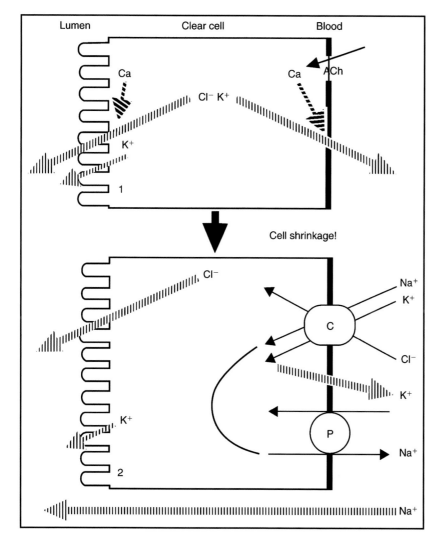

Figure 10.1 Mechanism of eccrine sweat secretion.
C = Na^+–K^+–$2Cl^-$ co-transporter;
P = Na^+–K^+–ATPase-dependent Na pump (modified from Sato[10] in Hölzle[9])

Figure 10.2 Mechanism of re-absorption of electrolytes from primary eccrine sweat. P = Na$^+$–K$^+$–ATPase-dependent Na pump (modified from Sato[10] in Hölzle[9])

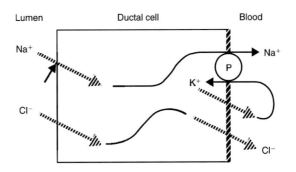

the basolateral membrane. The co-transporters carry sodium, potassium, and chloride ions into the cell in an electrically neutral fashion. In the steady state of secretion, potassium and sodium ions recycle across the basolateral membrane without further loss. In contrast, chloride ions enter the cell via the Na–K–2Cl co-transporters. The movement of chloride ions across the apical (luminal) membrane causes depolarization and generates a negative luminal potential. This then attracts sodium ions into the lumen across the Na-conductive intercellular junction. Thus, the sodium and chloride ions that enter the lumen form NaCl in the isotonic primary fluid.

In the coiled portion of the sweat duct, re-absorption of NaCl occurs to preserve electrolytes, creating the hypotonic sweat secreted at the skin surface. The absorption of NaCl by the duct is due to the active transport of sodium ions by the Na pump located in the basal ductal cell membrane (Figure 10.2). Chloride ions are also transported against the chemical gradient, but down a favorable electrical gradient. In cystic fibrosis, Cl channels in the luminal membrane are defective and those in the basal membrane are significantly decreased, resulting in excess chloride ions in the sweat secreted at the skin surface.

Topical treatments for focal hyperhidrosis

Antiperspirants

Only about 5 per cent of the approximately 3 million sweat glands distributed all over the body are active at any given time during rest or normal activity. This leaves 95 per cent of the 3 million sweat glands ready to become activated during stressful and abnormal situations. Body odors can be unpleasant to many observers; consequently much effort is put into stifling and removing them, chiefly by the use of antiperspirants or deodorants. Whereas deodorants act with fragrance and antibiotics, antiperspirants reduce the flow of sweat. In most deodorants, the active antibacterial agent is triclocarbon or triclosan. Antiperspirants have some degree of antibacterial activity, owing to their acidity[11].

Over the years, many theories have been suggested for the mechanism of action of antiperspirants. In 1967, Papa and Kligman summarized the efforts of more than 20 years of research with the words: 'Next to nothing is known concerning the way in which aluminium salts inhibit eccrine sweating'[12]. Sulzberger's theory that a periductal infiltrate of lymphocytes causes hypohidrosis has been abandoned, as has the suggestion of an increase in permeability of aluminum salts in the acrosyringium, leading to complete dermal re-absorption of the sweat. In 1981 Quatrale et al. used fluorescence microscopy to demonstrate the presence of a plug of electron-dense, amorphous material in the stratum corneum (Figure 10.3)[13]. Hölzle confirmed this by finding PAS-positive material in the upper part of the stratum corneum in the dilated

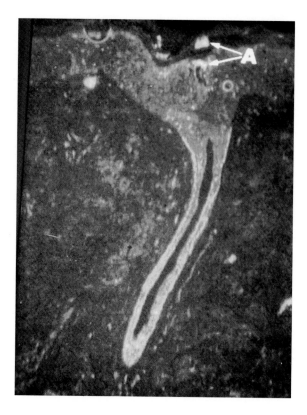

Figure 10.3 Fluorescent microscopy of the hydroxide containing gel in the very upper portion of the acrosyringium (A) leading to a plug of the duct due to slow neutralization of the acid metal[13]

lumen of secretory glands, with atrophy of the secretory cells. He concluded that sweat glands show a tendency to atrophy after long-term use of antiperspirants[14].

The most widely used ingredients for topical antiperspirants are aluminum salts. Aluminum chloride hexahydrate (AlCl-H), introduced by Stillians in 1916, is one of the most effective metallic antiperspirants. Unfortunately, AlCl-H has a high incidence for causing either irritant or even contact dermatitis. Aluminum hydrochloride is therefore preferred because this is less toxic, causes less skin irritation and allergic dermatitis, and is less corrosive to different fabrics. However, it is less effective than AlCl-H, and so aluminum hydrochloride is used in a concentration of 30 per cent. Aluminum salts in concentrations less than 20 per cent usually are not effective and are therefore only used in cosmetic products. Contrary to the manufacturer's recommendation, the solution or cream should be used every night before sleeping, and not every second or third night. In addition, it is very important to use the cream or solution in sufficient quantities only before bedtime, because for crystallization of the stratum corneum plug to occur, complete anhidrosis of the affected areas is absolutely necessary. Preparations containing zirconium salts have been abandoned, mainly because of their role in producing rare cases of skin granulomas, probably due to a delayed-type allergic reaction.

Anticholinergic drugs (parasympatholytics)

Anticholinergic drugs (postsynaptic ganglia blockers) are mentioned here for completeness. Anticholinergic medications work through the inhibition of parasympathetic postsynaptic membrane receptors on sweat glands. The receptors consist of three muscarinic subtypes: M1,

TABLE 10.3   SYSTEMIC ANTICHOLINERGICS COMMONLY USED TO SUPPRESS HYPERHIDROSIS

Medication	Dosage
Glycopyrrolate 1% cream	Apply 1% solution to affected area once daily
Glycopyrrolate (1 mg tablet)	1–2 mg PO bid/tid, titrate to effect
Oxybutrin	5 mg PO bid/tid; not to exceed 5 mg qid
Propantheline bromide	15 mg PO bid/tid 30 min ac initially; gradually titrate to effect
Benzotropine	1–2 mg/day PO; not to exceed 6 mg/day

M2, and M3. The M1 subtype is found on nerve cells and autonomic ganglia. M2 is found on heart, smooth, and skeletal muscle. The M3 subtype is found on smooth muscle, endocrine cells, and glands. While anticholinergics block all receptors non-specifically, the action at the M3 subtype reduces perspiration in patients with hyperhidrosis. Currently, hyperhidrosis approved medications include propantheline bromide (Pro-Bathine®), glycopyrrolate (Robinul®), oxybutynin (Ditropan®), and benztropine (Cogentin®) (Table 10.3). In addition, atropine is often used in a tap water mixture in iontophoresis, a therapy that uses electrical current applied to the skin to induce hypohidrosis. Glycopyrrolate is currently the only anticholingeric that can be found in a 1 per cent topical formulation. The other medications are systemic agents that must be taken orally.

Owing to their adverse effects profile, the use of anticholinergics is limited mostly to selected patients who manifest multifocal or generalized hyperhidrosis. These include patients with hyperhidrosis of different sites occurring in unison or separately such as the axillae, forehead, neck, and scalp. Systemic medication is best used in such cases because different sweating sites can be treated at the same time. Parasympatholytics are categorized as either tertiary (atropine, scopolamine) or quaternary nitrogen compounds (methylscopolamine, N-butylscopolamine, methantelin). The major indication for these antimuscarinic drugs is generally Parkinsonisms. The resorption of tertiary compounds is very good, the quaternary less so, being only 10–25 per cent resorbed. The list of side effects of these drugs is extensive and relatively severe. One of the most prominent side effects is the inhibition of perspiration. Other side effects include mydriasis, dry mouth and eyes, gastrointestinal disturbance, dizziness, blurred vision, tachycardia, urinary retention, and constipation. Because of the danger of glaucoma, parasympatholytics should not be prescribed without a prior ophthalmologic consultation. The half-life of postsynaptic ganglia blockers is relatively short (a few hours). This requires the consumption of medication by mouth three or four times a day, which easily and quickly becomes a compliance issue. In addition, owing to dose-dependent side effects, the dosage of the drug has to be titrated by increasing its strength slowly, until the desired degree of hypohidrosis is reached, while sustaining a modicum amount of other side effects. The dosage can therefore differ between patients, and patients usually are encouraged to titrate their medication up to a dose they can best tolerate. Many times these medications are not well tolerated by patients and are commonly discontinued after a short course.

Tap-water iontophoresis

The basis of iontophoresis was first described by Ichihashi in 1936[15], but therapeutic administration of electricity has been known for over two centuries. As early as 1740, Pivati used iontophoresis in the treatment of arthritis. The mechanism of iontophoresis is based on the principle of electricity: elements with the same charge repel each other, while oppositely charged ones attract. The penetration of charged molecules across the epidermis is therefore facilitated by the use of an external current. For many years, iontophoresis has been used to facilitate transport of molecules (mainly drugs), which otherwise would not penetrate the skin.

Levit was the first to introduce tap-water iontophoresis (TWI) into practical dermatotherapy[16]. The mechanism of TWI-induced anhidrosis has been much studied, but remains unclear. The suggestion that an obstruction high in the sweat duct leads to anhidrosis has been rejected, because no structural changes in the eccrine sweat glands are seen on light and transmission electron microscopy and because the low current densities are well below the threshold of damage to the acrosyringium. Wang et al demonstrated that the composition of neurotransmitters, the density of skin innervation, and the distribution of skin innervation do not change after iontophoretic treatment[17]. Sato et al confirmed that anodal current has more of an inhibitory effect than cathodal current and that water is superior to saline, but increased concentrations of electrolytes diminished the therapeutic effect. Sato also confirmed that the inhibitory effect is a function of the current used. He concluded that the strong acidity generated by the hydrolysis of water in the anodal bath, and the further accumulation of hydrogen ions in the sweat duct by the anodal current, may be responsible for the inhibition of sweating, due to an unknown lesion in the sweat gland duct and acrosyringium[18].

The widely used, direct current (DC) iontophoresis is increasingly being replaced by alternating current with direct current offset (AC/DC) iontophoresis. For DC TWI a current of 8–25 milliamps (mA) at a voltage of 20–40 V is used, whereas for AC/DC TWI the same efficacy is achieved with a lower current (8–12 mA) and a fixed voltage of 16 V[19]. In this mode, side effects such as burning and stinging sensations during treatment, erythema along the water surface, and especially electric shocks caused by abrupt changes in voltage (e.g. at removal from the bath) are minimized[20].

To achieve optimal results, TWI should be performed daily in the initial phase for about 10–14 days or until anhidrosis is achieved. At every treatment session, one extremity is bathed for 10 minutes in the anodal bath (Figure 10.4). Then the opposite extremity is bathed in the anodal pan for another 10 minutes. When palmoplantar hyperhidrosis is treated, both hands can be placed in one pan and both feet can be placed in the other pan. The polarity should be changed halfway through each therapy and not, as is sometimes recommended, every second session. After complete normhidrosis is reached, maintenance therapy is necessary on a weekly or twice-weekly basis.

Although TWI is effective in most cases, there are non-responders. For others, treatment with TWI is successful, but the patient's willingness to continue with maintenance therapy may vary. Regular treatment schedules (e.g. every Monday evening while watching the news on television) can help to improve patient compliance. Alternative therapies, such as botulinum toxin injections (see below), systemic anticholinergic drugs, or surgery should be provided as alternative modes of therapy for non-responders and for patients who are unable for various reasons to continue with therapeutic iontophoresis. There are a few contraindications for TWI,

Figure 10.4 Iontophoresis procedure for palmar hyperhidrosis. To achieve satisfactory anhidrosis on both hands it is important that both hands are treated in the anodal bath (red current). Therefore, after 10 minutes the red current plug has to be switched from one hand to the other and the treatment has be repeated in the same manner. For palmoplantar therapy the treatment principles remain the same, but both hands are bathed in one and the feet in the other pan

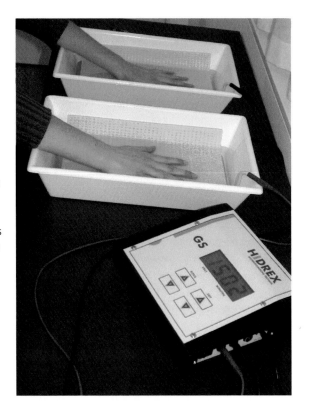

which include patients with pacemakers and metal orthopedic implants, and those who are pregnant[21]. These patients should be offered an alternative mode of therapy.

Surgical treatments for focal hyperhidrosis

Axillary sweat gland excision

Both eccrine and apocrine sweat glands are predominately located in the superficial subcutis and the dermal–subcutaneous interface; indeed, some eccrine glands are located entirely in the dermis. It is important to appreciate this anatomy, since abrasive surgery such as curettage will not completely remove the dermal sweat glands and is therefore not recommended[22]. Excision of the axillary skin and subcutaneous tissue en bloc represents the only comprehensive solution for severe cases of axillary hyperhidrosis that do not respond to botulinum toxin (see below).

Liposuction has the advantage of not leaving unsightly scarring but is much less efficient than excision, owing to the fact that it is a 'blind' technique with uncertain removal of all sweat glands. Because of this, the recurrence rate after axillary liposuction for hyperhidrosis is high, especially when many of the sweat glands reside in the lower dermis. In such cases, temporary anhidrosis is probably the result of physical damage to the fine superficial nerve plexi produced during liposuction, rather than because of the removal of the sweat glands. After several months the nerve plexi recover and the hyperhidrosis recurs.

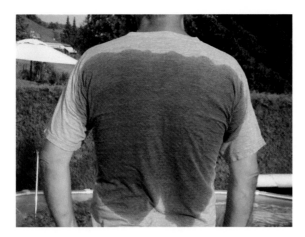

Figure 10.5 Increased sweating of the entire trunk after mild exercise or even after mental stress as a result of severe compensatory hyperhidrosis occurring after endoscopic thoracic sympathectomy for hyperhidroisis of the head

Endoscopic thoracic sympathectomy (ETS)

The aim of this treatment is to achieve anhidrosis by a surgical sympathectomy of the hyperhidrotic area. The indications should be evaluated very carefully, owing to the technical difficulties of the procedure, its invasive nature, and the high complication rate. Serious complications, such as Horner syndrome or pneumothorax, are relatively rare (0.1 per cent and 0.3 per cent, respectively); however, there are reports of intraoperative cardiac arrest during ETS for palmar hyperhidrosis[23]. Compensatory sweating is the most common side effect, occurring in up to 84 per cent of all cases, most of which are mild and unpredictable[24]. However, up to one-third of the patients suffer from moderate to severe sweating over their entire body, especially over the trunk and the proximal extremities (Figure 10.5). The risk of compensatory hyperhidrosis increases with the location and extent of the area treated. Consequently, the risk for compensatory hyperhidrosis is higher in those who undergo ETS for facial or axillary hyperhidrosis than for those who are operated for palmar hyperhidrosis. This is so because after ETS for facial and axillary hyperhidrosis, the entire area of the body above the upper trunk and shoulders becomes anhidrotic. In addition, for technical and other reasons, there is no standardized ETS procedure for plantar hyperhidrosis, which is performed by laparoscopy. Because of the potential for grave post-operative complications, ETS must be strictly reserved only for severe hyperhidrosis of the palms that does not respond to any other treatment.

Botulinum toxin for focal hyperhidrosis

The history of botulinum toxin: from poison to medicine

The first recorded case of food poisoning caused by the neurotoxin-producing bacterium *Clostridium botulinum* (botulism) is believed to have been in 1735. In 1817 Dr Justinus Christian Kerner (1786–1862) published a very precise description of the symptoms of patients suffering from botulism after eating uncooked, smoked sausages or ham[25]. The prominent clinical features of botulism include widespread parasympathetic symptoms such as blurred vision, diplopia, and dilated pupils, dry mouth with dysphagia, asthenia, constipation, nausea, vomiting, and abdominal cramps, followed by increasing muscle weakness descending from head to feet, and culminating in respiratory failure. Because very little was known about infections at that time, Kerner believed a fatty acid to be responsible for the illness. Pierre Emile van Ermengem (1851–1932), Professor of Bacteriology in Ghent, Belgium, isolated the responsible bacterium and refuted the fatty acid theory of Kerner. Before the First World War, Tchitchikine discovered the neurotoxin of *C. botulinum*, and it was Dr Hermann Sommer who first succeeded in purifying the exotoxin in 1920.

During the Second World War, much research was done in the Unites States at Fort Detrick, Maryland, principally by Edward J. Schantz[27,] who was searching for an antidote to counteract botulinum toxin, which was thought to be a potential biologic weapon ready to be used by several other countries. In 1949 Burgen showed that the block of acetylcholine release by botulinum toxin occurred in the presynaptic nerve endings and not, as previously believed, by postsynaptic blockage of receptors, like atropine. In the 1960s Alan Scott[28,29], an ophthalmologist, was searching for a non-surgical alternative for the treatment of strabismus. His idea to weaken the extraocular muscles with botulinum toxin brought him in contact with Ed Schantz. After several trials on monkeys, botulinum toxin, serotype A (BTX-A) was approved in 1989 by the Federal Drug Administration for the treatment of strabismus, blepharospasm, and hemifacial spasm. Other fields of medicine quickly became interested and BTX-A was used for a wide variety of indications, in particular for the treatment of hyperkinetic muscles. Bushara[30] was the first to suggest a possible indication for BTX-A in the treatment of hyperhidrosis. Since 2002, BTX-A has been approved for the treatment of axillary hyperhidrosis in many countries and most recently, in 2004, BOTOX® was approved in the USA by the FDA for axillary hyperhidrosis. There is little doubt that approval for the treatment of palmoplantar hyperhidrosis with BTX-A will soon follow.

Commercially available botulinum toxins

Botulinum toxin type A purified neurotoxin complex is presently available as BOTOX® (Allergan, Irvine, CA, USA) and as Dysport® (Ipsen Ltd, Wrexham, UK). Botulinum toxin type B neurotoxin complex is distributed as Myobloc® in the United States (or as Neurobloc® in Europe) and is manufactured by Elan Pharmaceuticals (San Francisco, CA, USA). BOTOX® is vacuum dried and Dysport® is lyophilized and both are distributed in the form of a dry, crystalline powder that must be reconstituted with 0.9 per cent physiological saline, whereas Myobloc®/Neurobloc® is distributed as an aqueous solution with a pH of 5.6. The biological activity for all three products is defined in mouse units (MU) or just units (U): one mouse unit is defined as the amount of neurotoxin that is lethal in 50 per cent of female, 18–22 g Swiss-Webster mice (i.e. lethal dose, LD_{50}) after an intraperitoneal injection (i.e mouse LD_{50} equals 1 mouse unit or U). It is very important to note that the equivalent units for the three products ARE NOT THE SAME, because the bacterial strain and the manufacturing process used to produce each individual product are entirely different from each other. The dose conversion factor between BTX-A (BOTOX®) and BTX-B (Myobloc®/Neurobloc®) according to the literature is 1:20[31]; and between BOTOX® and Dysport® it is 1:4[32] (see Chapters 8 and 9). However, this should not be construed as a confirmatory statement of a ratio, since this 'conversion' is in direct conflict with the labelling of these products. The package inserts of both BOTOX® and Myobloc®/Neurobloc® reads: 'Units of biological activity of BOTOX® cannot be compared to or converted into units of any other botulinum toxin or any toxin assessed with any other specific assay method'.

Before a physician uses any brand or serotype of botulinum toxin for a particular indication, it is wise for him or her to be familiar with the manufacturer's literature and specifications for its use. However, as a general principle, the potency of one 100 U vial of BOTOX® is roughly equal to the potency of one vial of Dysport®. Remember that any statement of a ratio of 'conversion' is in direct conflict with the labelling of these products, as stated above. There are currently studies underway in Europe and in the USA attempting to best define the conversion ratio between BOTOX® and Dysport® (see Chapter 8).

Birklein et al showed that BTX-B suppresses sudomotor function, effectively in a concentration-dependent manner[33]. They carried out sweat tests (the quantitative sudomotor axon reflex test (QSART) and the minor iodine starch test, see below) before treatment and at 3 weeks, 3 months, and 6 months. They showed that a threshold dose of 8 U BTX-B leads to anhidrotic skin spots (>4 cm^2) after 3 weeks and that the duration of anhidrosis was prolonged for 3 months with 15 U and for 6 months with 125 U of BTX-B. After 3 weeks, the QSART score had decreased to zero with doses of 62.5 U and more, and returned to 91 per cent of baseline after 3 months. After 6 months, recovery of sudomotor function was complete[33]. A similar study was performed by the same group using BTX-A (Dysport®) that showed doses of 2.5 U/cm^2 of Dysport® or more lead to clinically relevant hypohidrosis. A resulting decrease in sweating was maintained for at least 6 months if 12.5 U/cm^2 were injected. Complete suppression could be achieved with doses of 20 U/cm^2 and above[32].

The onset of improvement of hyperhidrosis is believed to be earlier with BTX-B than with BTX-A and the overall effect and duration of both products are comparable to that of BTX-A, but they both are strongly dose-dependent. To ensure delivery of the labeled volume of drug, commercially available vials of botulinum toxin type B (Myobloc®) are overfilled; the vial labeled as containing 2,500 units of botulinum toxin type B in 0.5 ml actually contains approximately 4100 units in 0.82 ml; the vial labeled as containing 5000 units of botulinum toxin type B in 1 ml actually contains approximately 6800 units in 1.36 ml; and the vial labeled as containing 10,000 units of botulinum toxin type B in 2 ml actually contains approximately 12,650 units in 2.53 ml. Therefore, drug solution should not be diluted in the vial since this may result in a solution with a higher concentration of Myobloc® than expected due to overfill.

Discomfort with injections of BTX-B is much higher, owing to its lower pH[34]. This disadvantage can be reduced by using preserved saline instead of preservative-free saline when further diluting BTX-B. Dilution of BTX-B is done only at the discretion of the physician, since a vial of Myobloc®/Neurobloc® comes already in solution[33]. Furthermore, autonomic side effects occur far more often after indications of BTX-B than after BTX-A. Systemic symptoms such as dry mouth, heartburn, and constipation suggest a systemic spread of BTX-B[35]. Myobloc®/ Neurobloc® may be useful in patients not responding to BTX-A, because of innate or acquired immunogenicity issues. However, to date there has been no report of secondary failure in patients treated with BTX-A for focal hyperhidrosis. Therefore current thought is that, due to the potential side effect profile of BTX-B, Myobloc®/Neurobloc® should not be used as the first-line treatment of focal hyperhidrosis.

Patient management and practical considerations

Before treating patients with BOTOX® a detailed patient history should be obtained, focusing particularly on clues for the presence of secondary hyperhidrosis, since the underlying primary disease must be addressed first. As with every other treatment, the potential side effects of the therapy, contraindications (Table 10.4), and the alternative treatments should be explained to the patient. It is also recommended that the patient understands the mechanism of action of BOTOX®, in particular, the need for re-injection after 6–9 months. All the different therapeutic

TABLE 10.4   BOTOX® TREATMENT FOR HYPERHIDROSIS: CONTRAINDICATIONS AND POSSIBLE SIDE EFFECTS

Contraindications

- Secondary hyperhidrosis due to underlying disease
- Neuromuscular disease (e.g. myasthenia gravis)
- Pregnancy/lactation
- Intake of aminoglycoside antibiotics
- Severe coagulopathies

Possible side effects

- Stinging and burning during injection
- Small hematomas at injection sites
- Infection at injection sites
- Weakening of underlying muscles (except when treating the axillae)

modalities (topical concentrated aluminum salt preparations, excision of the sweat glands, anticholinergic medications, or ETS) available should be explained to the patient. The example of a desk lamp can illustrate in simple terms the different therapeutic modalities available to treat hyperhidrosis. There are several different ways to prevent a lamp from casting light: either you take out the light bulb (sweat gland excision), or you cut through the electrical supply cord (ETS), or you temporarily insulate the light bulb contacts (BOTOX® injections).

It is very important that the patient understands the basic pharmacology of BOTOX® and possible side effects. The discussions should include the typical chronologic course required for

TABLE 10.5   CONSENT TO TREAT WITH BOTOX® FOR FOCAL HYPERHIDROSIS

I have been thoroughly informed about the above therapy by the doctor managing my treatment. I understand that the activity of my sweat glands will be decreased after the injection of purified botulinum toxin A (BOTOX®) into my skin. This effect will appear 3–7 days after the injections and last usually about 6 months, but its effect can last for a shorter or longer amount of time.

Additionally, I have received a leaflet about BOTOX® therapy that contains information that is complete and comprehensive, including alternative treatments. All my questions have been answered either by the treating physician or the nurse. I know that, owing to lack of evidence, BOTOX® should not be used in pregnancy or lactation. I am not aware that I am pregnant or have any significant neurological disease or systemic or local infection.

I understand that since 2003 BOTOX® has been approved by the FDA for the treatment of axillary hyperhidrosis only, but not for the treatment of palmoplantar or facial hyperhidrosis.

_____   _____   _____
Date   Physician signature   Patient signature

the clinical effects to become fully activated and the reasons and time for re-treatment. Patients should know not to be treated during pregnancy and lactation.

Many practitioners have the patient sign a written consent form that becomes part of the patient's permanent record (see example in Table 10.5). Good follow-up procedures and prompt response to any complaints after treatment are important. The potential risks in treating patients for focal hyperhidrosis with BOTOX® are comparatively small. However, clearly the treating physician must know the pharmacologic effect of the drug and the anatomic sites to inject. It is necessary to participate in one or two training workshops to learn the injection technique prior to initiating treatment. Every practitioner must know in advance how to manage patients with unsatisfactory results. Successful treatments are predicated upon choosing the right patient for treatment, injecting them with the proper technique and insisting on adequate follow-up visits in order to administer appropriate follow-up care.

Axillary hyperhidrosis

Axillary sweating is not a life-threatening disease, but nonetheless can have a substantial impact on the quality of the sufferer's life, both professionally and socially. Most patients with axillary hyperhidrosis have consulted many physicians in the past, most of the time without finding any substantial, long-lasting solution to their problem. In an open-label prospective study, we asked 251 patients about the impact of their focal hyperhidrosis on their lives (oral presentation at EADV, 2004, submitted); 68.5 per cent had to see more than two physicians (21.7 per cent more than three) before a correct diagnosis was made; 78.9 per cent suffered in their social and professional life due to their hyperhidrosis, 75 per cent were limited in their daily activity, and 50 per cent had to abstain from leisure activities. Naumann et al found similar data with 80 per cent of patients with at least a moderate limitation in daily activities and 72 per cent felt less confident or depressed (49 per cent)[36]. In fact, the negative impact of hyperhidrosis on a patient's quality of life is comparable to conditions such as severe atopic dermatitis, cystic acne, or mild to moderate psoriasis. Focal hyperhidrosis should therefore be viewed as a substantive illness and not simply regarded as a lifestyle disorder.

Hyperhidrosis is a chronic condition requiring a safe, long-lasting treatment. It is advisable that treatment should be approached in a stepwise manner[19]. In patients who do not respond to topical treatments – such as aluminum salt solutions or (for palmoplantar hyperhidrosis) tap-water iontophoresis – intradermal injections of BOTOX® can solve the problem in only a few minutes and on an outpatient basis. In contrast to invasive surgical procedures such as excision, curettage, liposuction, or endoscopic thoracic sympathectomy, injections of BOTOX® can be performed without any anesthesia, are easy and quick to administer, and give highly effective results without any scarring. Most importantly, the administration of BOTOX® is associated with high patient satisfaction and low morbidity[37].

Minor starch test

It is essential to assess axillary hyperhidrosis objectively before treatment. A patient's past medical history may not necessarily provide for a complete and accurate assessment of the severity of their hyperhidrosis. As mentioned above, an individual's subjective assessment of suffering can be over- or underexaggerated. It is the task of the treating physician to separate patients with moderate hyperhidrosis – manageable with aluminum salt solutions – from patients with severe hyperhidrosis – to be treated with BOTOX®. Each patient should undergo

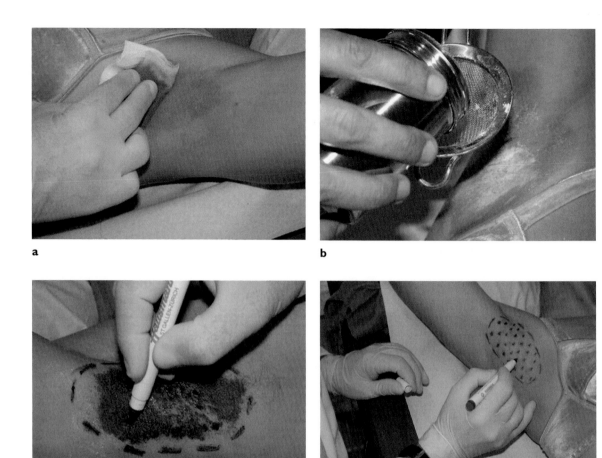

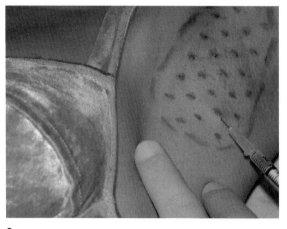

Figure 10.6 Performance of the Minor starch test. The hyperhidrotic area is doused with iodine solution (a) and after drying covered with starch powder (b). The hyperhidrotic area becomes clearly demarcated as a purple surface. Then the hyperhidrotic area is outlined (c). After removing the excess purple color from the center of the outline each injection site can be marked with gentian violet (d) to achieve the best results; (e) shows how the injections are placed

the Minor starch test before treatment with BOTOX® (Figure 10.6). First the hyperhidrotic area is completely dried and covered with an iodine solution (i.e. Lugol or Betadine solution) (Figure 10.6a) and then sprinkled with powdered starch (e.g. cornflower starch) (Figure 10.6b). It is important that as little powder as possible is used to achieve a good colorimetric response. If too much powder is used, the powder will absorb the moisture of the sweat and the intensity of the patient's sweating may not be assessed correctly.

A semiquantitative measurement of focal hyperhidrosis can be achieved using the Minor starch test, demonstrating the full extent of sweating in the affected area and, through the intensity of the purple coloration, the severity of sweating. Therefore, by performing a Minor starch test before each treatment, the treating physician can determine how many injection sites and how much BOTOX® is needed prior to commencing therapy. It is advisable always to measure the affected area and document the colorimetric response with photographs and retain them as part of the patient's permanent record. This will allow comparison of efficacy before and after treatment during follow-up visits, and will allay any misgivings or feelings of dissatisfaction that the patient may fallaciously come to have.

Low-dose BOTOX® therapy, dilution, and injection technique

After outlining the affected area with a marker (Figure 10.6d), the axilla should be cleansed of all iodine and starch, and a final wipe down with denatured 70 per cent isopropyl alcohol should be performed before initiating the BOTOX® injections. Generally, a total dose of 50 U of BOTOX® (250 U of Dysport®) per axilla is required to adequately treat a moderately severely hyperhidrotic axilla. Therefore, no more than a total dose of 1 vial (100 U) of BOTOX® (500 U of Dysport®) should be used per patient, which is currently being recommended in the literature. This is based on the manufacturer's guidelines that recommend a vial of BOTOX® be reconstituted with preservative-free isotonic saline. Consequently, once the vial of BOTOX® is reconstituted without a preservative, it should be fully used within 4 hours, owing to the possibility the solution may not remain sterile for an extended period of time. However, no studies to date have been performed to verify the sterility of a reconstituted vial of BOTOX® after more than 4 hours. The package insert however still advises the administration of BOTOX® within four hours after the vial is removed from the refrigerator and reconstituted. During these four hours, reconstituted BOTOX® should be stored in a refrigerator (2° to 8°C). Every treating physician therefore has become accustomed to using one whole vial of BOTOX® per patient for obvious economic reasons. Over the years, however, we have learned that there are no adverse events or significant loss of potency resulting from the storage of reconstituted BOTOX® for a few days and even a few weeks.

There is BOTOX® stability data before reconstitution, for 5 days up to 30°C with insignificant effect on potency. Additionally, a freeze/thaw cycle that might have occurred does not affect product potency (personal conmunication, Roger Aoki, PhD). Consequently, physicians should abandon this practice and use the exact amount of BOTOX® each patient needs, predicated upon the size and severity of the affected area as defined by the Minor starch test.

The number of injection sites, and consequently the total dose of injected BOTOX®, should no longer be defined as a total recommended dose for a given anatomic site (i.e. 50 U of BOTOX® per axilla), but by the number of units used per injection site (i.e. 2 Units BOTOX® for each injection point). This also depends upon the size of the colorimetric response exhibited by

TABLE 10.6 SUGGESTED DILUTIONS AND UNITS USED TO TREAT AXILLARY HYPERHIDROSIS

Dilution	BOTOX® 10 ml		Dysport® 10 ml		BOTOX® 5 ml		Dysport® 5 ml	
U/vial	100		500		100		500	
U/ml	10		50		20		100	
U/0.1ml	1		5		2		50	
ml/injection site	0.2		0.2		0.1		0.1	
Number of injections/axilla	10	20	10	20	10	20	10	20
U/axilla	20	40	100	200	20	40	100	200
Total U/patient	40	80	200	400	40	80	200	400

In general, the dilution and dosage are still subject to discussion. Note that the dosage should be defined by the dose per injection point (2 U) and not by the total dose per axilla, because depending on the extent of the affected hyperhidrotic area the total dose can vary considerably, whereas the dose per injection site always remains constant.

the Minor starch test, which in most patients is a surface area of approximately 8 × 4 cm to 10 × 5 cm (50 cm²). Since the diffusion capacity of BOTOX® is about 1.0 to 1.5 cm in diameter, 10 points injected at a distance of approximately 1.5 cm apart are sufficient to cover an area of 50 cm² (about a quarter of a vial of BOTOX® per side or half arial per patient respectively). If this area is larger than 50 cm², we consequently need more injections (in general 15 to 20 points of injection i.e. three-quarters to one vial of BOTOX® per patient, meaning for treatment of both axilla). With this technique generally only half a vial of BOTOX® is used (Table 10.6), with no loss of efficacy. This technique is referred to as the 'low dose, high volume botulinum toxin therapy'[38]. Higher doses (≥800 U) of BOTOX® have been used for therapeutic purposes, and they are associated with an increased risk of antigenicity and immunoresistance with the production of IgG-neutralizing antibodies[39].

The low-dose, high-volume technique has several advantages:

- Fewer injections
- Less painful treatment session
- Reduced incidence of neutralizing antibody production
- Reduced risk of immunoresistance
- Lower cost.

The optimal dilution of BOTOX® for the treatment of hyperhidrosis is still under discussion. Although the reconstitution of Dysport® with 5 ml of sterile saline is still widely accepted, Bigalke et al.[40] showed that the biologic availability of Dysport® could be enhanced by:

- Lowering the concentration of the BTX-A (Dysport®)
- Supplementing reconstituted Dysport® with additional albumin
- Increasing the dilution volume.

Since this study was performed with Dysport®, which has a higher protein content than BOTOX®, its conclusions cannot and should not be extrapolated to the use of BOTOX®[40]. The diffusion capacity of Dysport® was enhanced by increasing the volume of diluent used to reconstitute the product. Specifically, instead of reconstituting a 500 U vial of Dysport® with 5 ml of normal saline (which provides 50 U of BTX-A for each 0.1 ml of solution), Bigalke *et al*. recommended reconstituting a 500 U vial of Dysport® with 10 ml of solute (which provides 5 U of BTX-A for each 0.1 ml of solution) (Table 10.6)[39].

Further, to avoid immunoresistance, the following recommendations should be considered:

- Use the smallest possible effective dose
- Extend the interval between treatments as much as possible
- Avoid booster injections.

Therefore this author prefers to reconstitute a 100 U vial of BOTOX® with 10 ml of normal saline, instead of 5 ml, and inject 2 U of BTX-A (10 U Dysport®) per 0.2 ml injection site (see Table 10.6).

Although there are as yet no published data on the development of resistance to BOTOX® therapy in patients with hyperhidrosis, we should be concerned about the potential for its occurrence. Therefore, the use of BOTOX® should be based on the required dose needed to treat each individual patient so that an appropriate clinical response can be obtained. There are also economic considerations: BOTOX® is expensive and, by reducing the required therapeutic dose, costs are kept down – both for the patient and the health care industry.

Hyperhidrosis of the palms and soles

The dilution of BTX-A (BOTOX® or Dysport®) for the treatment of hyperhidrosis of the palms or soles can be the same as that for the treatment of hyperhidrosis of the axilla (see above). However, to avoid attendant muscle weakness after BTX-A injections, especially in the hands, the reconstitution volume for both BOTOX® and Dysport® can be reduced from 10 ml to 5 ml. Again, as the radial diffusion distance of BOTOX® is about 1.0–1.5 cm, the interval between two injection points should not exceed much beyond this diameter. Therefore, depending on the size of the hands or feet and the localization of the hyperhidrosis (sometimes not all the digits are involved), approximately 35–40 injection points should be planned for the treat-ment of one hand and 60–80 injection points for one foot, leading to a total dose of BOTOX® of approximately 80 U (320 U of Dysport®) per hand and 160 U (640 U of Dysport®) per foot.

In distinct contrast to the painless BTX-A injections of the axillae for hyperhidrosis, BTX-A injections of the palms and soles for hyperhidrosis require regional anesthesia.

Nerve block

Many trials of regional anesthesia have been reported, with differing results. Cooling sprays and topically applied EMLA® cream can provide limited skin surface anesthesia, but completely painless injections can only be achieved by nerve blocks, which commonly are poorly accepted by patients. The administration of nerve blocks requires careful and expert training. Nerve blocks can be painful and it is difficult to achieve a complete and total anesthesia in every patient. The risk of nerve injury and severe side effects (anaphylactic shock, cardiac problems) also should not be underestimated. Vasovagal syncopal episodes are common and the actual application of the procedure usually prolongs the overall time for the therapeutic procedure. Because of the effect of the anesthetic on motor muscle activity, patients are consistently inconvenienced (e.g. they are unable to drive or even shake hands for several hours or even days. To maintain the anhidrotic effect of BTX-A, the injections, and thus the nerve block, have to be repeated on a regular base. Because of the many disadvantages of BTX-A injections for nerve blocks in the palms and soles, particularly, the need for nerve blocks, many patients often postpone or even cancel the required second or subsequent treatment sessions, regardless of the excellent clinical outcomes they might have experienced previously.

A new anesthetic procedure for the treatment of palmoplantar hyperhidrosis therefore has been developed (see below). The use of nerve blocks then should be reserved for selected cases.

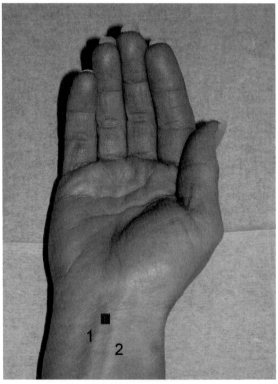

a

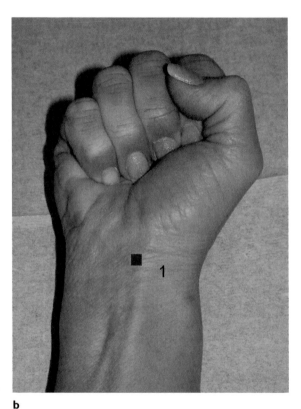

b

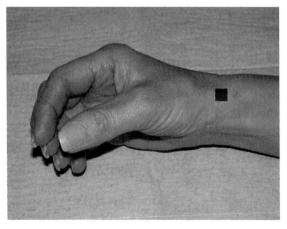

c

Figure 10.7 The different injection points for a nerve block of the hand; the red squares indicate the points of injection. (a) for an ulnar nerve block: 1 = tendon of the flexor carpi ulnaris, 2 = tendon of the pulmaris longus; (b) for a median nerve block: 1 = tendon of the flexor carpi radialis; (c) where to block radial nerve (over the tendon of the extensor carpi radialis and medial of the radial artery)

Hand block

To achieve complete anesthesia of the hand, all three nerves (ulnar, median, radial) have to be effectively blocked from transmitting a nervous impulse. To anesthetize the radial nerve, which lies in the superficial fascia at the wrist, 2–4 ml of 1–2 per cent lidocaine with or without epinephrine (1:100,000) is injected subcutaneously 1 cm parallel to the carpal bones on the dorsomedial aspect of the hand and over the tendon of the extensor carpi radialis and medial to the radial artery ventrally (Figure 10.7a–c). To anesthetize the median and ulnar nerves with or without epineprine 1:100,000 but approximately 2 ml of lidocaine 1–2 per cent (reduce the burning pain of injection with 0.5 per cent sodium bicarbonate) can be injected on both sides of the tendon of the flexor carpi ulnaris (the ulnar flexor muscle of the wrist and ulnar nerve) and the tendon of the palmaris longus (the long flexor muscle of the palm and median nerve), respectively (Figure 10.7). The needle should be inserted 0.5–1 cm perpendicular to the skin until firm resistance is felt and the deep fascia is pierced. It is then retracted about 2 mm before the lidocaine is injected (alternatively, xylonest 1 per cent or carbostesin 0.5 per cent may be used). After 15–30 minutes full anesthesia is achieved in the palm and the back of the hand. The totality of the block is discernible through loss of sensitivity, impairment of motor activity, and the hand becoming warm, red, and dry. This can be considered an advantage because the patient feels complete anhidrosis for the first time. However, because of the vasodilation, every injection site (30–40 per palm) tends to bleed copiously.

Foot block

The principle of a foot block is similar to the hand block (see above). The injection sites for the tibial nerve block are located on both sides of the tibial artery, dorsocaudal to the medial malleolus. The needle is inserted perpendicular to the skin and advanced 0.5–2 cm. Then 2 ml local anesthetic is injected (see above). For the saphenous nerve block, a subcutaneous infiltration of local anesthetic is made 2 cm above the ankles all around the lower leg. The fibularis profundus block is performed with an injection of 2 ml local anesthetic on both sides of the dorsalis pedis artery (Figure 10.8a–c). The foot block is relatively easy to perform, in many cases much easier than the hand block; however, the same disadvantages apply. Indeed, motor impairment is even worse than in the hand block, because at times the patient can experience much difficulty with walking after a nerve block of both feet.

New anesthetic procedure combining lidocaine iontophoresis with cryotherapy

Because of the long list of side effects associated with nerve blocks, many different modalities for regional anesthesia have been tried by the author, including cooling sprays and EMLA® cream under occlusion for one hour or more. The cooling spray technique produces an unpleasantly frozen hand, both for the patient and the treating doctor. Furthermore, there is only a moderate anesthetic effect, particularly for the burning pain experienced during the injection of the solution (it is less for the needle stick). EMLA® cream under occlusion for one hour or more gives an excellent anesthetic effect for the stinging of the needle, but only minimal relief from the burning experienced during the injection of the fluid. Moreover, the topical application of an anesthetic cream with occlusion for one hour produces maceration and swelling of the hand, which makes it extremely difficult to find the correct depth to inject the BOTOX®, which must be intradermal and not subdermal. It is imperative to remain intradermal with injections of BOTOX® for palmar hyperhidrosis, especially if muscle weakness is to be avoided.

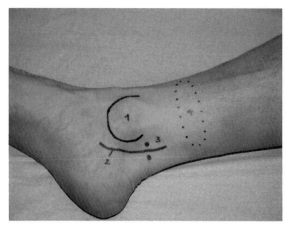

a

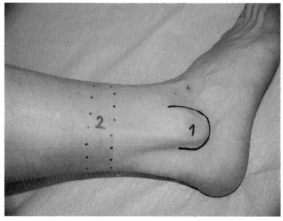

b

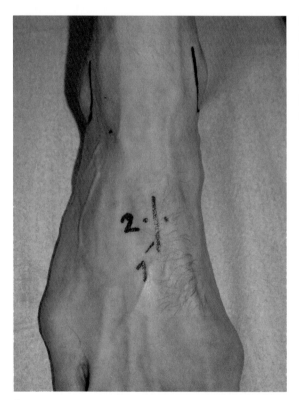

c

Figure 10.8 The injection points of tibialis. (a) Saphenous block, 1 = medial malleolus, 2 = posterior tibialis artery, 3 = injection points for tibialis block, 4 = area of subcutaneous infiltration for saphenous block; (b) Fibularis block, 1 = lateralis malleolus, 2 = area of subcutaneous infiltration for saphenous block; (c) Profundus block, 1 = dorsalis pedis artery, 2 = injection points for fibularis profundus block

A report on topical dermal analgesia induced by iontophoretic administration of 2 per cent lidocaine[41] led the author to perform a new form of anesthesia for the treatment of palmoplantar hyperhidrosis with BOTOX®[42]. This new technique achieves almost complete anesthesia with only slight stinging and burning, similar to what is felt during injections of BOTOX® for axillary hyperhidrosis[42]. Initially, this new technique was performed using only iontophoresis with 2 per cent lidocaine for 30 minutes (15 minutes for each extremity) (Figure 10.9). This reduced the stinging and burning sensation but did not abolish it completely, owing

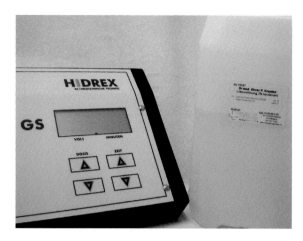

Figure 10.9 Before palmoplantar BOTOX® treatment, iontophoresis with 2% lidocaine for 30 minutes (15 minute for each side) is performed. With this procedure a very superficial anesthesia can be achieved. Thus the patient will tolerate much better the mild burning sensation caused by the following cryotherapy just before injection with BOTOX® (see Figure 10.11)

to the very superficial nature of the anesthesia. As this author's use of the new technique grew, a combined procedure was developed which now combines the spraying of a controlled amount of liquid nitrogen cryotherapy with the lidocaine iontophoresis (Figures 10.10 and 10.11). The lidocaine solution used for iontophoresis is ordered from a local pharmacy in large quantities (e.g. 5 liters of lidocaine hydrochloride 100 g in aqua conservans 4900 g). The iontophoresis unit used is the HIDREX GS (from HIDREX, Wuppertal, Germany), which can generate a current of 15 to 25 mA (Figure 10.9). The hand should be covered by the lidocaine solution until the back of

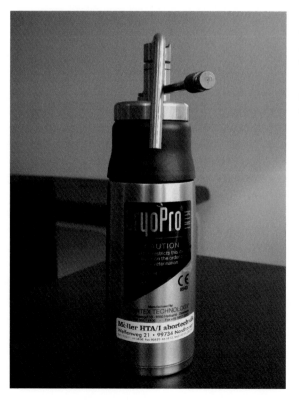

Figure 10.10 A cryotherapy unit commonly used for cryosurgery. After the container has been filled with liquid nitrogen the marked points on the skin are sprayed until frozen, leaving a white spot (see Figure 10.11)

Figure 10.11 Just before injecting BOTOX® for palmoplantar hyperhidrosis the injection point is sprayed with liquid nitrogen to achieve satisfactory analgesia

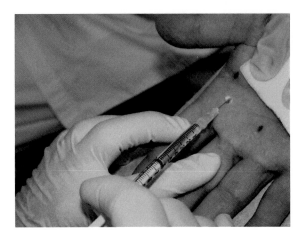

the hand is submerged, as is usually done for antihyperhidrotic iontophoretic therapy (Figure 10.4).

This new combination iontophoresis/cryotherapy technique has the advantage of specifically dosing a focus of liquid nitrogen cryotherapy in such a manner that it does not cause the entire hand to freeze. Just before BOTOX® is injected, the site to be treated is sprayed with liquid nitrogen cryotherapy until a faint white spot appears (Figure 10.11). The BOTOX® then is injected directly into this focus of partially frozen anesthetized skin (Figure 10.11). With this technique a pain-free vertical injection can be achieved, even on the fingertips.

This new combined iontophoresis/cryotherapy technique was used to produce anesthesia prior to BOTOX® injection in the palmo plantar surface in an experimental group of 36 patients. The technique resulted in an overall satisfaction rate in 92.3 per cent of all patients, compared to only 37.8 per cent in a group treated with EMLA® and 17.8 per cent in a group treated with the nerve blocks. The low level of satisfaction after nerve block is due not to the poor anesthetic effect, but to the severe side effect profile of this technique (see above). However, there is also an unpleasant side effect with the combined iontophoresis cryotherapy technique, i.e. liquid nitrogen often produces mild blistering at the application site when a small-one hole treatment cone is used (Figure 10.12). This blistering was never a severe medical problem, but was a source of embarrassment for some patients.

Different nozzles and cones are available for cryotherapy, but they all have a one-hole exit port. Moreover, the diameter of the cone or nozzle should be as small as possible to achieve precise anesthesia (Figure 10.12). However, it is inevitable that while this combined anesthetic technique is performed some sites will blister. Therefore the author has developed a new cooling system for liquid nitrogen cryotherapy using a 10-hole nozzle (Figure 10.13). This nozzle was initially produced to create a comfortably cool haze after laser therapy. The 10-hole nozzle produces a defocused iced spray that produces complete anesthesia without any blistering. Although this combined technique requires some training and an assistant to perform (the assistant cools, the physician injects), this technique is highly recommended owing to increased patient satisfaction.

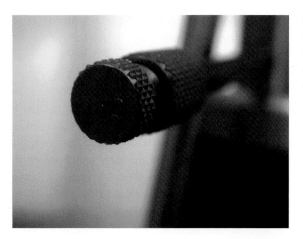

Figure 10.12 For local anesthesia the smallest nozzle is used to achieve the most precise anesthesia with as little damage as possible

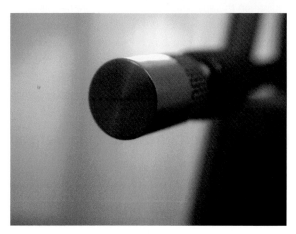

Figure 10.13 Improved freezing system with a 10-hole nozzle producing a cool haze instead of a white spot. With this system embarrassing blistering can be avoided

Applications for BOTOX® injections in rare forms of focal hyperhidrosis

Along with the common occurrence of primary localized hyperhidrosis of the palms, soles, or the axillae, there are rare forms of focal hyperhidrosis that can also be treated with injections of BTX-A. Some of these cases are classified as primary focal hyperhidrosis (hyperhidrosis of the forehead and inguinal area), some are associated with syndromes (Ross syndrome, Frey syndrome), and others are iatrogenic side effects and complications of surgical procedures, such as ETS (i.e. compensatory hyperhidrosis) and still others are idiopathic entities such as localized unilateral hyperhidrosis (LUH).

Primary focal hyperhidrosis of the forehead and anogenital area

Even though these localizations of focal primary hyperhidrosis are not as common as axillary or palmoplantar hyperhidrosis, it is very important to provide treatment for them. Patients can experience serious emotional stress and intense social embarrassment when they find themselves dripping sweat from their forehead down into their face, or when they find the need

285

to wear panty liners to prevent profuse sweating from saturating their pants and trousers caused by inguinal and perineal hyperhidrosis[43].

The principles of treatment of the anogenital area remain the same as in other localizations of focal hyperhidrosis. The first stage of therapy should be attempted with the application of aluminum salt solutions. This often achieves a satisfactory result and nothing else has to be done. ETS has been suggested for therapy-resistant severe focal hyperhidrosis of the forehead. However, this procedure is associated with an even higher risk of severe and widespread compensatory hyperhidrosis (see Figure 10.5), more so than with ETS for palmar hyperhidrosis. This is probably due to the huge area of attendant anhidrosis (of the head, back, breast, and shoulders) resulting from ETS. The treatment of compensatory hyperhidrosis is very complicated (see below). ETS for the lower limbs, including the inguinal area and perineum, is not recommended as a standard procedure, owing to technical difficulties in performing it laparoscopically. Systemic treatments such as anticholinergics, sedatives or tranquillizers – with or without combination therapy with beta-blockers – are neither very effective nor well tolerated by patients, because of the associated side-effects[44]. Therefore, if aluminum salts are not effective, BTX-A injections should be considered as a second-line treatment and surgical treatment reserved only for selected cases. However there are cases of huge areas of hyperhidrosis affecting not only the forehead, but the whole face, the back, the breasts, chest, and the shoulders, when oral anticholinergics may be effective before BTX-A injections are even considered.

Botulinum toxin injections for hyperhidrosis of the forehead and anogenital areas

In most cases of hyperhidrosis of the forehead, patients sweat profusely at the hairline. Owing to the involvement of the underlying frontalis, BOTOX® should not be injected within 1.5–2.0 cm of the eyebrows to prevent the occurrence of either brow ptosis, or blepharoptosis, or both. For the same reason, the dilution of the BOTOX® should be much less than that which is used for axillary hyperhidrosis. To prevent any diffusion beyond the target area, low doses (see above) and low-volume dilutions (2.5–5.0 ml) of BTX-A should be used. However, dilutions of 5 ml per vial of BOTOX® can be used without adverse sequelae if the proper technique is used. With such high-volume BOTOX® the risk of producing a 'heavy forehead' or brow ptosis for a few days or

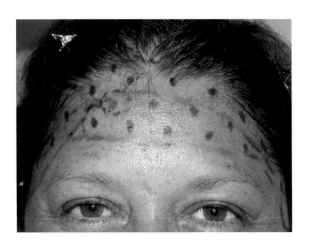

Figure 10.14 Marked injection points for treatment of frontal hyperhidrosis after a Minor starch test. The rings around an injection point indicating the estimated diffusion halo of BOTOX® after injection

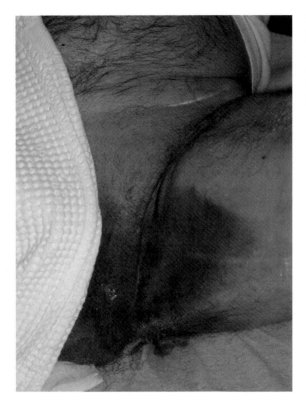

Figure 10.15 Hyperhidrosis of the left groin area after a Minor starch test. As shown the affected area can be extensive, which has to be considered before treatment

weeks is increased. However, a dilution with 4 ml or even 2.5 ml per vial of BOTOX® is recommended for treatment of the forehead. As with other areas, it is important to perform a Minor starch test before the injection points are marked on the surface of the forehead (Figure 10.14).

In sharp contrast to BOTOX® injections in the forehead, the dilution of BOTOX® when treating inguinal hyperhidrosis (Figure 10.15) should be as high as possible to achieve maximum diffusion, since the areas of hyperhidrosis in the anogential area can be quite extensive. However, the rule of injecting 2 U per site remains the same in this indication. The injection technique in principle is similar to the way other areas of focal hyperhidrosis are treated, but it is very important to perform the injections intradermally to prevent paralyzing the muscles of the pelvis. Therefore this procedure should only be performed by experienced practitioners.

Hyperhidrosis associated syndromes

Several rare syndromes associated with hyperhidrosis are described in the literature: POEMS syndrome, pachyonychia congenita, Apert syndrome, pachydermoperiostosis, Papillon–Lefèvre syndrome, nail–patella syndrome, etc.[45]. Only two syndromes that can be treated with BTX-A will be discussed here.

Frey syndrome

Gustatory sweating is a common complication following parotid gland surgery, infection, or trauma. It was first described by Lucie Frey in 1923[46]. The most likely explanation for the condition is a misdirected resprouting of postsynaptic salivomotor parasympathetic fibers that

Figure 10.16 Patient with Frey syndrome. Distinct hyperhidrosis of a confined area of the cheek during or after eating due to misdirected re-sprouting of post-synaptic salivomotor parasympathtic fibers after parotid gland surgery or infection

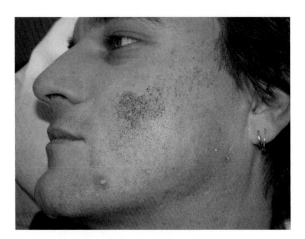

have lost their glandular target organ. Following gustatory stimulation, the clinical picture (Figure 10.16) includes pathological sweating of the preauricular area and sometimes a flushing reaction involving the superficial cutaneous vasculature. About 50 per cent of patients experience gustatory sweating after parotidectomy and 15 per cent consider their symptoms severe[47]. BTX-A (BOTOX®, Allergan Inc, Irvine, CA) is an effective therapeutic option for the treatment of gustatory sweating and it can be considered as a first-line treatment. The duration of treatment effect in patients with Frey syndrome is much longer than in patients treated for other indications, such as hemifacial spasm or blepharospasm or even hyperhidrosis in other areas (mean duration 17.3 months)[48].

Ross syndrome

Ross syndrome was first described by the neurologist Alexander T. Ross in 1958[49]. It is characterized by the triad of unilateral tonic pupils, generalized areflexia (Holmes–Adie syndrome), and progressive segmental anhidrosis with a compensatory band of excessive perspiration. Patients suffering from Ross syndrome usually do not perceive the hypohidrosis; instead, it is the compensatory segmental hyperhidrosis that is bothersome. In addition, many patients suffer from several symptoms of vegetative dysfunction, such as palpitation, stenocardia, orthostatic hypotonia, and irritable colon[45]. The pathogenesis of Ross syndrome is unknown. Multiple neuropathies of the autonomic nervous system or a failure in the synthesis or release of neurotransmitters have been suggested as possible causes[49]. There is no histologic evidence of nerve fiber destruction. Therefore Ross postulated a defect in acetylcholine cholinesterase activity, rather than the degeneration of sweat glands. The progression of Ross syndrome is very slow. There is no therapy for the segmental progressive anhidrosis. The bothersome compensatory hyperhidrosis can be improved, however, with systemic antimuscarinic drugs or with injections of BTX-A into the affected areas, usually the face. In 1992 Itin et al.[50] presented a case study of a patient suffering from Ross syndrome with a defined area of anhidrosis in the right hand, the right axilla, and the right side of the face. In follow-up, after 11 years the patient presented with additional anhidrotic areas in the right hemithorax and the underside of the left arm (Figure 10.17). Unfortunately the patient refused treatment with BOTOX®, even though the hyperhidrosis was so severe that electrolyte replacement was necessary (unpublished data).

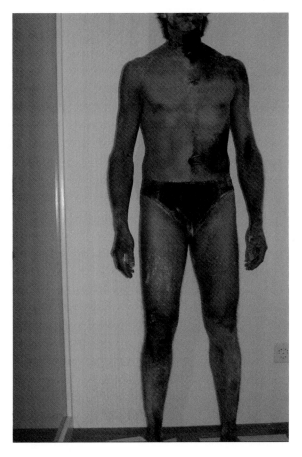

Figure 10.17 Patient with Ross syndrome characterized by progressive segmental anhidrosis with a compensatory band of excessive perspiration leading the patient to the physician. This is the very same patient 11 years after Itin *et al.*[45] first published their case study, showing extensive progression of the disease (unpublished data)

Treatment of compensatory hyperhidrosis after endoscopic thoracic sympathectomy (ETS)

Compensatory hyperhidrosis can be a very embarrassing, almost a disabling disease. The incidence after ETS is relatively high (see above); severe problematic cases with generalized severe sweating are fortunately rare. The treatment options for patients with copious sweating of almost the entire body are very limited. One possibility is the use of anticholinergic drugs, with their attendant adverse side effects. BTX-A treatment is limited by the potential toxic side effects associated with the high doses required (estimated LD_{50} of a human being is 3500–5000 U) and the expense of treating such large involved areas (Figure 10.5). BOTOX® therapy in such cases does not seem to be as effective as it is when treating focal hyperhidrosis, i.e. axillary or palmoplantar hyperhidrosis. A further limiting problem is suppressing excessive sweating without the risk of hyperthermia. Under these circumstances, the aim of each individual therapy should be to combine several therapeutic modalities to achieve the best outcome. The patient should be aware of the difficulties in treating such conditions and should be counseled to be satisfied with the reality of achieving moderate success. An algorithm that can be used in treating such cases is, first, the application of aluminium salt solutions, combined with the ingestion of anticholinergic drugs in an ever-increasing dosage, as the mandatory first line of

Figure 10.18 Typical Minor starch test of a patient with compensatory hyperhidrosis after endoscopic thoracic sympathectomy for hyperhidrosis of the forehead. Note the anhidrotric area of the upper trunk (no coloration) and the (compensatory) hyperhidrotic purple area of the chest

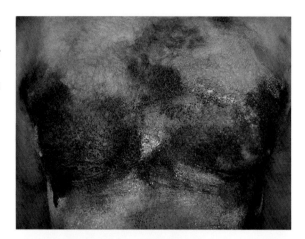

Figure 10.19 Same patient as in Figure 10.18. The most hyperhidrotic areas are marked for BOTOX® injections. The rings show the estimated diffusion halos of injected BOTOX® (unpublished data)

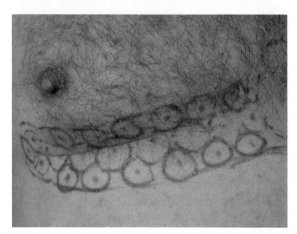

treatment. A few patients will need additional therapy for well-defined areas of intensely active sweating. Such cases will benefit from injections of BTX-A. Again it is most important to define the affected areas of hyperhidrosis by the use of the Minor starch test (Figure 10.18) Then BTX-A can be injected as described above (Figure 10.19).

Localized unilateral hyperhidrosis

Localized unilateral hyperhidrosis (LUH) is a rare form of idiopathic localized hyperhidrosis and is defined as a confined area of hyperhidrosis of less than 10 × 10 cm, mainly found on the forehead or the forearm, whose pathogenesis is unknown (Figure 10.20). Beside the unusual localization, the major difference from essential hyperhidrosis is that LUH has no typical triggering factor and occurs even while patients are asleep. The etiology of LUH is unknown but may be due to a misdirected reconnection of the sympathetic nerve fiber network after injury, similar to the Frey syndrome[1]. Before BTX-A, no treatment was available for this distinctive but enigmatic skin disorder. However, excellent results have been experienced following injection of 30 units of BOTOX® in a patient suffering from LUH[1].

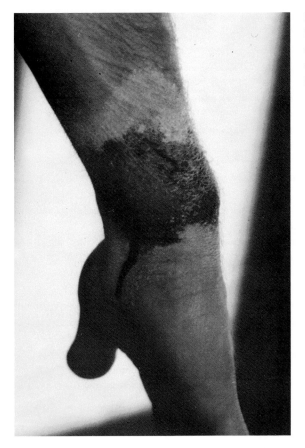

Figure 10.20 Patient with localized unilateral hyperhidrosis[1] on his right wrist, showing the dripping hyperhidrosis after the Minor starch test (from[1,45])

References

1. Kreyden OP, Schmid-Grendelmeier P, Burg G. Idiopathic localized unilateral hyperhidrosis. Case report of successful treatment with botulinum toxin type A and review of the literature. *Arch Dermatol* 2001;137:1622–5

2. Iwase S, Ikeda T, Kitazawa H *et al*. Altered response in cutaneous sympathetic outflow to mental and thermal stimuli in primary palmoplantar hyperhidrosis. *J Auton Nerv Syst* 1997;64:65–73

3. Glogau RG. Hyperhidrosis and botulinum toxin A: patient selection and techniques. *Clin Dermatol* 2004;22:45–52

4. Ro KM, Cantor RM, Lange KL *et al*. Palmar hyperhidrosis: evidence of genetic transmission. *J Vasc Surg* 2002;35:382–6

5. Sato K, Kang WH, Saga K *et al*. Biology of sweat glands and their disorders. II. Disorders of sweat gland function. *J Am Acad Deramtol* 1989;20:713–26

6. Kreyden OP, Heckmann M, Peschen M. Delusional hyperhidrosis as a risk for medical overtreatmnent: a case of botulinophilia. *Arch Dermatol* 2002;138:538–9

7. Groscurth P. Anatomy of sweat glands. In: Kreyden OP *et al*, eds. *Hyperhidrosis and Botulinum Toxin in Dermatology. Curr Probl Dermatol* Basel: Karger, 2002;30:1–9

8. Jarrett A, Morimoto T. Heat exchange between animals and their environment. In: Jarrett A, ed. *The Physiology and Pathphysiology of the Skin*. London: Academic Press, 1978;5:1597–609

9. Hölzle E. Pathophysiology of Sweating. In: Kreyden OP *et al*, eds. *Hyperhidrosis and Botulinum Toxin in Dermatology. Curr Probl Dermatol* Basel: Karger, 2002;30:10–22

10. Sato H. Biology of the eccrine sweat gland. In: Freedberg *et al*, eds. *Dermatology in General Medicine* New York: McGraw-Hill, 1993;5:155–64

11. Kreyden OP. *Über Körpergerüche und deren Bekämpfung – Deodoranzien und Antitranspiranzien unter der Lupe*. Hautnah, 2001

12. Papa CM, Kligman AM. Mechanisms of eccrine anidrosis. II. The antiperspirant effect of aluminum salts. *J Invest Dermatol* 1967;49:139–45

13. Quatrale RP, Coble DW, Stoner KL, Felger CB. The mechanism of antiperspirant action by aluminium salts. II. Histological observations of human eccrine sweat glands inhibited by aluminium chlorohydrate. *J Soc Cosmet Chem* 1981;32:107–36

14. Hölzle E, Braun-Falco O. Structural changes in axillary eccrine glands following long-term treatment with aluminium chloride hexahydrate solution. *Br J Derm* 1984;110:399–403

15. Ichihashi T. Effect of drugs on the sweat glands by cataphoresis and an effective method for suppression of local sweating. Observation on the effect of diaphoretics and adiaphoretics. *J Oriental Med* 1936;25:101–2

16. Levit F. Simple device for treatment of hyperhidrosis by iontophoresis. *Arch Dermatol* 1968;98(5):505–7

17. Wang L, Hilliges M, Gajecki M, Marcusson JA, Johansson O. No change in skin innervation in patients with palmar hyperhidrosis treated with tap-water iontophoresis [letter]. *Br J Dermatol* 1994;131(5):742–3

18. Sato K, Timm DE, Sato F *et al*. Generation and transit pathway of H⁺ is critical for inhibition of palmar sweating by iontophoresis in water. *J Appl Physiol* 1993;75(5):2258–64

19. Anliker M, Kreyden OP. Tap water iontophoresis. In: Kreyden OP *et al*, eds. *Hyperhidrosis and Botulinum Toxin in Dermatology. Curr Probl Dermatol* Basel: Karger, 2002;30: 48–56

20. Reinauer S, Neusser A, Schauf G, Holzle E. Iontophoresis with alternating current and direct current offset (AC/DC iontophoresis): a new approach for the treatment of hyperhidrosis. *Br J Dermatol* 1993;129:166–9

21. Atkins JL, Butler PE. Hyperhidrosis: a review of current management. *Plast Reconstr Surg* 2002;110:222–28

22. Hafner J, Beer GM. Axillary sweat gland excision. In: Kreyden OP *et al*, eds. *Hyperhidrosis and Botulinum Toxin in Dermatology. Curr Probl Dermatol* Basel: Karger 2002;30:57–63

23. Lin CC, Mo LR, Hwang MH. Intraoperative cardiac arrest: a rare complication of T2,3-sympathectomy for treatment of hyperhidrosis palmaris. Two case reports. *Eur J Surg Suppl* 1994;572:43–5

24. Lin TS, Fang HY. Transthoracic endoscopic sympathectomy in the treatment of palmar hyperhidrosis – with emphasis on perioperative management (1,360 case analyses). *Surg Neurol* 1999;52:453–7

25. Kerner JC. Vergiftung durch verdorbene Würste. *Tübinger Blätter Naturwiss Arz* 1817;1–45

26. Kreyden OP *et al*. Botulinum toxin: from poison to pharmaceutical. The history of a poison that became useful to mankind. In: Kreyden OP *et al*, eds. *Hyperhidrosis and Botulinum Toxin in Dermatology. Curr Probl Dermatol* Basel: Karger 2002;30:94–100

27. Schantz EJ, Johnson EA. Botulinum toxin: the story of its development for the treatment of human disease. *Perspect Biol Med* 1997;40(3):317–27

28. Scott AB, Rosenbaum A, Collins CC. Pharmacologic weakening of extraocular muscles. *Invest Ophthamol* 1973;12:924–7

29. Scott AB. Botulinum toxin injection of eye muscles to correct strabism. *Trans Am Ophthalmol Soc* 1981;79:734–70

30. Bushara KO, Park DM, Jones JC, Schutta HS. Botulinum toxin – a possible new treatment for axillary hyperhidrosis. *Clin Exp Derm* 1996;21:276–8

31. Dressler D, Adib Saberi F, Benecke R. Botulinum toxin type B for treatment of axillar hyperhidrosis. *J Neurol* 2002;249:1729–32

32. Erbguth FJ. Dose-dependent anhidrotic effect of botulinum toxin. In: Kreyden OP *et al*, eds. *Hyperhidrosis and Botulinum Toxin in Dermatology. Curr Probl Dermatol*. Basel: Karger 2002;30:131–40

33. Birklein F, Eisenbarth G, Erbguth F, Winterholler M. Botulinum toxin type B blocks sudomotor function effectively: a 6 months follow up. *J Invest Dermatol* 2003;121:1312–16

34. van Laborde S, Dover JS, Moore M *et al*. Reduction in injection pain with botulinum toxin type B further diluted using saline with perservative: a double-blind, randomized controlled trial. *J Am Acad Dermatol* 2003;48:875–7

35. Dressler D, Benecke R. Autoniomic side effects of botulinum toxin type B treatement of cervical dystonia and hyperhidrosis. *Eur Neurol* 2003;49:34–8

36. Naumann MK, Hamm H, Lowe NJ, Botox Hyperhidrosis Clinical Study Group. Effect of botulinum toxin type A on quality of life measures in patients with excessive axillary sweating: a randomized controlled trial. *Br J Dermatol* 2002;147:1218–26

37. Wollina U, Karamfilov T, Konrad H. High-dose botulinum toxin type A therapy for axillary hyperhidrosis markedly prolongs the relapse-free interval. *J Am Acad Dermatol* 2002;46:536–40

38. Kreyden OP. Low dose and high diluted botulinum toxin treatment in the indication of focal hyperhidrosis. Oral presentation at the 16 Lütfü Tat Symposium on behalf of the Turkish Society of Dermatology and Venerology, Anakara University, Ankara 2003

39. Wollina U, Karamfilou T, Konrad H. High-dose botulinum toxin type A therapy for axilliary hyperhydrosis markedly prolongs relapse free interval. *J Am Acad Dermatol* 2002;4:536–40

40. Bigalke H, Wohlfarth K, Irmer A, Dengler R. Botulinum A toxin: Dysport® improvement of biological availability. *Exp Neurol* 2001;168:162–70

41. Kim M, Kini N, Troshynski TJ, Hennes HM. A randomized clinical trial of dermal anaesthesia by iontophoresis for peripheral antravenous catheter placement in children. *Ann Emerg Med* 1999;33:395–9

42. Kreyden OP. Botulinum toxin A: new method for anaesthesia in the treatment for palmoplantar hyperhidrosis. Oral presentation at the European Academy of Dermatology and Venerology (ESCAD) on the occasion of the 12th Congress of EADV (European Academy of Dermatology and Venerology), Barcelona 2003.

43. Hexsel DM, Dal'Forno T, Hexsel CL. Inguinal or Hexsel's hyperhidrosis. In: Benedetto AV (ed.) Botulinum toxin in clinical medicine (Part II). *Clin Derm* 2004;22:53–9

44. Kreyden OP *et al*. Type A botulinum toxin: a new method in treating focal hyperhidrosis. A summary of various possibilities in hyperhidrosis therapy with special emphasis to type A botulinum toxin injections. *Schweiz Rundsch Med Prax* 2000;89:909–15

45. Kreyden OP. Rare forms of hyperhidrosis. In: Kreyden OP *et al*, eds. *Hyperhidrosis and Botulinum Toxin in Dermatology. Curr Probl Dermatol* Basel: Karger 2002;30:178–87

46. Frey L. Le syndrome du nerf auriculo-temporal. *Rev Neurol* 1923;2:97–104

47. Laskawi R, Ellies M, Rödel R *et al*. Gustatory sweating – clinical implications and ethiological aspects. *J Oral Maxillofac Surg* 1999;57:642–8

48. Laskawi R, Dobrik C, Schönbeck C. Up-to-date report of botulinum toxin type A treatment in patients with gustatory sweating (Frey's syndrome). *Laryngoscope* 1998;108:381–4

49. Ross AT. Progressive selective sudomotor denervation. *Neurology* 1958;8:808–17

50. Itin P, Hirsbrunner P, Rufli T *et al*. Das Ross-Syndrom. *Hautarzt* 1992;43:359–60

Storage of BOTOX®

BOTOX® and BOTOX® Cosmetic (botulinum toxin serotype A) purified neurotoxin complex is distributed in vials of 100 U of sterile, vacuum dried crystalline powder without preservative. The 100 U vials of BOTOX® are shipped frozen in insulated, styrofoam containers. When it reaches its destination it can be stored in its dry, powdered form in the refrigerator at a constant temperature of 2–8°C[1]. Once reconstituted, the solution of BOTOX® can be stored again in the refrigerator at a constant temperature of 2–8°C. DO NOT REFREEZE RECONSTITUTED BOTOX®. Although the package insert for BOTOX® recommends the reconstituted product be used within four hours, studies have shown that after reconstitution, the potency of BOTOX® should remain consistent and unchanged for up to 6 weeks, and can be used without any noticeable change in clinical efficacy[2,3].

Preparation of BOTOX®

The package insert for BOTOX® Cosmetic suggests that the 100 U vial be reconstituted with 2.5 ml of 0.9% non-preserved saline for a final concentration of 4 U/0.1 ml[1]. A report of a consensus conference of key physician injectors held in 2004 recommended that a 100 U vial of BOTOX® Cosmetic be reconstituted at a 'dilution that minimizes the likelihood of diffusion to neighboring muscle groups', and can be anywhere from 1 to 10 ml/100 U vial[4]. Anecdotal and published reports suggest that volume may influence duration of effect, in that the greater the volume, the shorter the duration of effect[5]. The 2004 consensus conference report also attested to the fact that the majority of dermatologic and esthetic physician injectors reconstitute BOTOX® Cosmetic with preserved normal saline instead of non-preserved diluent. The result of a bilateral, comparative prospective study has shown that there is less pain with injection when preserved isotonic saline is used instead of non-preserved isotonic saline[4–6]. There was no loss of efficacy nor duration of potency whether BOTOX® Cosmetic was reconstituted with preserved or unpreserved normal saline. Once reconstituted, the vial of BOTOX® should be clear, colorless, and free of particulate matter, regardless of diluent used[1].

Handling of BOTOX®

Concerns over a potential loss of potency resulting from rough handling, agitation and foaming during reconstitution were also addressed at the 2004 consensus conference[4]. Trindade de Almeida et al treated one side of six patients in the glabella and periocular area with BOTOX® Cosmetic that was reconstituted by agitation to the point of bubbling and foaming, and the opposite side with BOTOX® that was not agitated[7]. There was no difference in muscle relaxation between the two sides treated, and the duration of effect remained constant on both sides for approximately 16 weeks. Similar results were anecdotally confirmed by the majority of those present at the 2004 consensus conference[4].

Injection technique of BOTOX®

BOTOX® Cosmetic should be injected with sterile, plastic, single-use syringes. In order to minimize the pain and bruising of injection, tuberculin syringes with a 30–32-gauge needle are used to administer BOTOX® Cosmetic. For those injectors who want to reconstitute BOTOX® Cosmetic with a minimum amount of diluent (1 ml or less) and be able to control the minutest amount of solution injected, an insulin syringe with an attached 29- or 30-gauge needle can be used. Insulin syringes (0.5 ml or 0.3 ml) have no potential space at the hub where the needle is preattached, thereby minimizing any wastage of solution. In addition, the barrel of the syringe is scored with markings representing 0.01 ml that can be easily seen and which will correspond to 1 U of BOTOX® when a 100 U vial is reconstituted with 1 ml of diluent[8]. To further reduce some of the discomfort associated with any type of intramuscular injection, the application of either a topical anesthetic, ice, or both on the skin surface at the injection site can help provide a more comfortable, positive experience for some patients.

Although there are no controlled studies to support certain commonly prescribed post-operative recommendations made to prevent diffusion of the BOTOX® beyond the injection site (distant diffusion), many of the physicians at the 2004 consensus conference still recommend the following for their patients:

1. DO NOT massage the BOTOX® treated areas for 4–6 hours.
2. DO NOT bend over (e.g. to tie shoes or pick up something from the floor) for 2–3 hours after a BOTOX® treatment of the upper face.
3. LIMIT heavy physical activity, and lying down or sleeping for 2–3 hours after a BOTOX® treatment of the upper face.
4. DO contract treated muscles for 2–4 hours immediately after a BOTOX® treatment. This promotes the uptake of BOTOX® by the receptor sites at the neuromuscular junctions.

Current popular mode of preparing, handling, and storing BOTOX® Cosmetic

	Popular methods	Manufacturer's recommendations[1]
Storage		
● Before reconstitution	≤ 24 months at 2–8°C	≤ 24 months at 2–8°C
● After reconstitution	≤ 16 weeks at 2–8°C[3]	4 hours at 2–8°C
Preparation		
● Diluent	Preserved normal saline (0.9% saline with 0.9% benzyl alcohol)[6]	Non-preserved normal saline (0.9% saline)
● Concentration	Concentrations 1–10 ml/100 U vial as needed for appropriate uptake and diffusion[4]	2.5 ml/100 U vial
Handling	No special precautions[7]	Do NOT agitate or cause foaming
Injection technique	Insulin syringe with 30-gauge needle[8] or tuberculin syringe with 30–32-gauge needle[4]	None recommended

Adapted from Carruthers *et al.* Consensus Recommendations on the Use of Botulinum Toxin Type A in Facial Aesthetics, *Suppl Plast Reconstr Surg* 2004;114:2S.

References

1. Allergan, Inc. Botox Cosmetic (botulinum toxin type A) purified neurotoxin complex (Package Insert). Irvin, California: Allergan, Inc., revised May 2003
2. Garcia A, Fulton JE Jr. Cosmetic denervation of the muscles of facial expression with botulinum toxin: a dose-response study. *Dermatol Surg* 1996;22:39
3. Hexsel DM, de Almeida AT, Rutowitsch M *et al*. Multicenter, double-blind study of the efficacy of injections with botulinum toxin type A reconstituted up to six consecutive weeks before application. *Dermatol Surg* 2003;29:523
4. Carruthers J, Fagien S, Matarasso SL. Consensus recommendations on the use of botulinum toxin type A in facial aesthetics, *Suppl Plast Reconstr Surg* 2004;114:2S.
5. Klein AW. Complications and adverse reactions with the use of botulinum toxin. *Dis Mon* 2002;48:336
6. Alam M, Dover JS, Arndt KA. Pain associated with injection of botulinum A exotoxin reconstituted using isotonic sodium chloride with and without preservative: a double-blind, randomized controlled trial. *Arch Dermatol* 2002;138:510
7. Trindade de Almeida AR, Kadunc BV, Di Chiacchio N, Neto DR. Foam during reconstitution does not affect the potency of botulinum toxin type A. *Dermatol Surg* 2003;29:530
8. Flynn TC, Carruthers A, Carruthers J. Surgical pearl: the use of the Ultra-Fine II short needle 0.3 cc insulin syringe for botulinum toxin injections. *J Am Acad Dermatol* 2002;46:931–3

Rationale

I am aware that when a small amount of purified botulinum toxin (BOTOX®) is injected into a muscle it causes weakness or paralysis of that muscle. This occurs in 3–4 days or even later, and usually lasts 3–4 months but can last for shorter or longer amounts of time.

Frown lines between the eyebrows are due to contraction of small muscles around and between the eyebrows. Injecting BOTOX® into this area will temporarily paralyze or weaken these muscles causing a reduction or disappearance of the frown lines. Similarly, crow's feet and horizontal forehead lines can be improved by the injection of BOTOX® into these areas, weakening the muscles that cause the wrinkles on the forehead and around the eyes. Many other areas of the central and lower face, neck, and chest also can be treated successfully with BOTOX®, but treatment of any area other than between the eyes is currently not FDA approved.

Results and after treatment care

1. I understand that I will not be able to 'frown' while the injections of BOTOX® into this area are effective, but this will reverse itself after a period of months, at which time retreatment is appropriate.
2. I understand that I must stay erect and not lower my head (i.e. to tie my shoes, or pick up something), and I must not manipulate or rub the treated areas for 2–3 hours after my treatment session.
3. I understand I might experience quicker results if I repeatedly contract and use the BOTOX® injected muscles for the 2–3 hours after my treatment session.

Risks and complications

BOTOX® treatment of frown lines can cause a minor, temporary droop of one or both eyelids and eyebrows in less than 3% of those treated. This usually lasts 2–4 weeks and possibly longer. Bruising and a transient headache for a few hours after the treatment session can occur, or even numbness of a small area on the forehead lasting 2–3 weeks.

In a very small number of individuals the injections do not work as completely as they do in others nor do they last as long as they do in others. Everyone is affected by BOTOX® in their own way.

Photographs

I authorize the taking of photographs and their use for scientific and medical purposes both in publications and presentations. I understand that my identity will be protected.

Pregnancy and neurologic disease

I am not nursing nor am I aware I am pregnant nor do I have any significant neurologic disease.

Payment

I understand this procedure is cosmetic and payment is my responsibility and due at the completion of treatment. I have read the above and understand all of it. My questions have been answered satisfactorily by the doctor. I accept the risks and complications of this procedure.

_____   _____

Signed   Date

_____   _____

Name   Witness

Doctor's name and address

BOTOX® COSMETIC INJECTION SITE RECORD

PATIENT NAME:_____

CHART #:_____ **DATE:**_____

NOTES

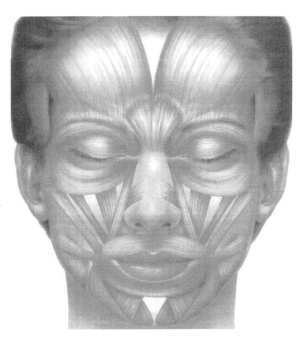

BOTOX® Lot # N. S. Lot #:	Dilution used: _____mL/100 U _____Units/0.1cc	Photos		Total Units/Site
Expires: Expires: _____ _____		Pre Rx Date	Post Rx Date	
Forehead				
Glabella				
Crow's feet				
Eyelids: (lower); (upper)				
Nose: bunny lines				
Nose: (flare); (tip)				
Mouth corners (DAO)				
Lips, upper; lower				
Lips, (G-smile)				
Chin: (apex); (M-line)				
Neck: (H-lines); (bands)				
Other:				
Total Units Injected				

The nature and purpose of the treatment have been explained to me and questions I had regarding the treatment have been answered to my satisfaction. I understand that these treatments may involve risks of complications both from known and unknown causes, and I freely assume these risks.

PATIENT SIGNATURE _____ WITNESS: _____

APPENDIX 4   MUSCLES OF FACIAL EXPRESSION

	Muscle	Origin	Insertion	Action	Function
I. Forehead	Frontalis (s)	Galea aponeurotica	skin of forehead and brow	raises eyebrow	wrinkles forehead; used in frowning and to express surprise and astonishment
II. Glabella	a. Corrugator supercilii (d)	medial superciliary arch (nasal process of frontal bone)	skin of in the mid portion brow	adducts and draws brow down	used to squint and protect eyes
	b. Orbicularis oculi, (s) i. orbital portion	medial and anterior orbital margin	surrounds orbital opening as a sphincter: fibers are over temple, cheek and into eyebrow	closes eyelid	wrinkles brow to produce a frown; used to squint and protect eyes
	ii. palpebral portion (s)	medial palpebral ligament	lateral palpebral raphe	closes eye involuntarily	produces sphincteric action of the eyelids
	iii. lacrimal portion (d)	lacrimal crest	upper and lower tarsal plates	draws eyelids posteriorly	facilitates the lacrimal pump
	c. Depressor supercilii (s)	nasal process of frontal bone	skin of brow	pulls down medial brow	pulls eyebrows down, closes eyelids, facilitates the lacrimal pump
	d. Procerus (s)	nasal bone and cartilage	skin of forehead between eyebrows	pulls down medial brow	wrinkles brow to produce frown; used to squint and shield eyes
III. Nose	a. Compressor naris (transverse nasalis) (s)	canine eminence of maxilla	nasal bridge aponeurosis	compresses nasal aperture	slows exhaled air
	b. Dilator naris (alar nasalis) (s)	maxilla above lateral incisor and alar cartilage	nasal tip and alar skin and cartilage	widens nasal aperture	prevents alar collapse in forceful breathing
	c. Depressor septi nasi (s)	incisive fossa of maxilla	lower nasal septum and under surface of lower lateral alar cartilage	draws nasal tip and alae downward	narrows the nostrils

	Muscle	Origin	Insertion	Action	Function
IV. Mouth	a. Orbicularis oris (s)	from many muscles that converge on mouth	forms a sphincter around lips	closes lips	protrudes, puckers and shapes lips
	b. Risorius (s)	fascia of masseter and parotid gland	angle of mouth	retracts angle of mouth laterally	used in smiling and laughing when present
	c. Levator anguli oris (d)	canine fossa below infraorbital foramen	angle of mouth and upper lip musculature	raises angle of mouth and lateral upper lip	used in smiling and laughing; it deepens nasolabial furrow as in contempt or disdain
	d. Zygomaticus major (s)	lateral surface of zygomatic bone	angle of mouth	draws mouth upward and laterally	used in laughing or smiling
	e. Zygomaticus minor (d and s)	malar surface of zygomatic bone (near maxillary suture line)	upper lip at angle of mouth into orbicularis oris and levator labii superioris	draws mouth upward and laterally	used in expressing sadness (see next above)
	f. Levator labii superioris (d and s)	lower margin of orbit, above infraorbital foramen	angle of mouth and upper lip	elevates and everts upper lip	used in expressing seriousness and sadness and deepens nasolabial fold
	g. Levator labii superioris alaeque nasi (s)	frontal process of maxilla	alar cartilage and lateral upper lip	dilates nares and everts and elevates lateral upper lip	deepens the upper nasolabial fold and used in scowling
	h. Depressor anguli oris (s)	oblique line of mandible	angle of mouth, upper and lower lip	depresses angle of mouth downward and laterally	used in grimacing and snarling; used in expressing sadness

Muscle	Origin	Insertion	Action	Function
IV. Mouth				
i. Depressor labii inferioris (d)	between symphysis menti and mental foramen; platysma	lower lip and orbicularis oris	draws lower lip downward and laterally	everts the lower lip, used in drinking and expressing irony; sorrow and doubt
j. Mentalis (d)	incisive fossa of mandible	skin of chin	raises and protrudes lower lip and wrinkles skin of chin	used in pouting and expressing doubt or disdain
k. Buccinator (d)	outer surface of mandible; alveolar process of maxilla; pterygomandibular raphe	angle of mouth; upper and lower lips; interdigitates with orbicularis oris	flattens cheek against gums; used when distending cheeks with air and compresses them to force air out of mouth	used in sucking and chewing; used to puff up cheeks and blow air out of the mouth; as when blowing up a balloon or playing a wind instrument
l. Platysma (s)	pectoralis fascia of 2nd to 4th rib and deltoid fascia	lower jaw, angle of mouth, lower mouth and parotid fascia	widens mouth aperture at commussures; pulls skin of neck taught	used in expressing horror; assists in shaving or in relieving pressure of a tight collar; and depresses lower lip

s = superficial
d = deep

Potential side-effects of BOTOX® Cosmetic injections*

I. Adverse effects of limited duration that are common, localized and not of a serious nature:
    Common with any percutaneous injection
    - Mild stinging, burning or pain with injection
    - Edema around injection site
    - Erythema around injection site
    - Mild headache, localized and transient

    Technique dependent
    - Ecchymosis lasting 3 to 10 days
    - Asymmetry
    - Oral incompetence and asymmetric smile
    - Lack of neck strength
    - Lack of intended cosmetic effect

    Rare and idiosyncratic
    - Numbness and paresthesias, localized and transient
    - Focal tonic movements (twitching)
    - Mild nausea and occasional vomiting
    - Mild malaise and myalgias (localized and generalized)

II. Adverse effects of longer duration that can be serious and are technique dependent:
    - Blepharoptosis
    - Brow ptosis
    - Diplopia
    - Diminished tearing and xeropthalmia with or without keratitis
    - Ectropion (can lead to xeropthalmia)
    - Lagopthalmus (can lead to exposure keratitis)
    - Dysphagia
    - Dysarthria

III. Adverse effects of longer duration that can be serious and are **not** technique dependent:
    Immediate hypersensitivity reactions
    - Urticaria
    - Dyspnea
    - Soft tissue edema
    - Anaphylaxis

307

Contraindications to BOTOX® Cosmetic injections

Patients should not be treated or treated with extreme caution who are:
- Psychologically unstable or who have questionable motives and unrealistic expectations
- Dependent on intact facial movements and expressions for their livelihood (e.g. actors, singers, musicians and other media personalities)
- Afflicted with a neuromuscular disorder (e.g. myasthenia gravis, Eaton-Lambert syndrome)
- Allergic to any of the components of BTX-A or BTX-B (i.e. BTX, human albumin, saline, lactose and sodium succinate)
- Taking certain medications that can interfere with neuromuscular impulse transmission and potentiate the effects of BTX (e.g. aminoglycosides, penicillamine, quinine, and calcium blockers)
- Pregnant or lactating (BTXs are classified as pregnancy category C drugs)

Potential beneficial effects of BOTOX® Cosmetic injections

- Relief of frontal or occipal "tension headaches"
- Relief of migraine headaches
- Compensary muscle strengtheining of the same muscles when segmentally treated (e.g. strengthening of the lower frontalis and elevation of the eyebrows when the upper frontalis is treated or improvement of posture and projection of breasts when the lower pectoralis major or minor are treated)
- Compensatory muscle strengthening of synergistic muscles (e.g. strengthening of the lip levators when the orbicularis oris is treated)
- Compensatory muscle strengthening of antagonistic muscles (e.g. strengthening of the lower frontalis and medial brow lift when the medial brow depressors are treated or lateral brow lift when lateral brow depressors are treated

References

1. Fisher NM, Schaffer JV, Berwick M, et al. Botulinum toxin type A injections: adverse events reported to the US Food and Drug Administration in therapeutic and cosmetic cases. *JAAD* 2005;53:07–415.
2. Gershon SK, Wise RP, Braun MM. Adverse events reported with cosmetic use of Botulinum toxin A. *Pharmacoepidemiology Drug Safety* 2001;10(Suppl):S135–136.

action mechanisms: pain   25–6
age: cosmetic treatment   3–4
Ahn, J.   211
Ahsan, J.   229
allergan   77
Alster, T.S.   252
anatomy: sweat glands   263–4
Ann, K.Y.   211
anticholinergics   267–8, 268
antiperspirants   266–7
anxiety   228
apraclondine eyedrops   76
Ascher, B.   238–41
asymmetric smile   145, 156, **157**, 159; treatment
   implications   161
asymmetry   54, 56, 79
Atamoros, P.F.   135

bands: vertical   192–3
Biddle, J.E.: and Hammermesh, D.S.   3
Bigalike, H.   278–9
Binder, W.J.: *et al*   70
Birklein, F.   273
blepharoptosis   75
body dysmorphic disorders (BDD)   7–10, 263;
   compulsive behaviours   9
BOTOX®: handling   295; injection technique
   295; preparation   295; storage   295; treatment
   274
BOTOX® effects   **51, 52, 53, 54, 55, 58, 59, 60,**
   174; asymmetric smile   **160**; chin puckering
   189, 190; crow's feet   **96, 98, 101**; deep
   mental crease   190; depressor anguli oris
   186; frown lines   **82, 83, 84**; hypertrophic scar
   228; lower eyelid   **112, 113, 114**; meloabial
   grooves   **142**; nasal tip drop   **136**;
   nasoglabellar lines 124, 125; orbicularis oculis
   74, 75; peribuccal rhytides   166; perioral
   rhytides   175, 176
botulinium neurotoxin: structure   **20**
botulinium neurotoxins: action mechanisms   **22**;
   manufacture   17–19, *18*, **18**
botulinium toxin: aesthetic use   250
botulism   271
breast asymmetry   231
breast lift   230–5
breast ptosis   231–2

breasts   232
brow elevation   **55**
brow ptosis   **35**, 48–9, **56**, 78
BTX-A: onset   257
BTX-A effects: calf recontouring   216
BTX-B: onset   257
BTX-B effects   256; frown lines   257
buccal sphincter incompetence   155
buccinator   166–171
bunny lines   40
Bushara, K.O.   272
Butzer, A.   211

calf recontouring: complications   215; functional
   anatomy   213; patient selection   213; results
   215; treatment implications   216
canine smile   149, **150**
canthal wrinkles   86–91
care: post-operative   299
Carruthers, J.D.A.   247
Catania, S.   229
central brow: frown lines   60–85
central lip levators   **152, 154**
cervical dystonia   249–50, 253
cervical dystonia patients   24–5
chest: wrinkling   200, 201, 202–3
chest wrinkling: complications   203
chin puckering 185–92; after BOTOX®   187;
   before BOTOX®   187; patient selection
   185–91; results   190
chinese moustache   179
Christian, Doctor J.   271
Clark, R.E.   252
complications 299; chest wrinkling   203;
   melomental folds   184–5
compressor naris   **126, 127**; injection sites **128**
compulsive behaviours: body dysmorphic disorders
   (BDD)   9
Conair Vibrating Massager   224
conjunctivitis   76
consent   299
Cordivari, C.   229
corrugator supercilii   46, **63**
cosmetic patients: psychological profile   5–7
cosmetic surgery   5–7, 11–12
cosmetic treatment   1–12; age   3–4; cultural
   influences   2–3; history   2; motivation   4–5

cranial nerve (fifth)   42
crow's feet   **86**, **88**, **94**, **95**, **99**, **101**, 243–4, 255;
    rhytides   38–40
cryotherapy   281–4; nozzle   285; unit   283
cultural influences: cosmetic treatment   2–3
cystic fibrosis   266

deep mental crease   185
depression   10–11
depressor anguli oris   41, 183
depressor labii inferioris   41, **156**, 170
depressor septi nasi   **134**
depressor supercilii   65, **66**, 71–2, 87
dilator naris   **132**
dilution   196; asymmetric smile   159; chin
    puckering   187; frown lines   66; hyperhidrosis
    277–9; melomental folds   181; nasoglabellar
    lines   **125**; perioral lips   172
Diplopia 78, 129
doasge: Dysport® 245
Doctors Scott: Carruthers   **17**
Dong, M.: *et al*   26
dosing   45, 91–5, 108–9, 134, 182–4, 253;
    asymmetric smile   159; chest wrinkling   201–2;
    chin puckering   187–9; jawline recontouring
    209; melomental folds   182; neck wrinkling
    196; perioral lips   173–5
drool grooves   179
dynamic wrinkles   93
dyshagia   199
Dysport   237–45, 272–3, 278–9; dosage   245;
    dosage test results   242; frown lines   241
dystrophy: reflex sympathetic   227–9

ecchymoses   80, 115, **116**
eccrine: sweat glands   263–6, 269
Ectropion   78
edema   80, 116
Edgerton, M.T.: *et al*   6, 11
Eisnbarth, G.   273
eklabion   184
EMLA   222; cream   281
endocytosis   21
endoscopic thoracic sympathectomy (ETC)   271,
    289
epiphora   115, 130
Erbguth, F.   273
erythema   **81**
eye wrinkles: lateral   **76**
eyelid: droop   257; injection sites   **110**; injection
    technique   **109**; lower   104–17, **106**

face: nerves   42–3
facial expression   33–4; muscles   121
Filippi, G.M. *et al*   22
Flynn, T.C. 252; *et al*   115
fold: melomental   179–86
foot block   281

forehead   243–4; injection sites   **51**
forehead lines: complications   56–60; functional
    anatomy   48–9; problem assessment   47–8;
    treatment implications   57
forehead wrinkles   **47**
French Study: results   239
frey syndrome   287–8
frontalis   **34**, **49**, 71–2, 252–3
frown lines   62–6; BOTOX® effects   **82**, **83**, **84**;
    dilution   66; glabellar   237–45; injection sites
    67, 68, **69**; problem assessment   60–2
frowning: before/after BOTOX®   **61**
functional anatomy   200; calf recontouring   213;
    chin puckering   186; forehead lines   48–9;
    melomental folds   180

Gajecki, M.   269
gastrocnemius   213–16
glabella: injection   85
glabellar lines   247, 251–5
Goin, M.K.   6
Goldberg, D.J.   252
Gooden, M.   252
Graham, J.A.   3
Grossbart, T.A.: and Sawyer, D.B.   7
gummy smile   148–56, **148**, **151**; asymmetric
    151

Hammermesh, D.S.: and Biddle, J.E.   3
hand block   281
handling: BOTOX®   295
headache   57, 240, 252
Hilliges, M.   269
history: cosmetic treatment   2;
    pharmacology/immunology   15–17
Hitachi Magic Wand   223, 224
Horn, C.   211
hyperalgesia   222
hyperesthesia   227–8
hyperhidrosis   261–90; axillary   275; dilution
    277–9; forehead   285–7; generalized   268;
    injection sites   290; onogenital   285–7;
    paloplanter   279–84; primary   261; secondary
    261, 273; treatments   266–90
hypersensivity   57

iatrogenic asymmetry   80
ideal brow   61, **62**
immunology   24–5
immunoresistance   248–9
incidental asymmetry   79–80
Increase in Palperbral Aperture   *110*
inferiors: depressor labii   181
injection   23–4, 45–6; corrugator supercilii   **70**;
    glabella   85; gummy smile   **152**, **153**; neck
    wrinkles   197, 198; orbicularis oculi   **71**;
    perioral rhytides   174; procerus   **72**

injection sites   254; compressor naris   **128**; elevating eyebrow   **73**; eyelids   *110*; forehead   **51**; forehead hyperhidrosis   286; frown lines   **67**, 68, **69**; lower crow's feet   **146**; nasaolabial fold   **144**, **145**; perioral rhytides   **177**; tibialis   282
injection technique: BOTOX®   295; eyelid   **109**
internal/external carotid   43–4
intradermal injections   24
iontophoresis   283; tap-water   269–70
Iten, P.   288

Jankovic, J.   229
jawline recontouring: complications   212; dosing   209; functional anatomy   208; patient selection   207–8; results   211; treatment implications   212
jelly rolls (festoons)   104, **106**, 107
Johansson, O.   269
Johnson, D.F.   3
Jung, D.S.   211

Kim, E.J.   252
Kisley, S.: *et al*   6
Kligman, A.M.   266

Lagophthalmos   78, 103, 115
laser resurfacing   **97**
Lask, G.P.   252
lateral canthal lines   85–104, **91**; treatment implications   105
levator anguili oris   141, **142**
levator labii superioris   **138**
levator labii superioris alaeque nasi   **138**, **140**, **155**
lidocaine   229, 281; iontophoresis   281–4
lip depressors   **41**
lip ptosis   146–7
liposuction   270
lips: perioral   164–79
localized unilateral hyperidrosis (LUH)   290
lopedine   77–8
Lowe, N.J.   252
lower crow's feet/lateral cheek rhytides   **139**
lower eyelids   104–17, **106**
lower face   40–1, 244
lower lip: adynamic   191
Lupton, J.R.   252

Maas, C.S.   250
McDougall, J.   9
Mckelroy, S.L.: and Philips, K.A.   8
mandibular branch (V3)   42
Manfrida, G.M.: and Micheli-Pelligrini, V.   6
manufacture of botulinum neurotoxins   17–19, *18*, **18**
Marcusson, J.A.   269
marionette lines   179, 182–4, 186
masseter   183, 208–12

masseteric hypertrophy: after BTX-A   210
mastication   33
maxillary division (V2)   42
Medline papers   219
melolabial grooves   137–48
melomental folds: dosing   182; results 184
Meningaud, J.P.: *et al*   6, 11
mentalis   189
Meyer, E.   6
Micheli-Pelligrini, V.: and Manfrida, G.M.   6
mid face   40
migraine   25
mimetic muscles   **122**
minor starch test   276, 287
Misra, V.P.   229
modiolus   40, 171
Mona Lisa smile   **149**
motivation: cosmetic treatment   4–5
muscle spindle structure   **23**
muscles: facial expression   33–4, 121, 303–5; gastrocnemius   214; hyperfunction   33–4; mastication   33
Myobloc   247, 249, 255, 272–3

Naphacon   78
Napolean, A.   6
nasal flare   131–3
nasal scrunch (bunny lines)   **123**
nasal tip drop   133–7, **134**
nasilis   40
nasoglabellar lines   123–30
nasolabial fold   **138**
Naumann, M.K.   275
neck   42; weakness   199
neck wrinkling   199; anterior   191; dosing   196–7; functional anatomy   193–6; problem assessment   192–3
Neo-Synephrine   78
nerve block   279–81, 284
nerves: face   42–3
neuralgia: post-herpetic   220–3
Neurobloc   247, 272–3
neuromuscular injection   23
nipple: projection   233–5
nose: muscles   **38**

oculi: orbicularis   168
open-eyed look   111
ophthalmic division   42
oral sphincter incompetence   99
orbicularis   163; oris   169–73
orbicularis oculi   **37**, 46, 63, 70–5; orbital portion   **87**
orbicularis oris   40
oris: depressor anguli   180–4, **184**; orbicularis   166, 169–73, 177–8
overdose: reversal   229–30

pain   219–29, 251; action mechanisms   25–6; gate control theory   223, 225
pain scale: patient   220; physician   221
pain score: PHN   222
palpebral orbicularis oculii   **89**
Papa, C.M.   266
Par, M.Y.   211
paresthesias: lip   178
pathogenesis: hyperhidrosis   262
patient: pain scale   220; selection   200
patient selection   47–8; calf recontouring   213; chin puckering   185–91; jawline recontouring   207–8
pectoralis major   231
pectoralis minor   230, 235
peribuccal rhytides   167; after BOTOX®   167; before BOTOX®   167
periocular lines   85–117
periocular wrinkles   **106**
perioral lips: complications   178; dilution   172; dosing   173–5; functional anatomy   165–71; problem assessment   164–5; results   176–7; treatment implications   178
perioral rhytides   174; Botox effects   175; injecting   174
pharmacology   20–4, 247–8; botulinium toxin   248
pharmacology/immunology: history   15–17
Philips, K.A.: and Mckelroy, S.L.   8
platysma   42, 192–203, 195; decussating   195
preparation: BOTOX®   295
procerus   64, **65**, 71–2
product comparison   237
pseudoblepharoptosis   79
pseudoherniation   115
pseudoptosis   **79**
psychiatric illness   9–12
psychological profile: cosmetic patients   5–7
psychology   1, 4–12
ptosis   243
ptotic upper lip   145

Ramirez, A.L.   250–1
Rankin, M.: *et al*   11
recontouring: jawline   207–12
Reeck, J.   250
results: calf recontouring   215; chin puckering   190, 190–1; melomental folds   184; neck wrinkling   197–8
Ringel, E.W.   4
risorius (laughter muscle)   **93**
ross syndrome   288
Rubin   149

Sato, F.   269
Sato, H.   265
Sato, K. II   269
Sawyer, B.B.: and Grossbart, T.A.   7
scars   225–7; Keloid   226

Schantz, Prof. E.J.   **15**, 272
Schengrund, C.L.: and Yowler, B.C.   27
Scott, A.   15–17, 272
selection: patient   164, 200
skull: anatomic photo   **53**
smile: adynamic   184; asymmetric   178, 184, 191; full denture   **150**
Spencer, J.M.   252
static wrinkles   86, 93, 95
Stevens, R.: *et al*   20
storage: BOTOX®   295
Sullivan, N.A.S.   2
superficial muscular aponeurotic system (SMAS)   33, 121
superficial punctuate keratisis   102
superficial punctuate keratosis   78
sweat: re-absorption   266; secretion   265
sweat glands: anatomy   263–4; apocrine   263–4, 270; eccrine   263–6, 269; excision   270
sweating   271, 287–90; pathophysiology   264–6

Tamuro, B.M.: *et al*   128
tear production   **107**
thermoregulation   264
Timm, D.E.   269
treatment implications: asymmetric smile   161; chest wrinkling   203; chin puckering   192; forehead lines   57; lateral cantal lines   105; melomental folds   185
turkey neck   193, 194

upper face   35–9
upper gum mucosa   148
upper lip levators   40, **116**
upper lip ptosis   113

vascular supply   43–4
vertical platysmal bands   193
vibration   223
Vuong, K.D.   229

weakness: neck   199
Wegelin, Doctor O.   230
Winterholler, M.   273
Wong, L.   269
wrinkles: canthal   86–91; crease   242; dynamic   93; facial   250, 253; forhead   252; furrow   242; line   242; lower eyelid   244; periocular   **105**; perioral   164; static   86, 93, 95
wrinkling: chest   200, 201, 202–3

xerophthalmia (dry eyes)   78, 115, 116

Yamauchi, P.S.   252
Yowler, B.C.: and Schengrund, C.L.   27

zygomatic arch   99
zygomaticus muscles   **90**, **91**, **92**, 99